Evidence of Harm

Evidence
of Harm

Mercury in Vaccines

and the Autism Epidemic:

A Medical Controversy

David Kirby

ST. MARTIN'S GRIFFIN ⚜ NEW YORK

www.stmartins.com

Library of Congress Cataloging-in-Publication Data

Kirby, David.
    Evidence of harm : mercury in vaccines and the autism epidemic : a medical controversy / David Kirby.
        p. cm.
    ISBN 0-312-32644-0 (hc)
    ISBN 0-312-32645-9 (pbk)
    EAN 978-0-312-32645-6
        1. Vaccination of children—Complications—United States. 2. Autism in children—Etiology. 3. Developmental disabilities—Etiology. 4. Organomercury compounds—Toxicology. 5. Vaccines industry—Corrupt practices—United States. 6. Pharmaceutical industry—Corrupt practices—United States. I. Title.

RJ240.K57 2005
614.4'7'083—dc22   2004051492

First St. Martin's Griffin Edition: March 2006

10   9   8   7   6   5   4   3   2   1

To my mother and father,

Barbara and Leo Kirby,

who never said no at the wrong time

Author's Note

The fact that an organization or Web site is referred to in this work as a citation and/or potential source of further information does not mean that the author endorses the information the organization or Web site may provide. Further, readers should be aware that Internet Web sites listed in this work may have changed or disappeared between when this work was written and when it is read. Many of the documents listed in the notes section of this book may be viewed at evidenceofharm.com.

In no way do I endorse the biomedical treatments for autism described in this book, nor could I. It is unlikely they would work for every child, and whether they work at all is unproven. There is not enough evidence. The point is that this avenue of research should be pursued with due haste. Only through double-blinded, placebo-controlled clinical trials will we know if these treatments provide any real benefit.

Contents

Introduction

July 9, 2004

DOES MERCURY in vaccines cause autism in children? A definitive answer has proven elusive, and it remains so to this day. No one can say with certainty that thimerosal, the vaccine preservative made with 49.6 percent mercury, helped fuel an explosion in reported cases of autism, attention deficit disorder (ADD), speech delay, and other disorders over the past decade. But no one can say for certain that it did not.

On May 18, 2004, the respected Institute of Medicine issued a much heralded report stating that the bulk of evidence "favors rejection of a causal relationship" between thimerosal and autism.[1] The independent panel, commissioned by the government to investigate alleged links between vaccines and autism, delivered a harsh blow to advocates of the thimerosal-autism hypothesis. But despite its authoritative certainty, the report failed to close the books on this simmering medical controversy. Indeed, recently published animal and test tube studies provide compelling biological evidence of harm (though certainly not proof) from thimerosal-containing vaccines.

Exactly five years ago, the federal government disclosed in a "Joint Statement" that some American children were being exposed to levels of mercury in vaccines above one of the federal safety limits. Since then, officials have moved to phase out mercury from childhood vaccines, and to determine if thimerosal exposure in infants could cause autism and other neurological developmental disorders. To date, neither goal has been fully attained.

Thimerosal has been removed from most routine vaccinations given to American children. But it is still found in the majority of flu shots, which the U.S. government now recommends for pregnant women and children between six months and twenty-three months of age.[2] In 2004, the Centers for Disease Control and Prevention (CDC) declined to state a preference for mercury-free flu shots in infants.[3] Mercury is also found in some tetanus, diphtheria-tetanus, pertusis, and meningitis vaccines, which are sometimes, though not routinely, given to children. It is also used in many over-the-counter products, including nasal sprays, ear and eye drops, and even a hemorrhoid treatment.[4]

Meanwhile, the CDC has been unable to definitively prove or disprove the theory that thimerosal causes autism, ADD, speech delays, or other disorders. Several studies funded or conducted by the agency have been published in the past year, all of them suggesting that there is no connection between the preservative and the disease. The CDC insists that it has looked into the matter thoroughly and found "no evidence of harm" from thimerosal in vaccines.

But "no evidence of harm" is not the same as proof of safety. No evidence of harm is not a definitive answer; and this is a story that cries out for answers.

Many have asked why a trusted health agency would allow a known neurotoxin to be injected into the bodies of small babies—in amounts that exceed federal safety exposure levels for *adults* by up to fifty times per shot? It's a disturbing question, and there are no satisfying answers.

But a small group of parents, aided by a handful of scientists, physicians, politicians, and legal activists, has spent the past five years searching for answers. Despite heavy resistance from the powerful public health lobby, these parents never abandoned their ambition to prove that mercury in vaccines is what pushed their children, most of them boys, into a hellish, lost world of autism.

Of course, there are two sides to every good story, and this one is no exception. For every shred of evidence the parents and other researchers have unearthed linking thimerosal to autism, public health authorities have produced forceful data to the contrary.

The parents and their allies accuse public health officials and the pharmaceutical industry of negligence and incompetence, at best, and malfeasance and collusion at worst.

On the other hand, the mercury-autism proponents have been greeted with contempt and counterattack by many in the American health establishment, which understandably has an interest in proving the unpleasant theory wrong.

Each side accuses the other of being irrational, overzealous, blind to evidence they find inconvenient, and subject to professional, financial, or emotional conflicts of interest that cloud their judgment. In some ways, both sides are right.

Some children with autism were never exposed to thimerosal, and the vast majority of people who received mercury in vaccines show no evidence of harm whatsoever. But if thimerosal is not responsible for the apparent autism epidemic in the United States, then it is incumbent upon public health officials to mount a full-scale quest to identify the actual cause. At the very least, the thimerosal debate has compelled the scientific community, however reluctantly, to consider an environmental component to the disorder, rather than looking for a purely genetic explanation. Autism, by most accounts, is epidemic. And there is no such thing as a genetic epidemic.

Something in our modern world is apparently pushing a certain number of susceptible kids over the neurological limit and into a befuddling life of autism and other brain disorders. Several potential culprits beside thimerosal have been mentioned, though there is no hard evidence to link any of them to autism. Possible environmental "triggers" include: mercury in fish, pesticides, PCBs, flame retardants, jet fuel, live viruses in vaccines or some as-yet unidentified virus, and even rampant cell phone use. It is plausible that any combination of the above, with or without thimerosal exposure added into the mix, might cause harm to some fetuses and infant children.

But so far, thimerosal exposure has received the most studies (though the measles-mumps-rubella vaccine, or MMR, has also been studied). This book looks at evidence presented on both sides of the thimerosal controversy, but told from the parents' admittedly subjective point of view. Perhaps this story will be told one day from the opposing view, that of the doctors, bureaucrats, and drug company reps who claim nothing more than the laudable desire to save kids from the ravages of childhood disease.

But many of the public health officials who discount the thimerosal theory were unwilling to be interviewed for this book (or prohibited from speaking by superiors). Readers are invited to reach their own conclusions on the evidence.

Did the injection of organic mercury directly into the developing systems of small children cause irreparable harm? It's a plausible proposition, and a hugely important question. If the answer is affirmative, someone will have to pay to pick up the pieces.

Why did the CDC and the Food and Drug Administration (FDA) allow mercury exposures from childhood vaccines to more than double between 1988 and 1992 without bothering to calculate cumulative totals and their potential risks?

Why, for that matter, was there a corresponding spike in reported cases of autism spectrum disorders (ASD)? Why did autism grow from a relatively rare incidence of 1 in every 10,000 births in the 1980s to 1 in 500 in the late 1990s? Why did it continue to increase to 1 in 250 in 2000 and then 1 in 166 today?[5] Why are rates of ADD, attention deficit/hyperactivity disorder (ADHD), speech delay, and other childhood disorders also rising, and why does 1 in every 6 American children have a developmental disorder or behavioral problem?[6] And why does autism affect boys at a 4-to-1 ratio over girls?[7]

Autism has traditionally been a disease of industrialized nations, at least until recent years. But not all Western countries have autism epidemics. Autism spectrum disorder in the United States, with 60 per 10,000 (1 in 166) kids now affected, is much more prevalent than it is in northern European countries such as Denmark, which removed thimerosal from vaccines in 1992 and now reports just 7.7 per 10,000 children (or 1 in 1,300). The UK, meanwhile, which just announced that it would remove mercury from vaccines in September 2004, reports exactly the same prevalence of ASD—1 in 166 children—as the United States.[8]

This is not an antivaccine book. Childhood immunization was perhaps one of the greatest public health achievements of the twentieth century, and vaccines will continue to play a crucial role in our lives as we enter an uncertain age of emerging diseases and potential bioterrorism.

Some parents, fearing harmful effects, have been tempted not to vaccinate their children. Most people would agree that this is foolhardy and dangerous. Few of us are old enough to remember the great epidemics of influenza, pertussis, smallpox, polio, diphtheria, and measles that once swept entire populations—until the advent of vaccines reduced those maladies to abstract, unthreatening concepts, at least in America. These diseases, all of them preventable, can kill children. When vaccination rates fall, disease rates rise.

Neither should this book be viewed as partisan in nature. While some named in this book raise harsh criticisms of the Bush administration or Republicans in the Senate, two of the leading protagonists—from these parents' point of view—are among the most conservative members of Congress. Moreover, it is important to remember that much of the story takes place during the administration of President Bill Clinton.

Parental fear of vaccines has threatened the viability of the U.S. National

Immunization Program. But if scientists prove that mercury in vaccines was at least partly to blame for much of the autism epidemic—and that the culprit has been largely (or one day entirely) removed—then confidence in childhood immunization should return to comfortable levels.

But most health officials insist that mercury in vaccines is harmless, even as warnings go off about the toxic effects on infants and fetuses from mercury in fish. This mixed message is doing nothing to bolster faith in the immunization program.

Most vaccines come in multidose vials and cannot be sold without a preservative, such as thimerosal. Because of its mercury content, thimerosal prevents bacterial and fungal contamination in vials that undergo repeated puncturing of the seal by needles. Thimerosal is not required for single-dose vials, nor is it found in vaccine preparations, including MMR, that contain live organisms.

Thimerosal was marketed for vaccines in the 1930s and remained the preservative of choice in the United States throughout the twentieth century. Mercury-free preservatives were developed, but never widely used. The main reason is thought to be economic.

Developing alternative preservatives and having them tested and approved by the FDA is a costly proposition. Switching to single-dose vials, another option, is feasible, but it is also expensive and more cumbersome for transportation and storage. Finally, thimerosal is often used in vaccine manufacturing itself, to preserve sterility in the production process. Since it was already in vaccines, it didn't make much sense to seek out an alternative. And at any rate, the FDA and CDC never said that thimerosal might be hazardous.

Curiously, autism was not identified as a disorder until the early 1940s, a few years after thimerosal was introduced in vaccines. It was described by psychiatrists Leo Kanner and Hans Asperger, who independently coined the terms *autism* and *autistic* respectively. The term comes from the Greek word for self, *autos*.

In the late 1940s, Austrian-born psychologist Bruno Bettelheim proposed that autistic children came from backgrounds of aloof mothering by women who could not or would not provide the warmth and emotional support needed for the normal development of a child. He labeled these women *refrigerator mothers,* a term that stuck until the 1960s.

In 1964, Bernard Rimland, a psychologist and father of an autistic son, wrote a groundbreaking book called *Infantile Autism: The Syndrome and Its Implications for a Neural Theory of Behavior.* The book is widely credited with debunking the refrigerator mother theory, which today seems both laughable and insulting to many parents. The book helped convince the psychiatric community that autism was not an emotional problem at all, but rather a biological one.

In the 1980s, suspicions began to surface among some parents of autistic children that vaccines were somehow involved in the disorder. In 1985, Barbara Loe Fisher, cofounder of the National Vaccine Information Center, coauthored a book (with H. L. Coulter) called *A Shot in the Dark*. In the course of her research she found many children who developed brain damage after a reaction to the diphtheria-tetanus-pertussis (DTP) shot.

Vaccines continued to remain on autism's radar screen, and were raised to new notoriety when a young English doctor named Andrew Wakefield said that the MMR live-virus vaccine (which does not contain thimerosal) might be contributing to regressive autism in children.

Then in July 1999 came the U.S. government announcement—the "Joint Statement"—about mercury levels in childhood vaccines.

Now the stakes could not be higher. Perhaps billions of dollars in legal claims are pending against drug companies involved in vaccine production. The deep-pocketed pharmaceutical industry has extended its financial largesse to politicians and scientists around the country, in open pursuit of indemnity against lawsuits and, some charge, in a darker effort to suppress evidence of thimerosal's toxicity.

Meanwhile, the reputation of American public health is on the line.

The jury is still out on thimerosal, but deliberations are well under way. One side will emerge vindicated, and the other will earn eternal scorn in the medical history books.

In November 2003, the father of an autistic boy in North Carolina, an antithimerosal activist and a believer, approached a well-known pediatrician after the doctor had delivered a lecture on the safety of vaccines in general, and thimerosal in particular.

"You know something, Doctor?" the father said. "If it turns out that you are right, then I will personally come down to your office and apologize to you with every fiber of my being.

"But if it turns out that you are wrong," he added, "then you are going to hell."

Evidence of Harm

Prologue

LYN REDWOOD got the call from a lawyer friend only an hour before the vote. The prospects were bad, he told her. It was too late to do much about it now.

The news came like a kick in the gut. Lyn almost dropped the phone into a pot of pasta on the stove. "Damn!" she shouted. Her cry was loud enough to startle her eight-year-old, Will, who sat quietly at the kitchen table in the Redwoods' expansive house south of Atlanta. The boy nearly burst into tears.

It was the evening of November 13, 2002, and the House of Representatives was about to approve the historic Homeland Security Act. Lyn was all for security in this age of Al Qaeda. But she never dreamed it would come with such a price tag.

The lawyer told Lyn that some unnamed agent had secretly inserted a last-minute provision into the bill, adding two brief paragraphs onto the massive document before the roll call. The provision would dismiss hundreds of civil suits filed by parents against Eli Lilly and other drug companies for allegedly allowing dangerous levels of mercury into their kids' vaccines. Very few members of Congress knew it was there.

The stealth rider would change everything, wiping out years of struggle that Lyn and many others had endured to get their day in court.

Will Redwood had autism, and Lyn blamed it on the mercury in his shots. The toxic heavy metal was used as a vaccine preservative called thimerosal. Thimerosal had been developed by Eli Lilly & Company in the 1920s, though Lilly no longer made the product. But the company still licensed it to other producers, reportedly earning a profit in the bargain.

Lyn and her husband, Tommy, had filed a thimerosal lawsuit in Georgia state civil court. The Redwoods and other parents had spent three years compiling evidence of mercury poisoning in their children. Many were preparing to present this evidence in individual and class-action lawsuits filed in courts of law across the country.

But now, with the stroke of a computer keyboard, all those lawsuits would be thrown out. The Redwoods and others would be left in the legal lurch, without due process or any further recourse. Now there would be no day in court.

The surreptitious rider essentially funneled all thimerosal lawsuits into a little-known federal claims court that had been created by Congress in 1986 to compensate damages for vaccine injuries or death. The "Vaccine Court," as it is known, shields drugmakers from liability by having awards paid out of a taxpayer-funded account, rather than by the companies themselves.

But there was one hitch. The Vaccine Court had a statute of limitations of three years. If your child had allegedly demonstrated signs of injury before that period, as was the case with Will Redwood and tens of thousands of other autistic children, you were plain out of luck. You could not enter the federal compensation program.

For this reason, the Redwoods had brought their claim to civil court. Here, the burden of proof was higher, but so were the potential payouts. Parents of autistic children were facing lifelong bills estimated at over two million dollars per child. The families were neither greedy nor litigious, as some politicians had charged. They were desperate. And now the only door left open—civil court—was being slammed shut, perversely, by an antiterrorism bill.

The irony was punishing. Congress was approving a colossal reorganization of the bureaucracy to fortify the nation in the perilous post-9/11 world. It was all being done in the name of liberty, as President Bush had said. But what liberty was there, Lyn thought, when greedy hands blithely rewrote laws and slapped justice in the face?

The language in the rider dismissing the lawsuits was nothing new. It had been drafted the year before—written as part of a larger vaccine injury bill crafted by a senator from Tennessee named Bill Frist, a conservative Republican with strong ties to the drug industry, and the only M.D. to serve in the

upper chamber. Lyn Redwood and many other parents had fought fero-
ciously all summer against the Frist vaccine bill. Their Democratic allies, who
controlled the Senate at the time, had prevailed. It was one more battle in the
ongoing thimerosal war, but at least the parents had won this round. Or so
they thought.

But Republicans had just swept the midterm elections on November 5,
2002, and recaptured control of the Senate. Someone in the party, it is safe to
assume, was feeling cocky and confident enough to pull this off. But they
hadn't reckoned with the wave of outrage they were about to unleash.

Lyn Redwood ran to the computer in her large comfortable home and
fired off an urgent communiqué to several comrades across the country: good
friends like Liz Birt, an attorney from Chicago with an autistic son, Matthew;
and Sallie Bernard, a successful marketing executive out in Aspen, Colorado,
with an afflicted boy of her own, named Bill.

For three years, since the government had admitted that most American
kids vaccinated between 1990 and 2000 were exposed to mercury levels in
excess of federal safety limits, Lyn, Liz, and Sallie had been drawn to each
other in common cause. They grew united in the belief that thimerosal had
damaged their kids and hurled them into the shuttered hell of autism. They
had formed an influential advocacy and research group called the Coalition
for Safe Minds (Sensible Action for Ending Mercury-Induced Neurological
Disorders). Largely self-taught in the complexities of biochemistry, toxicology, and epidemiology, the three mothers and dozens of their allies had taken
on science, business, and government with their radical new mercury-autism
hypothesis.

Many parents of autistic children applauded the women and bestowed on
them an affectionate nickname, the "Mercury Moms." But on the other side
of the equation, within the inner circles of their powerful opponents, the
women had earned themselves ridicule and scorn.

"Well, it looks like they caught us unaware," Lyn wrote to Liz, Sallie,
and a handful of other parents that evening. "I just received a phone call that
parts of the Frist bill dealing with thimerosal are being added to the Homeland Security Bill that is being voted on tonight! Please, if possible, try to
contact your local representative by e-mail and ask that they specifically exclude anything related to the vaccine compensation bill being included in
Homeland Security."

Everyone who got the message tried desperately to do something to alert
lawmakers. But it was too late, of course. Even some of the parents' staunchest
allies were about to vote away their rights, however unwittingly, in the name
of freedom.

One of the people most devastated by the news was Laura Bono, the mother of a twelve-year-old boy, Jackson, who had been diagnosed not only with severe autism, but also with mercury poisoning. Laura and her husband, Scott, an insurance salesman in Durham, North Carolina, were about to file a civil suit of their own. It had been several years since Jackson's diagnosis, and they were ineligible to file in Vaccine Court. Jackson's medical and educational care had already cost over seven hundred thousand dollars, and much of it was not covered by insurance. The Bonos had depleted their savings simply struggling to provide for their very sick boy.

Scott and Laura Bono had fought side by side with other parents against the Frist bill, and were ardent believers in the mercury-autism connection. And the Bonos had connections in Washington. Scott had known since high school a bright, conservative young woman named Beth Clay. In recent years, Beth had gone to work on the Republican staff of the House Committee on Government Reform. By chance, the committee's colorful chairman was the controversial Republican congressman Dan Burton of Indiana—a man with his own suspicions of thimerosal.

Burton, it turned out, has a grandson named Christian, who had become desperately ill after receiving multiple vaccinations against several childhood diseases in one day. Most of them contained thimerosal. Within days, Christian became completely unaware of his surroundings. He would run aimlessly around the house, screaming indiscriminately, flapping his arms and banging his head against the walls. Doctors diagnosed autism. Dan Burton blamed thimerosal.

When Laura Bono got Lyn Redwood's e-mail, she called Beth Clay on her cell phone. "Beth, they've stuck a rider in to protect Lilly from lawsuits," Laura said. "You have to alert Burton." Beth leapt to action. She knew that the congressman, had he known about the "Lilly rider," would have gone ballistic and scrambled to the House floor to raise hellfire among his colleagues. But Beth was unable to reach Burton before he cast his lot to protect the homeland.

The next day, Dan Burton was fuming. There was only one person in Washington, he thought, who wielded the power, and had the gall, to commit such an act. It was the Republican Majority Leader, Richard Armey, who was set to resign at the end of the year. Burton and a few staffers marched over to Armey's office and confronted the politically powerful Texan with the slow, folksy drawl.

"I'm told the two of them almost got in a fistfight," Beth told Scott Bono later that day. "I have never seen the chairman so angry in my life. And believe me, I have seen him pretty damned steamed before. But nothing like this. If only I had gotten to him, maybe we could have stopped this."

"But what did he say?" Scott asked anxiously. "Armey, I mean. What did he say about the Lilly rider?"

"Armey did it," Beth said. "He said the request came from the White House." It would be weeks, however, before Dick Armey would admit—and then deny—the legislative mischief.

In the meantime, the mystery over who had inserted the controversial provisions (three other unrelated riders were also clandestinely stapled to the bill) had become, as the *New York Times* put it, "A Washington whodunit worthy of Agatha Christie."[9]

"On Capitol Hill, Congressional aides-turned-detectives have traced the emergence of the provision to the Veterans Day weekend," wrote the *Times*'s Sheryl Gay Stolberg. "Flush from their party's victories on Election Day, and with a mandate from President Bush to pass a domestic security bill, Republican negotiators in the House and Senate holed up for three days in the Capitol to hammer out the details."

One aide told the paper that the language "mysteriously appeared in the House version of the bill in entirely different type than the rest of the measure, as though someone had clipped it out of Mr. Frist's legislation and simply pasted it in." All the negotiators apparently supported the move, but no one would say who was responsible.

Critics of the provision, the *Times* noted, were "quick to point out that the White House has close ties to Lilly. The first President Bush sat on the Lilly board in the late 1970's. The White House budget director, Mitchell E. Daniels, Jr., is a former Lilly executive. The company's chairman and chief executive, Sidney Taurel, was appointed in June by President Bush to serve on a presidential council that will advise Mr. Bush on domestic security."

The White House denied having any hand in the rider. So did Eli Lilly.

" 'I personally had no involvement whatsoever with these provisions,' Mitch Daniels protested. 'I spoke to no one, either inside the administration or outside the administration. I did not have any communications with anyone from Eli Lilly regarding the issue. Indeed, I had not even heard of thimerosal until [now], which is not surprising because Eli Lilly stopped making thimerosal a decade before I began working there.' "[10]

To many observers, what seemed "surprising" was that Daniels, who had been Lilly's senior vice president for corporate strategy, had not known about a product that was licensed by his own company.

Lilly executives also feigned ignorance. " 'We made absolutely no contact with Mitch or anyone in his office about this,' " company spokesman Rob Smith said at the time. " 'It's a mystery to us how it got in there.' "[11]

On November 18, Dan Burton went to the House floor and demanded that the rider be removed before the Senate voted on the act. "These provisions don't belong in this bill," he said. "This is not a homeland security issue. This is a fairness issue."

"We have an epidemic on our hands," Burton warned in a statement released the same day. "More and more parents believe that the autism affecting their children is related to a mercury preservative used in numerous vaccines given to their children. These provisions in the Homeland Security Bill will cut off their recourse to the courts, and that's just wrong. Instead of passing legislation to take away the rights of families with vaccine-injured children, we should be passing legislation to try to help them."[12]

Senate Democrats agreed, and offered a motion to kill the Lilly rider before voting on the legislation. The move was opposed by none other than Senator Bill Frist.

"We are a nation at risk," Frist intoned gravely in the Senate. "The threat of liability should not become a barrier to the protection of the American people."[13] The implication was that thimerosal liability protection was essential if companies were going to develop vaccines against bioterrorism weapons like smallpox and anthrax. But Frist failed to mention that these vaccines contain no thimerosal whatsoever.

Lyn Redwood's phone was ringing off the hook. *Good Morning America* wanted to talk to her, and so did Bob Herbert, columnist for the *New York Times*.[14]

Herbert went on the offensive against the Lilly rider. "Buried in this massive bill," he wrote, "snuck into it in the dark of night by persons unknown (actually, it's fair to say by Republican persons unknown), was a provision that—incredibly—will protect Eli Lilly and a few other big pharmaceutical outfits from lawsuits by parents who believe their children were harmed by thimerosal. . . . There's a real bad smell here. Eli Lilly will benefit greatly as both class-action and individual lawsuits are derailed. But there are no fingerprints in sight. No one will own up to a legislative deed that is both cynical and shameful. The politicians with their hands out and the fat cats with plenty of green to spread around have carried the day. Nothing is too serious to exploit, not even the defense of the homeland during a time of terror."

As for Lyn Redwood and the Safe Minds advocacy group, Herbert wrote, "They're at a slight disadvantage, wielding a popgun against the nuclear-powered influence of an Eli Lilly."

The effort to kill the rider failed, despite intense lobbying by parents and their allies on Capitol Hill. The next day, the Senate passed the House version of the bill in its entirety. The same day, Bush administration lawyers quietly filed a motion in the federal Vaccine Court to permanently seal the records on all thimerosal-related material handed over by the government.

But the furtive move was also a blessing in disguise, Lyn thought. So many people had dismissed the mercury-autism theory as pure nonsense. Despite all their efforts to connect the scientific dots between thimerosal and neurological disorders, the parents had been unable to gain much attention, let alone support.

Now that was changing. If government and industry had nothing to fear from thimerosal lawsuits, many observers were asking, what was the need for all this secret maneuvering and rush to liability protection?

1. Mothers on a Mission

LYN REDWOOD KNEW she was pregnant at the first sip of white Zinfandel. In her previous two pregnancies, the taste of alcohol had taken on an unpalatable, almost metallic quality, and now, here it was again. Lyn gagged and set down the frosty wineglass. Her husband, Tommy, looked at her with a slight note of alarm. But Lyn just closed her eyes and waited for the nausea to subside. Then she stood up and smiled.

"I'm fine," she said quietly to Tommy. "Everything is just fine." It was Memorial Day Weekend, 1993, and the couple had driven from their home outside Atlanta across the steamy deep South to the hamlet of Columbus, Mississippi, for a visit to Tommy's parents. On the five-hour ride home, Lyn could think of nothing but the taste of that wine. She was excited, but wanted to make sure before saying anything to Tommy.

Lyn smiled at the prospect of a new child. She knew that Tommy adored her children, Drew and Hanna, from her previous marriage. But she also knew that it must be difficult at times to raise someone else's kids.

When they got home, Lyn ran upstairs to the master bathroom where she kept some pregnancy tests. The Zinfandel had not deceived her. She really was pregnant.

Lyn went downstairs to tell Tommy the news. He was overjoyed. Now he would have a child who would call him Dad instead of Tommy. The new baby would complete the happy picture.

Lyn was an attractive woman with cocoa-colored hair and soft, almost catlike brown eyes. She met Tommy in 1986, in Birmingham, Alabama, where she was completing her MS in nursing and he was a young med student from the University of Mississippi with a handsome smile, dark hair, and an athletic physique.

The two were married in 1987, and Tommy wholeheartedly accepted Lyn's children, Hanna and Drew, as his own. In 1991, the young family moved to Atlanta, where Lyn began work as a family nurse practitioner, and Tommy got a job in the ER at Newnan Hospital, outside Atlanta.

The past six years had been almost dreamlike for the Redwoods. They had recently put the finishing touches on a three-story, wood and stone contemporary home on nine acres of hardwood forest in tiny Tyrone, Georgia, thirty minutes south of Atlanta. A rural small town, Tyrone looks a lot like Mayberry from the *Andy Griffith Show* (except for the Confederate symbol on the old Georgia state flag that still flutters above the American Legion hall).

The kids had never been happier. Hanna and Drew were excelling in the gifted program of the local school, where Drew entered kindergarten at the third-grade reading level. Life was sweet in the new house, with its free-form pool and flat stone terraces, its hiking trails through Georgia pines and open pastures, and the covered wooden bridge that Lyn and Tommy built over Trickum Creek, which meanders lazily across their land.

Lyn's third pregnancy was perfectly normal, by all measurements. The only thing to set it apart from the first two was that Lyn, whose blood type is RH-negative, was given two injections of Gamalin brand Anti-Rho(D) globulin, at fourteen weeks and twenty-eight weeks of gestation. About 15 percent of all women have an RH-negative blood type and, if the fetus is RH-positive, as was the case with Will, the mother could produce antibodies against the child's blood type. This in turn could create potentially deadly complications in subsequent pregnancies. Anti-Rho(D) globulin staves off that disaster. (Lyn received a third injection immediately after Will was born, in case there had been any undetected mix of blood during delivery.)

In Lyn's third trimester, she was told the pregnancy was breech. When she entered labor, in February 1994, a baby boy appeared with two feet sticking out. It was Groundhog Day, and the Redwoods would later joke that their son had seen his shadow and tried to run back in. The doctors ordered a C-section and the procedure went well. A beaming baby boy, named Will Redwood, arrived into the world happy and healthy.

Will, with his brown hair and cool, gray-blue eyes, was an exceedingly good baby. Rarely fussy and almost always smiling, he seemed alert and engaged in his new world. Will chuckled and grinned whenever Lyn tickled him, and he loved to play tag with the family cat, crawling around the living room and squealing with delight whenever he "caught" the kitty. He was an unusually inquisitive and adventurous boy. At eight months, he learned to use his baby walker, and wandered around the ground floor of the house exploring every corner he could get into.

Will breast-fed without trouble and met, or exceeded, normal developmental landmarks. He began speaking right on schedule, and learned new words like *mama, daddy,* and *kitty cat* almost daily. By twelve months, he could play Little Tykes basketball with his brother, Drew. Lyn and Tommy watched in awe as Will toddled to the hoop and slam-dunked the ball home. Each time, he turned to his parents, clapped his little hands, and cried, "Yea!!"

Lyn, the experienced nurse, made sure that Will received every vaccination on the U.S. Childhood Immunization Schedule. She couldn't help but notice that kids were getting a lot more shots now than Hanna and Drew had received in the 1980s. At two months, four months, six months, and one year, Will was brought in for a "well-baby" visit, each time receiving multiple injections against dangerous diseases like hepatitis-B, *Haemophilus influenzae* type B (Hib), or diphtheria-tetanus (DT).

Shortly after Will's one-year visit, he developed strep throat, which is rare in young infants. Then he developed rotavirus, a gastrointestinal bug that can cause severe pain and discomfort in a child. One Saturday, while Lyn had a good friend visiting for the weekend, Will vomited on the living room floor. Lyn didn't think too much about it, but a few hours later Will vomited again, and it quickly got to the point where he couldn't keep food down at all. Worried, Lyn called her pediatrician, who prescribed an antinausea suppository. The pediatrician said that rotavirus was fairly common in children. He was not unduly alarmed.

The next day, the diarrhea began. It quickly got so bad it would fill the toddler's diapers and run down his legs in burning, acidic streams. But there was no treatment for rotavirus, and the only remedy Lyn could think of was to give Will rice-and-glucose water every hour or two, to replace the electrolytes he was losing. The diarrhea drained from him like foul floodwaters and the vomiting wracked his small body. Even though the worst symptoms abated after a week or so, Will never really made a recovery to full health. He ran periodic and unexplained fevers. He seemed under the weather all the time.

At around seventeen months, Will developed an upper respiratory infection, like a very bad cold, and began wheezing uncontrollably. The Redwoods rushed him to Peachtree Regional Hospital, where he was immediately admitted and given IV antibiotics, steroids, and other medications. Lyn stayed with her son for two days, sleeping with Will inside his misty respirator tent.

Will also lost an alarming amount of weight. He had, for all practical purposes, stopped eating. Lyn put him on a strict regimen of vitamins and supplemental nutritional treatments. And even though she had weaned him from the bottle, she found it was now the only way to get real food (in the guise of meal-replacement shakes) inside the boy.

Once spritely and impish, Will now sat motionless in his infant seat, gazing at videos in dogged, unnerving repetition. And there was something else, something ominous that transpired during this period—something that Lyn and Tommy noticed only gradually, and didn't pay much mind to because Will had been so darned sick.

But there was no denying it. Will had stopped talking.

"Oh, don't worry about that," Lyn was told by friends and family. "Boys always talk late." Tommy, for instance, hadn't started speaking until he was three, and he turned out to be a skilled physician. Lyn's first son, Drew, hadn't been a late talker. So maybe it was something in Tommy's genes.

There were other signs of trouble, of course, signs that Lyn only realized several years later. One weekday morning, when Will was in his infant seat, staring at space, Lyn walked directly in front of him, bending down until her face met his, her deep brown eyes just inches from Will's. She smiled, she waved. But Will just sat there, looking straight through his mother.

"My," she marveled. "You have incredibly intense concentration!"

Years later, Lyn would scoff at her own naïveté. Loss of speech and lack of eye contact are classic symptoms of autism. But the disorder, still so rare at the time, was way off her maternal radar screen. Despite her medical background, Lyn had never met an autistic kid in her life.

AUTISM CONTINUED to be the last thing on their minds as Lyn and Tommy witnessed Will's increasingly baffling behavior. He grew acutely sensitive to sound, and would cover his ears and yelp in pain if the TV were turned up. Going to Drew's basketball games was always an ordeal. When the buzzer went off, Will threw his hands to his ears and screamed loudly enough to pierce the crowd's roar. Lyn learned to watch the timer and cover Will's ears in advance.

Then there was the incident at the Little League game. One muggy evening in Tyrone, the Redwoods were at the local ballpark taking in one of Drew's games. Will, the restless toddler, kept trying to get up and wander around the bleacher area. Finally, after several attempts at trailing her son and returning him to his seat, Lyn decided to let Will go, just to see what would happen.

"I'm going to just sit here and see how far he goes before he realizes he's out of the ten-foot radius or so," she said to Tommy. Will just kept wandering aimlessly away, far from the stadium lights. He was a good fifty feet away from his parents, heading nowhere into the night, before she ran to fetch him. At that point the Redwoods knew: if they didn't keep an eye on him every second of the day, Will would be gone.

Will's hearing continued to deteriorate. In September 1995 he was referred to a pediatric ear-nose-and-throat specialist at Emory University, who poked and prodded the boy like some pet science project. He said fluid had accumulated behind Will's eardrums, and the pressure was causing severe hearing loss. Will would need tympanostomy tubes surgically implanted in his eardrums in order to drain the fluid, relieve the pressure, and restore hearing.

On the morning of the operation, Lyn arrived at 5:00 A.M. with a very nervous, hyperactive little boy. The nurses slipped Will into a pale blue gown and Lyn let them walk him up and down the hall. Even at that early hour, Will could not sit still.

The procedure went well. But the doctor remarked on how little fluid he found behind the eardrums. It perplexed him. The surgery might not have been enough to address Will's difficulties, he said. Perhaps Will's problems were not related directly to hearing. There might be a deeper problem with his communication abilities. Will would need speech therapy immediately.

In October 1995 an assessment confirmed that Will's language skills were exceedingly low. At the time, all he could do was make baby sounds. He could verbalize, but none of it made any sense. It came out all garbled. His speech and language skills at twenty months were those of a six-month-old. On expressive language, he scored at the level of a five-month-old. Will was examined by a neurologist, who ordered an MRI, EEG, and chromosome studies, all of which returned normal. But the boy was not making any real progress. No one had any idea what was wrong.

Mostly, the Redwoods felt relieved. Their biggest fear had been that a brain tumor or some other type of malignancy had caused Will's regression. But nothing was wrong. There were no brain abnormalities, no damaged chromosomes that might cause mental retardation. Will's speech delay was just a fluke, an easily denied sign of things to come.

When Will was two, Lyn enrolled him in a new nursery school program run out of the local New Hope Baptist church. She assumed that leaving him in a classroom with other toddlers would naturally help his speech develop. But when she took Will in on the first day, she discovered that most of the other kids in the program weren't talking, either.

"My God," Lyn muttered sadly under her breath. "What on earth is going on around here? So many kids who aren't talking. Is there something in the water?" Lyn never found out what was wrong with the kids, but seeing children who were not unlike Will, for the first time ever, left her with an odd, slightly guilty sense of comfort.

When Will was three, in 1997, he entered a special program run by the local county school system for kids with advanced developmental disorders. It was held in a public elementary school, a modern, clean, brick-and-steel affair that had been built just two years before, where the "typical" kids went. There were six kids in Will's classroom, all of them with developmental disorders. One afternoon, about a week into school, Lyn came by to pick up Will. She'd arrived early and decided to peek through the window. What she saw horrified her.

A teacher had strapped Will into a wooden chair with plywood panels going up the sides. It looked like something from *One Flew over the Cuckoo's Nest,* Lyn thought. She had no idea that such contraptions existed. She rushed into the school to hear Will's spine-chilling screech echoing from the walls. She tore down the hallway and burst into the classroom, fuming.

"What are you doing!? I don't want him in that chair! Get him out, right now."

"But Mrs. Redwood," the teacher sputtered. "He won't sit still for circle time."

"Fine," she snapped. "I will come and hold him, every day if need be. He can sit on my lap." Lyn was working weekend shifts in order to free up time to look after Will. For the next several months, she came to school every day for circle time.

One day while collecting Will at class, Lyn struck up a conversation with the mother of another boy enrolled in the program. The woman regarded Will intently, one eyebrow arched. "You know something?" she said, wary but kindly. "Will looks and behaves very much like my son. He has the same demeanor."

Lyn was intrigued, even a bit heartened. Perhaps this mother knew the secret to unlocking Will's locked-in world.

"Really. And do you know what's wrong with your son?"

"Sure," the woman said, matter-of-factly. "He has autism."

THERE WAS NO WAY that Will had autism, Lyn still believed. He didn't flap his arms, didn't run in circles or bang his head on the walls like the autistic kids she had seen in some of the more graphic news programs. But the mother at Will's school gently persisted. She told Lyn that a new behavioral therapy was helping children with developmental disorders.

"There's this really great program on the north side of Atlanta," she informed Lyn. "They're doing amazing things with our kids. You really have to come see for yourself." Lyn agreed to go. She was so desperate by now, she would do anything for an effective therapy, even if her son didn't have autism.

The program employed a treatment method called Applied Behavior Analysis (ABA), which was developed by Dr. Ivar Lovaas in the 1980s. Based on the revolutionary theory that autism is treatable, ABA has shown remarkable success in children with autism and severe developmental disorders. Some of the children treated with this method go on to achieve normal intellectual and cognitive functioning. Lyn went to sit in on an ABA session being held in the private home of an Atlanta mother with an autistic son. He was two years older than Will, and seemed to be doing extraordinarily well. Lyn watched, dumbfounded, as the boy recited his ABCs and read aloud from a storybook.

Proper ABA therapy requires a team of experts to work one-on-one with the affected child for hours at a time. The treatment is rigorous, exhausting, and prohibitively expensive; the cost for one year can reach a hundred thousand dollars. The Lovaas method uses behavior modification principles to encourage "good" and appropriate behavior—proper language, communication, and play skills; better observation; and outward affection—while repressing and discouraging problematic behavior like withdrawal, aggression, inattention, and temper tantrums. ABA therapists then break down each desired skill into small, discrete steps. This "discrete trial training" systematically drills each step into the child's psyche through endless hours of painstaking, repetitive conditioning. Teachers warmly reward children for good behavior, ignore them when they exhibit bad behavior, and remove them to "time-out" when things get out of hand.

The method is not without its critics, who say it is little better than training a dog. But many parents have claimed complete success with ABA therapy, and it is the only nonmedical autism treatment endorsed by the U.S. Surgeon General. Lyn was now genuinely excited, for perhaps the first time since Will got sick. She returned home and immediately called the woman in her school district who handled special services, to request that they provide ABA therapy to Will.

"Well," the woman said, "we can only do that for children with autism."

"But, but . . ." Lyn interjected.

"Don't worry. Will's eligible."

"What do you mean?" Lyn asked. "You're saying he's autistic?"

"Mrs. Redwood, to be honest, we have sort of thought that all along."

Lyn was stunned. "Why didn't you tell me?"

"As teachers, we can't diagnose," the woman said. "The children must be diagnosed by the school psychologist, but they don't do exams until the kids are five."

"You know," Lyn said, "this is like someone having cancer, but no one wants to tell you because they don't want to upset you."

"I know, Mrs. Redwood. I'm sorry. But Will *is* eligible."

In November, the school met with Will and Lyn. All the specialists were brought in: Will's speech and language pathologist, his two teachers, the school district's autism coordinator, its director of special education services, and the principal.

"Mrs. Redwood, what are your goals for your son?" the director asked.

"I want him to know his name," she replied. "That is my first goal."

"And your second goal?"

"By the time he starts kindergarten," she said, smiling, "I want him to be indistinguishable from his peers."

Heavy sighs broke the silence, but Lyn held fast. Her son did not have an official diagnosis, and she was going to cling to her faith that his dire condition might only be temporary. The group agreed that the school would provide ABA therapy to Will, and train some of its teachers in the unfamiliar method.

Within weeks, Lyn began delivering Will to school an hour early every day for intensive one-on-one therapy with teachers. He received another hour of ABA at school after class, then came home, ate, and completed another two hours of therapy.

By this time, Lyn's denial about Will's autism was beginning to crumble. Lyn and Tommy purchased a copy of a Lovaas handbook written by Catherine Maurice, who also wrote the groundbreaking book *Let Me Hear Your Voice,* in which she detailed the amazing story of curing not one, but two of her children with autistic disorders. Lyn would later come to refer to the handbook as her "autism bible." Lyn learned that parents aren't always the most suitable ABA therapists for their own children, though some parents have tried. So the Redwoods used the manual to train two other people to take on the task, a local unemployed college graduate and a teacher's aide at a school for children with developmental disabilities. For Lyn, it was often difficult to watch. Will wasn't always the best student. "He does some of it for a while very well," she told Tommy, "but he needs it to be very fast-paced, and he needs the rewards all the time." When that didn't happen, Will would wail like a trapped animal.

Will began to log modest progress with his ABA home-style therapy. During the next few years, he would learn his name, as Lyn had hoped. Eventually he started to learn his colors, and then the alphabet.

And just as slowly, Lyn and Tommy came to accept that their son was afflicted with some form of autism. Despite all the experts who had examined him, ultimately it was the medically trained Redwoods who diagnosed Will themselves. One night in mid-1998, they got out the DSM-IV (*Diagnostic and Statistical Manual of Mental Disorders*—Vol. 4) and compared Will's symptoms with those listed in the book of mental maladies. Lyn and Tommy concluded that Will had pervasive developmental disorder, not otherwise specified (PDD-NOS), a moderately severe neurological illness that lies within a constellation of diseases known as autism spectrum disorder, or ASD.

ASD, which includes "classic" full-blown autism, PDD-NOS, Rett syndrome, and Asperger's syndrome (the so-called Idiot Savant malady popularized in the film *Rain Man*), is a neurodevelopmental disorder that emerges early in life. Children with ASD exhibit an assemblage of seemingly unrelated features, with wide variation in symptoms and severity. In the most notable cases of classic autism, children flap their arms, bang their heads, walk on their toes, line things up in rows, or spin in endless circles.

Will showed none of those traits. But many ASD symptoms described him well, such as severe social impairment, verbal and nonverbal communication problems, repetitive behaviors, movement disorder, sensory dysfunction, and cognitive impairments. In many children, and Will was no exception, there are also unusual gastrointestinal difficulties and immune abnormalities.

Onset of the disorder, as in Will's case, occurs before thirty-six months of age. Some children are clearly autistic from birth. But today, most cases appear only after a year or more of normal development—followed by clear regression or failure to progress.

Autism was long thought to be purely genetic in origin. But there is now an emerging belief that many cases are the product of an interaction between some type of genetic predisposition and early exposure to environmental triggers, called "insults."

Like most Americans at the time, the Redwoods assumed that autism was an extremely rare disease. Lyn was soon to learn otherwise, however. From the 1940s, when autism was first described in the literature, until the late 1970s, it had indeed been rare. The U.S. incidence was just 1 to 3 births per 10,000. But by 1998 the figure had climbed to 20 to 40 births per 10,000. Today, there are accounts of 60 to 80 cases per 10,000 children (or 1 in 166) reported in some states, including New Jersey and California, making it more common than multiple sclerosis, cystic fibrosis, or childhood cancer.[15] Could there have been something in the water, as Lyn had joked to herself back at the Baptist church, or was there something else at play? Had some other "insult" damaged Will and so many other kids?

SALLIE McCONNELL met Thomas Bernard in 1975 when they were freshmen at Harvard. The Bernards married in 1979 and eventually settled into a loftlike apartment on East Twenty-third Street in Manhattan. Tom landed a handsomely paid job on Wall Street, at Salomon Brothers, while Sallie got work with TMP Worldwide, an ad agency that specialized in regional Yellow Page directories. The Bernards were on their way to building significant wealth.

In 1986, Sallie took her business skills and started a market research firm, Advertising Research Corporation, now called ARC. Based in Cranford, New Jersey, the twelve-employee operation manages a network of focus groups, telephone studies, shopping mall questionnaires, and surveys through the mail and on the Internet.

In 1987, Sallie learned she was pregnant—with triplets. The Bernards went shopping for a real house outside the city, with trees and a lawn and a garden for the new arrivals. They purchased a large Tudor in the affluent suburb of Summit, New Jersey.

The triplets were born five weeks premature in September 1987, at Manhattan's Lenox Hill Hospital. All three were underweight, but Bill was born perilously so. Fred weighed in at 5¾ pounds, and Jamie was 4¾ pounds, but Bill tipped the scale at just 3 pounds. Healthy Fred went home right away. Jamie, who needed to gain just a few more ounces before release, stayed a couple of days longer.

Bill was less fortunate. Diagnosed with anemia, he was given a blood transfusion and remained in the hospital for nearly four weeks. It was a trying time for Sallie; even with hired household help, the young mother and businesswoman found herself torn between the clamors for attention from two babies at home, demanding clients at work, and a very sick boy in the hospital.

When all three sons were safely at home, Sallie began to notice that Bill was developing a bit more slowly than Fred and Jamie. She kept track of the boys' milestones. Fred and Jamie vied to be the first to raise his head up, first to roll over, first to stand up, and first to fall down. "It was always within days of each other," remembered Sallie, who retains a youthful freshness, with sea-green eyes and honey-colored hair. But Bill was always at least two weeks behind the other boys. He couldn't seem to catch up.

By the time the Bernard triplets turned two, they were beginning to speak, and Sallie kept track of the exciting progress. But as usual, Bill lagged behind his brothers. In one typical week, Fred would log in twelve new words, and Jamie would learn maybe eleven. But Bill, though he was learning, typically would have a new word list of five.

Sallie also made sure the boys completed their well-baby visits, and had their full range of required vaccinations. But given their small birth weights, the pediatrician decided to push back the first round of shots, from two months to four months.

Over the Christmas holidays in 1989, when the boys were around two and a half, Tom's parents flew to New Jersey for a visit. On a snowy night when the extended family was enjoying a roaring fire in the large living room, Tom's father, Fred, was horsing around with the triplets. Jamie and little Fred were squealing with glee, but Bill seemed distant, losing interest. Later, when Sallie got out the Tinker Toys to settle the boys down, Bill had a tough time inserting the sticks into the wooden wheels. He grew inconsolable until one of his brothers came to help him out.

"I must tell you," Fred confided in Tom and Sallie later that evening, after the boys went to bed, "I think something might be wrong with Bill. He's a little different than the other boys. He doesn't play with the same intensity they do."

The young couple brushed aside Fred's concerns, having convinced themselves that Bill would eventually catch up with his siblings. He just needed some time, that's all. Bill would be fine.

But Bill wasn't at all fine. By New Years, 1990, he began to withdraw from the world. He began screaming and tearing around the house as if he'd been set on fire. He quickly went downhill from there.

The Bernards, now aching with worry, brought Bill in for a full battery of neurological and cognitive tests.

"Mrs. Bernard," the doctor said, "I'm afraid we've found a number of things wrong."

"I'm ready, Doctor," said Sallie, whose trademark was a cool and calm demeanor, regardless of the situation. "Go ahead."

"The primary dysfunction we found was dysphasia. Do you know what that is?"

Sallie said she did not.

"It's a rather severe type of language disorder," he announced. The doctor went on to discuss some of the other problems he had diagnosed in Bill, including hyperactivity and attention problems.

A few days later, when Sallie received the full written report in the mail, she noticed that the doctor had scribbled in his notes: "Possibly watch for autistic-like tendencies." But the official diagnosis stood at language disorder. Sallie was concerned, but not overly alarmed. "Language disorder" sounded serious, but surely nothing that could not be overcome. Then she went to look up the definition of *dysphasia* in the dictionary. What she read was unsettling: the disease, it said, is "An impairment or loss of speech or ability to understand language, caused by brain disease or injury."

SALLIE COULDN'T GET those dreadful words, "brain disease or injury," out of her own restless mind. Bill had never been seriously injured, she thought, and certainly there was nothing catastrophic that could have injured his brain. But brain *disease*? Could such a thing have afflicted Bill, yet leave his brothers, with whom he shared the womb, unscathed? Sallie spent the next several months combing the libraries and bookstores of northern New Jersey, buying every book she could find about speech disorders, attention deficit/hyperactivity disorder (ADHD), brain disease, and aphasia. But she didn't buy anything on autism. Despite the doctor's note to "possibly watch for" autistic tendencies, nobody else had mentioned the disease. It never occurred to Sallie, until Bill was officially diagnosed, that the source of her son's distress was autism.

Evidence of that distress began presenting itself daily as Sallie and Tom frantically tried to figure out what was racking their son. Bill's speech problems only grew worse. He stopped learning new words, and the words he did know quickly became unintelligible. Sallie couldn't understand him anymore. Bill wanted to talk, she could see that, but his articulation was so poor she could no longer make out a word.

The bad news just kept coming. Bill began losing fine motor control. Then his eating habits became downright ungainly, even for a three-year-old. Sallie snapped photos of the triplets sitting around the kitchen table after a meal. Fred and Jamie cleaned their plates, keeping themselves reasonably tidy. But Bill looked as if he'd dumped his food on his head, staining himself with the bright hues of a childhood dinner, which splattered down his bib and onto the table. The poor kid, obviously floundering, had a hard time getting food to his mouth.

Not long after that, playing with building blocks, something Bill had always loved to do, became impossible for the painfully clumsy child.

Bill's visual perception was next to falter. Sallie noticed that when Bill was climbing stairs with gaps between the steps, he would freeze in fear. She wondered if maybe he couldn't make out the spatial difference between the gaps, because it seemed to panic him.

By the summer of 1990, Bill had grown somewhat distant and often sad. During the first months of preschool, he really started to deteriorate. By December he had grown squirrelly, distracted, disruptive, even aggressive in class. He was asked to leave.

One day in the late winter of 1991, when the snow had melted and crocuses sprang from the warming earth, the triplets were out back playing catch. Sallie watched and smiled as they tossed the baseball around. But when it came time for Bill to catch, it seemed as though he wasn't seeing the ball until the last second, when it was suddenly in his face. He put his hands to his face and sobbed. After that incident, it was many years before he enjoyed playing ball with his brothers again.

Years later, Sallie learned that autistic kids often suffer from a variety of vision troubles. One trait that Bill exhibited was to avoid making eye contact with people or objects directly in front of him, as though facing the world head-on were too daunting a task.

Bill also began displaying the distinct lack of social skills found in most autism cases. He no longer expressed much emotion in his face, as though his eyes and mouth were frozen by some permanent Botox. This apparent lack of emotion is often attributed to a deep social "aloofness" on the part of autistic children. But Sallie, like many parents of afflicted kids, wondered if something else was at work here. She didn't think Bill was socially aloof; in fact, like many autistic kids, he showed exceptional signs of affection. Instead, Sallie thought there was something medically wrong with him. He was too sick to function in a social environment. If someone were recovering from heart surgery and didn't hop from bed to greet you, she thought, would you call them aloof? Sallie didn't think so.

Sallie would also learn that autistic kids, because they can't form words and can't control their body language, find it extraordinarily difficult to interact with "typical" children. She began noticing this with Bill. It wasn't that he didn't like other kids, he did. But in a group situation, Bill felt more comfortable, and less bewildered, quietly wandering off into his own little realm.

The next several months were spent at endless appointments with speech therapists, special ed teams, and four or five neurologists. During each visit, Sallie heard the same thing: her son had developmental problems that were "pervasive." But she had no idea what the hell *pervasive* meant. She plowed through the indexes of every book she had bought. In those days, there was nothing under the heading *pervasive*.

What the specialists were trying to tell her, she only realized years later, was that Bill's problems were autistic. Yet no one wanted to use that word. If anything, Bill's teachers, his child study team, and his therapists said things like, "Oh no, don't worry about that. He doesn't have that. He doesn't have *autism*."

In late February 1992, during yet another visit to yet another child psychologist, this time at Columbia University in Manhattan, Bill was diagnosed with PDD-NOS. Sallie and Tom struggled home through rush hour traffic on the Jersey Turnpike, discussing the news. They were, in an odd way, slightly elated. Not that autism was a good thing, but at least it was *something*, a logical explanation, a solid diagnosis. "Tom, this is a good step," Sallie said. Tom looked at her as if she'd gone off the edge. How could there be anything good about autism? "Because," she said, "now we have something to work with. Now we can form a plan of attack."

The upbeat emotions the tough businesswoman brought to bear on the situation that evening were short-lived. Sallie went out to scour the book-stores again (there was no Internet to speak of yet), buying up everything on the subject she could find. What she read depressed her. Autism was genetic, according to all the books. Onset was believed to occur early in pregnancy, after which time the damage was already done. And the damage, she read over and over again, was acute, irreversible, incurable. Autistic children could look forward to a lifetime of struggle, isolation, and failure. They would re-quire lifelong specialized care, at great cost. Many ultimately would face insti-tutionalization, where they might live out their days in their own mystifying worlds. Sallie could not stop imagining such an atrocious future for her little boy. That night, as Tom held his wife gently in bed, the unflappable executive cried herself to sleep.

SALLIE BERNARD was not one to give up. There were autism parent support groups, autism research organizations, and autism medical societies out there. Sallie wanted to join them all. She became a member of the New Jersey Center for Outreach and Services for the Autism Community (COSAC), and the Autism Society of America (ASA), a national network founded in 1965 and now a leading source of autism information and referral, with some two hundred chapters nationwide.

Within weeks, Sallie found out about ABA therapy and the pivotal work of Dr. Lovaas. She was thrilled by its promise. But she was also filled with dread. By then, Bill was getting a little too old to derive any significant bene-fit from the therapy. All the published research indicated that ABA therapy should commence before the child was five, and ideally by three. Bill was al-most four and a half.

Sallie and Tom wanted to try anyway. They engaged the services of a Liv-ingston, New Jersey, psychologist trained in the Lovaas method. He worked with the couple on Bill's ABA therapy at home. They focused on stopping "bad" behavior more than on academic pursuits, such as teaching Bill his ABCs.

Sallie knew that Bill would have to return to school. But first she would have to find a place that would take him, "quirks" and all. In New Jersey, in the early 1990s, that was no easy task. Eventually they found the Develop-mental Learning Center in nearby Madison, an attractive bedroom commu-nity on a low-rise ridge. Bill made minor progress there. But he was still disconnected from others, and still not speaking.

When Bill was six, his parents transferred him to the local school to see if he might do better around large numbers of typical kids. The school had a special ed teacher trained in the ABA approach, a situation that worked out remarkably well. But within two years, the ABA teacher became pregnant and left.

The next year or so was awful as Bill tried to adjust to a public school special ed class. It didn't work. The thoroughly untrained teacher barked at him or banished him to a small corner of the room, when she wasn't ignoring him. Sallie returned her son to the Developmental Learning Center.

But there was something very different about the place now. When Bill first went there, he was one of a few dozen kids in a very small school. Now the Center had mushroomed to encompass three large campuses. It provided education services to hundreds of newly diagnosed autistic children. Where on earth, Sallie wondered, had all these kids come from?

By the fall of 1996, Sallie began to suspect there might be some medical explanation for Bill's autism. She was beginning to wonder if genes could be the only explanation. If autism were purely genetic, then why would Bill's learning center have seen such explosive growth in students in just a few years? To Sallie, autism was starting to look like some kind of epidemic. And she knew there was no such thing as a genetic epidemic.

From that point on, Sallie's reading list became increasingly technical. She hunted for medical journals and other published scientific papers on the biology of autism. She was especially keen on investigating its "etiology," or cause.

In late December 1996, while bracing for another New Year of upheaval, Sallie sat down for a rare moment of peace, clutching a glass of Chardonnay and a copy of *Time* magazine. It was the "Man of the Year" issue, honoring AIDS researcher Dr. David Ho. The scientist was selected for his ground-breaking work in lifesaving drugs, such as protease inhibitors to halt the replication of HIV. Damn, Sallie thought. If they can do that for AIDS, then they can do it for autism.

By early 1997, Sallie had been invited through her fledgling autism network to attend a meeting of a new group called the National Alliance for Autism Research. She was also mailed a flyer from yet another neophyte group. It was the state branch of Cure Autism Now (CAN), a national alliance of parents and researchers who raise money for biomedical research, education, and outreach. Founded in 1995 by Portia Iverson and her husband, Hollywood producer Jon Shestack, CAN has granted more than twenty million dollars to date.[16] Among its earliest projects was to amass a gene bank from thousands of autistic individuals.

Sallie thought that the concept of parents raising money to pay for their own scientific research was revolutionary. On the day of the CAN meeting, she gathered many of the books and papers on autism she had acquired and drove down the Garden State Parkway to the Day's Inn Hotel in Kenilworth, New Jersey.

It was an electric gathering. Sallie realized she had walked into a nest of comrades-in-arms. She immediately took to the man who was organizing the chapter, Albert Enayati, an Iranian immigrant with an autistic son living at home.

Albert supported the genetic research efforts of CAN, of course. But he also held that the scientific establishment needed to be jostled from what he thought was a myopic stupor. Albert had bigger plans than holding a bunch of ice cream socials for the benefit of lab researchers at faraway universities.

Despite his soft features and gentle voice, Albert seemed to Sallie like some fiery preacher. He exhorted the parents to demand answers from the scientific establishment. "Why are there so many autistic kids all of a sudden?" he cried. "Where did they all come from? Who is going to care for them? Who is going to find treatments to mend their agony?"

Sallie was buoyed by Albert and his hot rhetoric. She signed up for Cure Autism Now on the spot. When the long day ended, she drove back up the parkway and into the green hills of Summit. She was so excited she had trouble navigating the winding roads. Soon after, Tom arrived home from work to find a keyed-up wife bursting to tell him something. "I've got the most exciting news! I'm going to be an agitator!"

Tom regarded his handsome young wife in her well-tailored suit and executive bob. He couldn't repress a chuckle. "You're going to be *what*?"

"An agitator, Tom. I signed up for autism. You know, activism, advocacy, tearing down the halls of government. That sort of thing."

"Oh fine," Tom muttered. A soft smile showed he was at least partly kidding. "Our own home-grown agent provocateur. *That* should go over big in Summit."

THINGS DID NOT GET OFF to a great start when Liz Birt gave birth to her second child, Matthew, in January 1994. It was one of the coldest days on record in Chicago, with icebergs forming on windswept Lake Michigan. Getting to Rush Medical Center with her husband had been difficult. Now Liz's doctor was telling her she would need a C-section. Liz, the steely attorney with straw-colored hair and soft brown eyes, did not hesitate for a second. She signed the papers and went under the knife.

But halfway through, something went wrong.

"Oops," she distinctly heard the ob-gyn say over the beeping machinery.

"What's that?" Liz asked, groggy but awake. "What happened?"

"Oh, not to worry," the doctor said. "Listen, we're going to call a surgical resident in here to fix this. Perhaps you'd like to go to sleep now?"

Liz trusted her doctor, and she trusted modern medicine. Whatever "it" was that needed fixing, it was best not to be awake for it.

"Sure, Doctor," she said. "Sleep. That would be great."

During the extraction, Liz's bladder had stuck to the infant. It was partially lifted up with him, and Liz required a second surgery to fix the mess. A few days later, on the day of her discharge, when the temperature had dropped to 21 degrees below zero, the hospital staff was more fretful about Liz than about Matthew. Liz's husband,[17] a business executive, bundled his wife and baby in down covers and hurried them into the car. It was an awful and glorious day. Matthew seemed like the happiest baby on earth, oblivious in his mother's warm arms to the icy tempest that howled outside. No one, of course, had any idea that Matthew would be coming back to the hospital many times.

Liz spent the next six weeks sick at home, hauling around a catheter and urine bag. It was a painfully sluggish recovery. With the bladder mishap to heal, and two active infants to care for, Liz was taxed from the start.

When Matthew was eight weeks old, and Liz was still regaining her strength, she went outside, bundled up against the 62-degrees-below windchill factor. She dug her car out from a solid mountain of snow and drove with Matthew through the Siberian landscape and downtown to the pediatrician's office.

Liz's husband had been called to South America on business. But Matthew was due for his first round of childhood inoculations. "I'm a good mom," Liz told herself. She felt like crap and it was bitterly cold. But she was determined to get her baby vaccinated.

Over the next several weeks, Liz improved and so did the weather. Matthew continued on his normal infant trajectory, and never had any serious medical issues. Liz and her husband were deliriously happy. The first time Liz breast-fed Matthew, she sighed happily and thought, My God, what a miracle. What a life we're going to have—raising our kids, watching them grow. She dreamed of high school and first cars; college and weddings. Liz thought she was ready for everything that was to come.

From an early age, Elizabeth Ann Birt had demonstrated a fierce streak of determination and independence. At fifteen she announced her intention to spend a year in Switzerland, to learn French and supplement her already fluent Italian and Spanish.

Liz came from a solid, loving family in Kansas City, Missouri. Hers was a quintessential Middle American upbringing. "Stand up for what you believe in," she was told. "Always try to do the right thing."

Liz married her husband in 1989, and soon after the wedding she chased her dream of getting a law degree. Eventually the couple settled in Chicago, where Liz finished her studies at DePaul University. In 1990 they bought a two-bedroom condo on the top floor of a brownstone in bustling Lincoln Park.

Liz was pregnant with her first child before she finished law school. In May 1992, right after her last final exam, she gave birth to daughter Sarah, who weighed in at a healthy 7 pounds 10 ounces. While still in the maternity ward, Sarah was given a "birth dose" of hepatitis-B vaccine. The shot had just been added to the federal list of childhood immunizations by the CDC. Liz gave it little thought, even though hep-B is transmitted almost exclusively through sexual contact and IV drug use.

Two years later, Matthew was born in that unfortunate C-section. Despite the rocky beginning, little Matt met all his infant milestones. He was crawling, sitting up, walking, and talking right on schedule. He learned to say *momma* and *dada* early, and just after his first birthday, he could count to ten.

Liz would walk him up and down the stairs, and they would count together as they went. Everyone was impressed with the bright little boy. He was extremely playful and social and engaged in the world around him. Matthew loved doing peek-a-boo with his mom, and cried whenever she left the room. His vocabulary grew as fast as he did, quickly expanding to thirty words or more. He learned to say "Sassa" for his big sister Sarah. He learned *ball* and *hello* and *bye-bye* in no time. His favorite game was to shout "Ready-set-go!" and tear around the house, with his mother close behind.

Liz made sure that Matthew was taken to the pediatrician on schedule for all his routine visits and vaccinations. Then, at fourteen months, he was brought in for another round of shots, including his first of two scheduled vaccines against measles-mumps-rubella (MMR). Almost immediately afterward, Matthew began to fall apart.

The first night after his shots, Matthew developed a fever that spiked to over 101 degrees. The doctor had told Liz he might get a temperature. He recommended Tylenol, which she gave him. The fever broke a few days later. Before Matthew could fully recover, he erupted in a rash of little red spots all over his torso.

Then came the ceaseless and violent diarrhea.

On Thanksgiving Day of 1995, the family babysitter, a sixty-year-old Polish woman with a thick accent named Margaret, told Liz: "Something is very wrong with baby. I know this." Matt was no longer paying attention to her, she complained. But Liz dismissed Margaret's worries, despite the nanny's dogged insistence. It wasn't until shortly before Christmas that Liz began to see the signs for herself.

One day Liz came home from work to find Matthew staring up at the light fixtures, spinning like a top on the floor. In the next few days, she realized that Matthew did not always recognize her right away when she entered the room. A few months before, he couldn't bear to be apart from his mother. Now he often regarded her as an object of curiosity, at best.

Liz also noticed that Matthew had stopped learning new words. Not long after that, he stopped talking altogether.

Liz and her husband thought that Matthew must have developed a hearing problem. That would explain his sudden lack of communication. As for the chronic diarrhea, they attributed that to too much orange juice. Still, Liz was crestfallen: her son was going deaf.

By the time Liz's third child, Andrew, was born in June of 1996, Matthew was worse than ever. The spinning went on for hours. He would laugh uncontrollably at nothing at all. He was not the same little boy his parents once knew.

Liz brought Matthew back to Rush Medical Center for a full battery of childhood psychological evaluations. The therapists diagnosed "pervasive delay." Nobody uttered the word *autism* until many months later, when the official diagnosis was made: Matthew suffered from PDD-NOS, an autism spectrum disorder.

By January of 1997 Matthew had stopped sleeping through the night. He would wake at 3:00 A.M., miserable and screaming, unable to go back to sleep. At night, frantic, Matthew would scoop diarrhea from his shorts and smear it in his hair, the bedding, and the carpeting.

"I can't live like this," Liz muttered to herself and anyone else who was around to listen. Chronically drained, she would fall dead asleep at her desk. More than once, her secretary walked in to find her drooling over legal papers. Worse, Liz's husband had started a new job in St. Louis, where he spent the workweek, coming home to Chicago only on weekends. The fragile state of their family was hard on both parents. Her husband worried that the other two kids, Sarah and Andrew, were not getting the attention they deserved.

Liz was stressed and wounded by the state of affairs. She knew the other children felt neglected. Awash in guilt, Liz would buy them whatever they wanted, whenever they wanted it. She wished the kids all the things in life they deserved. What they really wanted, however, was their mom.

But there was rarely a moment away from autism. Liz was overwhelmed by the constant responsibility for Matthew. She didn't know how to care for a child with autism. And no one was around to help: no support system, no relatives within hundreds of miles.

SOMETIME DURING 1997, she can't remember exactly when, Liz hopped on the Internet and began to connect with others in her situation. Like many parents of autistic kids turning to the net for information and advice, Liz had heard the early rumblings about a possible link between developmental disorders and vaccines, including hep-B, diphtheria-tetanus-pertussis (DTP), and MMR. But Liz did not pay much heed to the chatter. Vaccines were harmless; everyone knew that. Miracles of modern medicine, they were to be disregarded only at great peril to the individual child and the public health. Failure to vaccinate was criminal, Liz Birt had always believed.

But Liz's faith began to waver one chilly March morning in 1998, when she drove out to Chicago's western suburbs for a conference on autism sponsored by the local chapter of Cure Autism Now. She was impressed by the talk of a neuroimmunologist from the University of Michigan, Dr. Vijendra K. Singh, who said that autistic kids suffered from an apparent adverse reaction to the three live viruses in the measles, mumps, and rubella vaccine.

Singh believed that autism was an autoimmune disorder linked to some type of viral exposure, probably from vaccines. He identified a "hyperimmune" response (exaggerated increase of antibodies) to measles virus in many autistic kids. This incorrect immune response created "autoantibodies" in the child's brain.

"I have found," the doctor announced in his formal south Asian accent, as Liz furiously scribbled notes, "that up to eighty percent of autistic children have autoantibodies to specific brain structures, in particular a brain protein known as myelin basic protein, or MBP, of the myelin sheath. This is a fatty coating that insulates nerve fibers and is absolutely essential for higher brain functions."[18]

Liz's faith in vaccines was crumbling, but it was neither an easy nor a natural process. The lawyer in her told her to keep an open mind, but she had a hard time grappling with the thought that vaccines could have caused Matthew's torment.

Liz turned her legal research skills to investigating all viral autoimmune disorders and their possible link to neurological dysfunction, especially in children. But it wasn't until September 1998, the day before she was scheduled to bring Matthew in for his second MMR shot, that Liz found an article in a British medical journal that was causing shock waves of alarm—and derision—on both sides of the Atlantic.

The study had appeared in the Lancet, perhaps the world's preeminent scientific journal. Its principal author was Dr. Andrew Wakefield, a young specialist in pediatric gastroenterology at the Royal Free Hospital in London. Wakefield had examined 12 children (11 of them boys), referred to him with a history of normal development followed by loss of acquired skills, including language, together with diarrhea and abdominal pain. The children were given thorough neurological, developmental, and GI exams, including colonoscopy and biopsy, MRI, and EEG. All 12 had intestinal abnormalities, and 11 showed "patchy chronic inflammation" in their colon. Onset of symptoms was associated (by the parents, it's important to note) with MMR vaccination in 8 of the 12 children, who fell ill shortly after immunization.[19]

Liz read the description and thought, "My God, this sounds like Matt." Then she remembered that Matthew had received his first MMR vaccine at fifteen months. Within hours, he'd developed that soaring fever and, a week later, the red body rash and his still-endless battle with diarrhea. At the time, it never occurred to Liz to connect the vaccination dots to her son's illness. Now, she vowed to pursue the question with haste.

Matthew was so physically ill that, at four and a half years, Liz refused to allow him to get his second MMR. His stools were abnormal and at times were green with mucus or pasty yellow in color, as if he were no longer digesting any food. Matthew was perpetually listless, like a hapless dope addict. Liz knew there was something terribly wrong. But the doctors weren't helping, and nobody else seemed to know what to do, either. She was on her own.

The day after reading the *Lancet*, Liz brought Matthew to the pediatrician for his regular visit, which quickly devolved into a heated confrontation. Her refusal to let Matthew get his MMR shot left the doctor livid. "Matthew has been ill with fever and diarrhea for two years," Liz said. "He hasn't slept a full night for eighteen months, and neither have I. There's no way in hell that he's getting that booster. I hope that's clear."

"Mrs. Birt," the exasperated doctor said, "if you don't let him get this shot, you're crazy. Do you have any idea what measles can do to a child?"

"At this point, Doctor, he's so badly off I'm not sure it would make a difference," Liz said flatly. "He's too sick for another MMR. I'm not going to do it."

LYN REDWOOD TREMBLED as the specialist spoke to her on the phone.

"Mrs. Redwood," he said, "there's nothing I can do for your son Will. Why don't you just take him fishing?" The words were heartless and devastating. Lyn had a difficult time steadying the phone as she listened to the doctor—the latest in a succession of overpriced experts who had examined her struggling four-year-old. Lyn was getting used to gloomy prognoses. But this was too much.

She looked down at Will. He stared through the plate glass windows straight out at nothing at all. His mouth slightly ajar, his eyes glazed over, Will seemed more out of it than normal this morning. Lyn kept silent.

"Mrs. Redwood?" the doctor said. "Did you hear me?"

Lyn heard, but wouldn't let herself speak. She wanted to growl and slam down the phone. But years of courteous southern upbringing kept her thoughts and words at a safe distance from each other.

"Fishing, Doctor?" she said finally. "That's the best you can do? Fishing?"

"Or some other activity the boy wants to do. It doesn't have to be fishing."

"What I think Will wants to do," she said, "is be a normal kid."

Lyn thanked the doctor as politely as she knew how, though she felt like demanding a refund of the five hundred dollars that she and Tommy had shelled out for his useless counsel.

She walked over to Will and scooped him up in her arms. He refused to meet her gaze. He neither giggled nor smiled. Today, he seemed to barely move at all, though some days he never stopped moving for a second. Tears welled in Lyn's eyes as she spoke to her son, trying to see if the words were registering behind that faraway face.

The boy kept his gaze out the window, as if something were stirring in the garden. But in the late September afternoon, all was still. "We're going to find out what happened, Will," Lyn vowed. Her voice tripped with emotion. Will didn't notice. "We're going to make it better. That doctor doesn't know what the hell he's talking about."

Doctors be damned, Lyn thought. She could no longer place blind hope and faith in the American medical establishment she had once revered.

It was a radical change. Lyn was now a member of her county Board of Health. And Tommy was doing his second residency in the ER at Grady Memorial Hospital, among the busiest trauma centers in the burgeoning New South. The Redwoods were believers in modern medicine. They had built their careers in the same public health establishment that Lyn was about to challenge. She did not relish the thought of battling her own profession. But the doctors had come up with no better answer than a day of fishing. What choice was there?

That afternoon, Lyn ventured downstairs and into the basement. It was crammed with dusty boxes of toys, trophies, and old schoolbooks—mementos from the childhoods of Hanna and Drew. Lyn picked through the morass until she found the computer that Tommy had bought when Will was born. At the time, Lyn could not think of a single use for such a contraption. She didn't know the first thing about computers. She had barely turned one on, let alone navigated the Internet. The whole thing seemed as mysterious and complicated as an instruction manual to a nuclear power plant.

Lyn found a disk for an Internet dial-up service that came with instructions. "I can do this," she said aloud. She lifted the computer and hauled it up two flights to her private office, perched in an aerielike loft above the living room floor, where she could work while keeping vigil over Will down below. It took Lyn the rest of the day to get online. One hour before Tommy got home that night, she discovered the Alta Vista search site.

Lyn typed in "a-u-t-i-s-m," and hit the enter key. That night, she learned she was far from alone.

2. Injecting Fear

ANDREW WAKEFIELD'S THEORIES about MMR vaccine were circulating on the Internet as public debate over vaccine safety grew louder and more vitriolic. Wakefield was now reviled among medical opinion-makers of the British and American establishments. They dismissed the London doctor as a grandstanding zealot and regarded his MMR hypothesis with ridicule and alarm. Officials fretted that Wakefield's paper would send nervous English parents away from the MMR "jab" (British term for a shot) in dangerous droves. The rhetoric could have been moderated, however, if more attention had been paid to the disclaimer Wakefield published in the same study.

"We did not prove an association between measles, mumps, and rubella vaccine and the syndrome described," he noted in the *Lancet*. "Virological studies are underway that may help to resolve this issue."

Even so, Wakefield had no intention of being silenced. Following his article, the specialist defended his work in a series of media appearances that detractors dismissed as fatuous. Wakefield was unbowed. "When you're taking on something like the establishment," the young doctor said, "you are inevitably going to come up against this kind of issue."[20]

The establishment was demanding proof, and so far Wakefield had none to deliver. "Urgent further research is needed to determine whether MMR may give rise to this complication in a small number of people," he wrote in his study. Still, many doctors attacked his premise and methodology. The number of children examined was too small to approach statistical significance, for one. Wakefield had also failed to include data on "control" subjects (healthy kids). Even if he had demonstrated an "association" between MMR, bowel disease, and regressive developmental disorder, it was hardly proof of a connection. After all, some children had GI distress before receiving their MMR vaccine.

In the following month's issue of the *Lancet*, two officials from the CDC's National Immunization Program, Dr. Robert Chen and Dr. Frank DeStefano, wrote a scathing editorial about the MMR hypothesis and chastised Wakefield for his ideas. They said the English doctor would lead the public and the media to "confuse association with causality." Vaccine safety concerns, they warned, "may snowball," leading parents to shun immunization.[21]

Another counterweight to Wakefield's study came out of Finland and was also published in the *Lancet*, in May 1998. The National Public Health Institute of Finland had detailed results from a fourteen-year study of that country's use of MMR (a triple live-virus shot that does not contain mercury). Out of three million Finnish children who had received the MMR, only 31 reported gastrointestinal distress, such as vomiting or diarrhea, within two weeks of immunization. The Finns concluded that, despite all efforts to count every adverse effect associated with MMR, they could find no data "supporting the hypothesis that MMR causes pervasive developmental disorder or inflammatory bowel disease."[22]

But the damage, in Britain at least, had already been inflicted upon the public's confidence in MMR. The "jab" garnered alarming headlines in the tabloids. Reports of parents refusing the shot began to surface. British health officers warned of measles outbreaks where vaccination rates fell below the crucial 90-percent "herd immunity" level (the point at which disease can spread more readily from one unvaccinated individual to another). UK parents with the means to do so quietly shuttled their kids across the Channel to France, where the three shots were given separately.[23] (It didn't help matters a few years later when members of Parliament alleged that Prime Minister Tony Blair refused to allow his son Leo to get the MMR vaccine—an allegation that Blair never confirmed or denied.)[24]

IN AMERICA, in late 1998 and early 1999, much of the nation was fixating on the impeachment and ultimate acquittal of Bill Clinton for his dallyings with an intern. But many parents of autistic children faced a far more intimate distraction. Had live vaccine virus wrecked their kids' GI tracts, they wondered?

Had MMR upended their children's immune systems and rewired their brains for mental regression?

It became a hot topic on new Internet message boards. News of the MMR controversy was posted several times each week.

Lyn Redwood, Liz Birt, and Sallie Bernard kept current with Wakefield's ideas and the effort under way by public health officials to undermine his theory. But Sallie, for one, was less than impressed with Wakefield. She knew there had been rumors for years about a connection between vaccines and autism, as well as other diseases. But most experts wrote it off as a coincidence, and she was inclined to agree. "This is so ridiculous," she said to Tom one night after reading about Wakefield's work. "How could vaccines do that? They couldn't possibly cause *autism*."

Not far away in New Jersey, Albert Enayati, the head of the Cure Autism Now chapter who so impressed Sallie at the Day's Inn, was less skeptical. Albert, who has an autistic son, Payam, speaks in gentle tones, with a decidedly Persian lilt. He grew up in a Jewish family in Tehran until 1973, when he left for America to get a degree in chemical engineering. Eventually Albert found work with Howmedica, a medical devices division of Pfizer Corporation, in Rutherford, New Jersey, in the vast pharmaceutical manufacturing belt that stretches south from Newark along the New Jersey Turnpike. Albert met and married his wife, Sima, an Iranian exile, in 1985.

Their first son, Babbak (who goes by the name Bobby), was born in 1987, and their second son, Payam, arrived in 1990. The Enayatis made sure their boys received the required vaccinations of the day. It was important to the couple, who worked for the high-tech pharmaceutical industry of their adopted homeland. Looking back, Albert wished he hadn't been so trusting.

"I'll never forget the day," he said. "My son was three days old or so. And my wife says, 'They're going to give him hepatitis-B vaccine.' And I asked the nurses if it was required. Wasn't that a disease transmitted through sex or IV drug use? And they said, 'Yes, but it's required for children, too. We have to give it to him.' "

Bobby and Payam developed normally during the first years of their lives. But shortly before Payam was two, in 1992, his mother brought him in for his booster diphtheria-tetanus-pertussis (DTP) shot. That day, he developed acute diarrhea. A week later, Payam was back at the doctor, who prescribed medication for the runs and, while he was there, gave the ailing boy his MMR vaccine.

The diarrhea did not settle down for months. When Payam began feeling better, he started uttering his first words, in both English and Farsi, the language of Iran, which he picked up from his parents. His parents considered him to be a very bright boy.

One evening in 1993, Albert came home to find a worried Sima fretting over Payam. "He's stopped talking," she said. "All of a sudden, Albert, he's just become mute!" A trip to the doctor reassured the anxious Enayatis. He told them not to worry about Payam's speech loss, even if he had been bilingual. It happened sometimes. But Payam continued on a downward track. He stopped making eye contact with his parents.

Then he began the horrible banging of his head against the wall.

Within months, the boy was biting his hand to the point of profuse bleeding. He ran amok through the house without cessation. When Albert got home from work, a time of day that used to send Payam into fits of delight, the boy would flatly ignore his father. He was hyperactive, wouldn't sit down, not for a minute. "Running, running, running!" Albert said to Sima. "Oh God, what is this? I've never seen anything like it." Albert was devastated. He cried almost every night.

Desperate over Payam's decline (he still wasn't speaking and had grown even wilder), the Enayatis turned to traditional Persian herbal medicine. Then they took Payam to see a Chinese medicine practitioner. Nothing worked. Finally, their pediatrician put Payam on the antidepressant Zoloft.

When his son was finally diagnosed with autism, in late 1993, Albert began attending medical conferences and parents' meetings about the disorder. His first conference, in New York, was sponsored by Cure Autism Now. There he met the group's founders, Portia Iverson and John Shestack.

Greatly inspired, the New Jersey father offered to start a state chapter of the national organization founded by the powerful Hollywood couple. John and Portia agreed, and Albert became president of New Jersey CAN. His first self-appointed task was to attend the next stockholders' meeting at Pfizer. Standing up and keeping his emotions in check, Albert made a pitch for the company to cough up some research money. Within days, he landed a commitment of two hundred thousand dollars for the CAN organization.

Then Albert assembled a group of ten New Jersey parents with autistic kids and boarded the Metroliner for Washington. They held a series of meetings with members of Congress who controlled the national research purse strings, including John Porter (R-IL), chairman of a house appropriations subcommittee on health. In 1997 and 1998 Albert attended meetings between CAN members and officials at the National Institutes of Health (NIH) and two of its agencies, the National Institute of Child Health and Human Development and the National Institute of Mental Health. But it wasn't easy trying to get research money, even in the booming economy of the late nineties.

By 1998 Albert had seen all the vaccine rumors whirling about the Internet, and he would bring up the subject during late-night phone calls with Sallie, who had become active in New Jersey CAN and very friendly with

Albert. But Sallie was still unmoved. She was inclined to dismiss the idea as the ravings of simple-minded conspiracy theorists who wouldn't know scientific proof if it landed on their front lawn.

Undaunted, Albert kept reading. He was struck by the personal account of Barbara Loe Fisher, of the National Vaccine Information Center. Her son became terribly ill, and then developed severe learning disabilities, after receiving his DTP vaccine. Albert remembered how sick Payam became after his own DTP shot. He started to give grudging credence to the crazy vaccine theory.

One day, Albert found a brochure he had been given at work about the benefits of hepatitis-B vaccination, published by Merck. Albert remembered that most of Payam's vaccines came from that company. On a whim, he called the 800 number listed on the brochure.

"Hello, Merck product information," a young man said.

"Thank you, sir," Albert said in his polite English. "I have some questions, please, about your vaccines. May I ask what is in them?"

"Sure," the man said. "Which vaccines?"

"Well, how about DTP. What are the ingredients of that?" Albert could hear the man click away on a computer. Then he listened intently to the list of nearly unpronounceable components. "Is it possible," he asked, "that any of those things could cause neurological damage?"

"Absolutely not, sir," the man said. "All our vaccines were tested for safety and approved by the FDA. They've been shown to be completely safe."

"Okay. What about MMR? Or hepatitus-B? Anything that causes neurological damage?"

"No, sir. Nothing at all. I told you, they are FDA approved."

"And there's nothing else at all in the vaccines?"

"Some do contain an additive. Let's see. It's called thimerosal."

"What is that, please?"

"It's a preservative."

"Could that cause neurological damage?"

Albert could hear the man chuckling.

"My goodness, no!" he said. "It's harmless. Like what you use to keep food safe. It's like lemon juice."

"Lemon juice? Do you have any other information on it? How do you spell that?"

"Capital T," said the man, slowly, "H-I-M-E-R-O-S-A-L. It's pronounced thigh-MARE-iss-sol, I think."[25]

Albert thanked the man and hung up, curious about this preservative. Lemon juice? In vaccines? Was that even possible?

The next morning, Albert headed straight for Pfizer's medical library and its computerized access to MedLine, which can call up thousands of published studies within seconds. He typed the name of the preservative into the search engine, but nothing came up. He double-checked the spelling, but still nothing was found. Albert walked down the hallway to his lab. He was relieved he could check off at least one item from his list of fatherly worries. Nothing's in the literature about this thimerosal stuff, he thought. Nobody's working on it. It must be safe.

That night, Albert came home to phone messages from parents following the Internet conspiracy theories. They all wanted to go on about vaccines. Albert rolled his eyes. There was also a call from Sallie. It was the one call Albert returned.

"You know something?" he said. "I think you're right about this vaccine thing. There's nothing to it. And now I have to come home to all these messages from parents screaming about vaccines. I'm starting to think they're out of their minds."

"I'm glad you see the light on this one," Sallie said.

Albert told Sallie about his phone call with Merck, though he didn't mention the harmless, lemon juice–like preservative. And he told her about the close scrutiny that FDA officials pay to the medical device industry. He said the agency kept an eagle eye on his own workplace. "They're relentless about it. They inspect everything, make sure the numbers are correct," he said. "They check our notebooks to make sure everything's calibrated properly. And if you get a warning letter, your life is ruined."

THE VACCINE-AUTISM THEORY may have seemed preposterous to mainstream medicine, but it was gaining traction among some parents' groups. In early March 1999, Cure Autism Now and the San Diego–based Autism Research Institute joined with the National Vaccine Information Center to demand that one billion dollars from the federal vaccine budget be earmarked for independent studies by "non-governmental researchers" into the possible link between vaccines and autism.[26]

CAN President Portia Iverson said that roughly half of the hundreds of calls to the foundation each month were from parents reporting children who became autistic soon after vaccination. She conceded that some criticism of Wakefield was valid, given that certain developmental disorders become apparent only around the same time as routine MMR vaccination. But, she added, "Isn't it the responsibility of the government to take a proactive position on behalf of these children rather than a defensive one?"

Sallie and Albert were thrilled to hear such combative words coming from their group's president. CAN also called on federal officials to adopt a "more consumer protective response" by funding research that "proves or disproves the association (with vaccines) rather than to discredit the preliminary report of such an association."[27]

Barbara Loe Fisher, cofounder and president of the National Vaccine Information Center, said her group had told the government for years about children who "are dying and getting very sick after being vaccinated." A seasoned vaccine activist who knew how to play ball within the inner sanctum of American public health, she was also a frequent and vocal thorn in the side of the immunization establishment. "It is tragic," she said, "that vaccine policymakers in the government and the private sector would prematurely condemn independent clinical and basic science research which could identify children who are genetically or otherwise at high risk of vaccine injury. We need more science and less stonewalling. Parents are outraged and they should be."[28]

The parents didn't get very far in their early push for federal funds. In late 1998, Albert Enayati attended a meeting sponsored by two NIH agencies, which had gathered some of the country's leading geneticists together with groups including CAN. "They brought in all this evidence, and all these experts who presented it to the geneticists to decide if autism is genetic," Albert told Sallie afterward. "There was this real push to call autism a genetic disease, because there were reports of families with two or three autistic kids in them. They said autism almost *had* to be genetic. There were no other satisfactory explanations."

In the middle of the meeting, a professor from Utah State University got up to ask a provocative question. "He said, 'Maybe this is environmental,' " Albert remembered. " 'Maybe this has something to do with vaccines. Has anyone looked into that?' Suddenly every geneticist there started attacking him. They were yelling and screaming, telling him he was crazy. I'll never forget that." It was the first time Albert heard anyone mention autism and vaccines in public.

One doctor in particular, a geneticist, grew purple and his eyes bulged with annoyance. "Professor," he said to the Utah renegade, "you are out in left field. You are, in fact, skating on very thin ice." Albert had been puzzled. American slang still escaped him. Left field? he asked himself. Skating? What does he *mean*?

AFTER LIZ BIRT'S SHOWDOWN with her pediatrician over Matthew's second MMR vaccine, the Chicago attorney began arming herself with reams of medical literature on the shot, and on the rationale behind giving children a second "booster" immunization. After the first injection, she learned, 95 percent of all kids develop a proper immune response: they produce an appropriate level of antibodies to measles, mumps, and rubella. But the remaining 5 percent require a second injection in order to achieve the desired response. Liz discovered there were tests that measure antibody levels, or "titers" in the blood, to see if the first shot took. But it is more expensive to do the titers than it is to give everyone the second shot.[29]

"If Matthew already has immunity," she informed the pediatrician, "there's no need to give him a second vaccination." The doctor reluctantly agreed and gave Matthew the antibody test. It came back positive; he had his immunity. The pediatrician relented. "As long as there's a way to get this done so that legally I'd be covered," he said, "then I don't really care."

Liz's faith in modern medicine was beginning to collapse. A few months before the fight with her pediatrician, Matthew had contracted shingles, which is exceedingly rare in children. It usually implies some form of serious immune dysfunction. Liz secured an appointment with a leading immunologist at Children's Memorial Hospital. She watched apprehensively as he examined Matthew's painful, pussy bumps.

"Well, he's got shingles," the doctor finally announced.

"That's all you can say?" she snapped. "Doctor, I *know* what he has. What I want to know is why does he have it? Shouldn't you do an immune system profile?"

The specialist fired a withering look at Liz. She didn't flinch. Reluctantly the doctor drew some blood and agreed to send it in for an immune analysis. Then he showed her the door. Liz never went back for the results, and never heard from the doctor again.

Liz was slowly coming to the conclusion that if nobody in the medical profession was going to help her, she would have to figure out what to do about Matt, about the diarrhea, the shingles, the spinning. Something was going haywire inside his body. But no one else seemed the least bit alarmed about it.

THE MAIN CONDUIT of online parental discourse about autism had become the Families for Early Autism Treatment (FEAT) list. It was launched in March 1999 by Lenny Schafer, the father of an autistic boy, Izak, from Sacramento, California. Now called the Schafer Autism Report, the Web site is a comprehensive compilation of autism news, research, and opinion.

One article, posted on June 1, 1999, captured the collective mood of many parents during that disconcerting spring. The Scripps Howard News Service story, written by Joan Lowy, explored the growing antivaccine movement and its implications. Among the diseases being attributed to vaccines were SIDS, multiple sclerosis, and autism.

"Doctors and public health officials are worried about a growing backlash against vaccinations that they fear will lead to outbreaks of preventable childhood diseases and even deaths," Lowy reported. She said that more parents, "citing information they heard on television talk shows, found on the Internet, or read in news stories," were openly questioning vaccine safety.[30]

In fact, the American Academy of Pediatrics was so alarmed over falling hepatitis-B vaccination rates that it embarked on a public relations and lobbying campaign in partnership with the drug companies to defend the hep-B vaccine. Meanwhile, the rhetoric of vaccine opponents had "taken on a decidedly hard edge." Phyllis Schlafly, president of the conservative Eagle Forum, likened the shots to "authoritarian rule in Communist China."

The other hot topic was the staggering increase in autism cases being reported in California and the nation as a whole. Was the jump explained by improved diagnostics, wider awareness, and/or more accurate reporting, as many in the medical establishment contended? Or was there really a genuine and alarming increase in the actual numbers? In other words, was America in the midst of an actual autism epidemic? It was a crucial question. If autism had become epidemic, then how could it be genetic?

Evidence for an epidemic was powerful. On March 1, 1999, the California Department of Developmental Services issued a report to the state legislature, which had requested an update on the numbers of people living with autism and pervasive developmental disorders in the state. (California has long tracked the number of cases and is considered to be the gold standard of American autism epidemiology.)

The growth had been explosive.

"In the past 10 years, California has had a 273 percent increase in the number of children with autism who enter the developmental services system—1,685 new cases last year alone," said the report, which did not examine factors behind the increase.[31]

The spike was not necessarily evidence of an epidemic. Rather it showed a "huge increase" in the number of reported and diagnosed cases. Autism had long been considered a rare disease, however, on the order of 4.5 cases per 10,000 births. Now, in California, the rate had leapt to 15 to 20 cases per 10,000, or nearly 1 in 500 kids, the report said.

The following month, the FEAT Report posted data from the U.S. Department of Education's "20th Annual Report to Congress on the Individuals with Disabilities Education Act." IDEA provides services to young people with developmental problems and keeps a registry of schoolchildren classified according to disability.

In just four years, between the 1992–1993 and 1996–1997 academic years, reported cases of autism in U.S. public schools had rocketed from 12,238 to 34,082, or an increase of 178.6 percent. Some states reported even more stunning numbers. Maryland and Nevada saw rates go up more than 2,000 percent and Oregon and Washington had increases over 3,000 percent. In Illinois, the spike in cases seemed impossible: cases shot up *21,920 percent.* But on closer inspection, in 1992 the state had reported just 5 autism cases, compared with Pennsylvania, with the same population, where there were 346 cases. Four years later, the Illinois number had risen to 1,101, and Pennsylvania's to 1,109.[32]

Such drastic increases invited skepticism about the Department of Education numbers. Surely Illinois had somehow missed most cases in the early years of the IDEA program. Illinois was at least partially "catching up" with states like Pennsylvania in terms of counting and reporting its own numbers. Anyway, IDEA was radically revamped and expanded in 1992, when autism spectrum disorders were added to the list of disabilities covered. Of course it would take a few years to count all the new cases.

The statistics sparked an outcry on both sides of the autism controversy, pitting those who believed in an epidemic—and thus an environmental cofactor—against those who saw no true increase at all—allowing for a purely genetic explanation. Dr. Edward R. Ritvo, a professor emeritus at UCLA Medical School, wrote a letter posted on FEAT, headed "No Epidemic of Autism." "My research efforts to identify mild forms of the disease which began in the 1970s is paying off," he wrote. "We now diagnose a spectrum of severity ranging from the 'classical' description of the most severe cases, to the mildest forms, called 'Asperger's Syndrome.' In other words, milder forms of autism had simply gone undiagnosed until very recently." Increased case finding, Ritvo said, was mainly due to "education of doctors and the public on the nature of autism so that more cases are identified; availability of agencies to provide autism services that would attract previously uncounted children; and closure of 'warehouses' where many autistics were improperly diagnosed and housed."[33]

LYN REDWOOD, like Sallie Bernard, Liz Birt, and Albert Enayati, had become an avid reader of the FEAT newsletter. One day in early 1999 an e-mail popped into her box announcing a meeting on "biological treatments" for autism and PDD. The conference, sponsored by Great Plains Laboratory, a "holistic" biochemical and medical testing outfit in Lenexa, Kansas, was scheduled for Mother's Day weekend in Orlando, Florida. "This sounds like a winner," Lyn thought. That night at dinner, she told Tommy and the kids why she wouldn't be around for Mother's Day. "It's about intervention and treatments," she said, pleading for understanding. "They think we can *do* something for Will. I have to go to this."

Lyn flew to Tampa, where her mother lived, and borrowed her car for the ninety-minute drive to Orlando. She arrived a little late on the first day to find a hotel ballroom jammed with hundreds of people, half of them doctors and researchers and the rest parents, each one full of questions. Lyn was overwhelmed by the gathered force. So many parents, she thought. So many damaged kids. But she was also heartened; she and Tommy weren't alone in this anymore.

Lyn sat down and took out her notebook. Parents were standing up and talking about all sorts of immunological implications in autism. They had candid discussions with the M.D.'s about a dizzying array of experimental treatments designed to improve immune function, increase nutritional uptake, even enhance cognitive ability. Lyn's head was spinning. The information came fast and thick. Her hand throbbed as she struggled to take notes.

For the next two days, Lyn absorbed as much information as she could on autism and vaccines, on immune dysfunction, gut problems, and dietary interventions. She returned home to Atlanta with the elation of a lottery winner, bursting with news to share with Tommy. That night after dinner, the two sat down at the table. Lyn gave her husband a thorough debriefing.

She spoke admiringly about Dr. Vijendra Singh, for example, the University of Michigan immunologist who had impressed Liz Birt at the CAN conference in Chicago. According to his account of things, autism was an autoimmune disorder. Something had triggered the body to attack itself. He had spoken about the myelin autoantibodies that attack the protective coating on nerve cells.

"He is finding the autoantibodies in up to 90 percent of the autistic kids he's looked at," Lyn recounted as Tommy listened intently. "He thinks this plays a major role in their developmental dysfunction. And there might be potential therapies for this, things to boost the immune system, like steroids and IV immunoglobin."

Lyn was also intrigued by a youthful doctor from Palm Bay, Florida, named Jeffrey Bradstreet, a family physician and Christian activist with his own radio show, *The Good News Doctor*. Bradstreet was the father of a young son with autism named Matthew.

"He said that autism is a multisystem disorder, but the root cause is an immune system that is somehow suppressed and overactivated at the same time," Lyn said. Even more intriguing, Bradstreet surmised that autism was caused by some as yet unknown combination of genetic predisposition and "environmental insult." And, he said, autistic children were more likely to have severe gastrointestinal distress, extremely poor absorption of food, and a disorder known as "leaky gut syndrome."

"Everything he talked about sounded just like Will," Lyn said. "I think Will has leaky gut. It pierces tiny holes in the intestinal tract. Bradstreet thinks it's caused by viral infection, perhaps from MMR. Or it could be from yeast infection, or a reduction of phenol sulfur transferase," a sulfur-based enzyme that protects the intestines. (Low sulfur levels in autistic kids would later play a major role in the mercury-autism theory.)

The intestinal system breaks down proteins into peptides, which in turn are converted into basic amino acids. Bradstreet believed that peptides from two of those proteins—gluten, from grain, and casein, from dairy products—were leaking through holes in the intestines and into the bloodstream, rather than being absorbed through the normal GI tract. Both peptides, he said, act like morphine in the body. They can cross the blood-brain barrier (a highly complex structure of blood vessels that helps prevent toxins and microbes from entering into brain tissue), and thus damage brain development and affect behavior.

"Now I see why autistic kids crave wheat and dairy, Tommy," Lyn said. "Maybe they're addicted to the high they get from the morphins. They're doping themselves up on bread and milk. That's why Will seems so out of it so often."

Then there was the powerful MMR presentation from Dr. Andrew Wakefield. "When he started talking about these poor kids, and how damaged their guts were from measles virus, he brought most of us to tears. We were sobbing," Lyn recounted.

Wakefield had also put forward the possibility that a genetic predisposition, combined with the insult of live vaccine virus, had pushed the immune system of autistic children over the edge. Chronically high levels of "opioids" in the blood (from gluten and casein) were impacting behavior, causing constipation, and possibly the disturbing trait of "toe walking," when children walk on tiptoes. He urged a diet free of gluten and casein.

"He calls the syndrome a new phenomenon, and he has a name for it," Lyn said. "Autistic enterocolitis. It's being detected in 97 percent of the autistic children that he and his team looked at. And he found measles virus protein in biopsies taken from the inflamed intestines of autistic children, kids whose only exposure to measles had been through vaccination." By contrast, Wakefield had not made similar findings in children with Crohn's disease (chronic inflammation of the bowels believed to be caused by bacteria or a virus). Nor did he uncover evidence of live mumps or rubella virus, the other components of the MMR vaccine.

The theory fascinated Lyn, though she and Tommy questioned how it might apply to Will's own particular case. He'd been given MMR, but he had started showing signs of neurological impairment a good three months before the shot. Could there be something else about the vaccine schedule that was making kids sick?

"These doctors," Lyn told Tommy, "they have an entirely different take on autism. They're from another planet than that jerk who told me to take Will fishing."

Lyn was not the only one impressed with Wakefield. Also in the audience that weekend was Mark Blaxill, a young Massachusetts father of an autistic girl named Michaela. Blaxill, a partner at the Boston Consulting Group, possessed remarkable aptitude for statistical analysis and complex theory. He thought the MMR vaccine-autism premise had merit. After the conference he posted his own account on the FEAT list:

"I came away from Orlando absolutely blown away," he wrote. "I am mobilized to do measles vaccine titers [measurements] for our daughter. I want to get more data myself before I start going ballistic, but if what Wakefield is saying is true, then we have a very dramatic and simple story: The epidemic has been created by a massively misguided public health initiative, the MMR vaccine. What an incredible tragedy this would be if it is proven to be true; how careless they have been with our children! The epidemic has yet to be recognized by the CDC and the official medical establishment. To the extent that progress has been made, it has been made or motivated by parents. Fortunately, there are many parents who are medical professionals, too."

The medical establishment, Mark predicted, "will move swiftly to defend its vaccination program, but will move incredibly slowly to accept effective therapies that are not developed through their own processes. Meanwhile, every day, thousands more children are put at risk with enormous human, social and economic costs. This is a preventable tragedy. Am I overreacting to the conference, fellow attendees? By nature, I am not a revolutionary, but . . . finding it hard to think about anything else. Mark."[34]

THE AUTISM-VACCINE HYPOTHESIS was about to take a new turn. Few parents knew it, but the FDA had ordered a review of mercury-containing vaccines and biologics, as mandated by the Food and Drug Modernization Act of 1997. Among the products being reviewed was thimerosal, the "lemon juice"–like vaccine preservative that Albert Enayati had researched without success in 1998. What Albert did not discover then is that thimerosal is a potentially toxic mercury-based preservative.

The FDA unit charged with investigating thimerosal was the Center for Biologics Evaluation and Research, or CBER. In December 1998, CBER published a notice in the *Federal Register* (a national diary of bureaucratic activity) asking manufacturers to provide details on thimerosal use in their products. Then, on April 29, 1999, acting director William Egan dispatched a letter to the companies, inquiring about their future "plans" for thimerosal use in vaccines. Removal was far from obligatory. "If you intend to remove thimerosal from your product(s), please discuss the following," Egan wrote, asking for details on the impact that removal would have on vaccine sterility and potency, and plans for finding alternative preservatives. If the companies opted not to eliminate or reduce thimerosal, they should "provide a rationale for this decision."[35]

Thimerosal was a major topic among much of the American public health bureaucracy in 1999. The CBER officials had added up the total amount of mercury that children were receiving in their vaccines, and were disturbed to find that small children were being exposed to much more mercury than anyone had imagined.

One week before the government went public with the news, word was leaked to a conservative Internet columnist who goes by the name Jon Christian Ryter. On July 1, his warning appeared on a right-wing site called FreeRepublic.com.

"Warning on Thimerosal Will Be Played Down by National Vaccine Program Office of the CDC on Friday," his headline said. Ryter claimed to have a document implicating the CDC in a "cover-up" in order to "play down the danger of the chemical thimerosal, simply because the government can't afford to dispose of its inventory containing this substance." The CDC "would rather play with words in order to minimize the danger to both mothers and infants."[36]

According to Ryter, the European Agency for the Evaluation of Medicinal Products had recently called thimerosal a "well-recognized problem" that can cause nerve damage. But the "sluggish wheels of the US federal government speedily chugged into action—not to issue a national alert of their own," he said. "The risks are acceptable to them. Are the risks acceptable to you? The choice is yours, even though the CDC seems to think the choice is theirs." The feds would release a statement on thimerosal the following Friday afternoon, he said, when official Washington dumps its most dismal news, knowing that few Americans pay attention on Saturday. He was right.

3. Mercury Rising

RIDAY, JULY 9, 1999, began typically enough across the United States, another summer day with many people away on extended July Fourth holidays. It was, as Ryter had predicted, a great time to release bad news.

At precisely 4:15 P.M. media outlets were issued a document called "Thimerosal in Vaccines: A Joint Statement of the American Academy of Pediatrics and the Public Health Service." It got little pickup in the mainstream press. But if the PHS thought that parental activists would be caught unawares, they were mistaken. Within hours, the news unleashed a wave of anxiety in homes around the nation. Copies quickly found their way onto the autism Web sites. Parents were stunned to learn that children had been exposed to mercury levels above federal safety standards.

"Some children could be exposed to a cumulative level of mercury over the first 6 months of life that exceeds one of the federal guidelines on methyl mercury," the statement said.[37] It did not provide details on which federal standard had been exceeded, nor by how much. But it emphasized that all "acceptable" limits provided for a "significant safety margin" in any case. And there was no data or evidence of harm "by the level of exposure that some children may have encountered." Nor was there any need for kids to be tested for mercury exposure.

In crafting the statement, the authors weighed "two different types of risks." On one hand, there was the "known serious risk of diseases and deaths caused by failure to immunize." But these far outweighed the "unknown and probably much smaller risk, if any, of neurodevelopmental effects posed by exposure to thimerosal-containing vaccines over the first 6 months of life."

The reassuring claim was followed by a rather unsettling disclaimer: "Because any potential risk is of concern, the USPHS, AAP, and vaccine manufacturers agree that thimerosal-containing vaccines should be removed as soon as possible."

In their far-flung corners of the country, parents like Liz, Lyn, and Sallie read the statement and arrived at similar conclusions. The government and the AAP were posing an extraordinary contradiction. If thimerosal exposure had been so minimal, and if there was no evidence of harm, then why call for its removal "as soon as possible"?

According to the statement, the PHS would take several "key actions" on thimerosal, including a formal request for drug companies to furnish a "clear plan to eliminate or reduce [mercury content] as expeditiously as possible." It called for a review of thimerosal data "in a public workshop" and more studies to "better understand the risks and benefits of this safety assessment." The FDA would also accelerate the review of applications by drug companies to produce thimerosal-free vaccines. (The next month, with notable haste, it approved a request by Merck to sell a thimerosal-free pediatric vaccine for hepatitis-B.)

Despite the cautionary note, the government and the AAP urged doctors and parents not to waver from the list of childhood vaccinations, citing the "safety margin" built into the mercury exposure calculus. There was little reason for concern. There was no need to do anything at all. Curiously, though, the statement added that parents could postpone the birth dose of hepatitis-B until two to six months of age, "when the infant is considerably larger" (with the exception of infants born to women with antibodies to hepatitis-B, or whose status was unknown).

Sallie read the Joint Statement and called Albert.

"Did you see this?" she asked.

"I saw it." There was no need to specify what "it" was.

"Basically what they're saying is 'Hey, we've totaled up the thimerosal and we're giving your kids too much mercury,'" she scoffed. " 'So let's just reschedule the hepatitis-B shot and everything will be okay.'"

"Those bastards," Albert fumed. "Do they really think we're so stupid? Why would they postpone the birth dose if it is so 'harmless'?"

"Because they know there's something seriously wrong here," Sallie said. "They wouldn't just reschedule a vaccination unless they knew there was a real danger."

. . .

THIMEROSAL IS A WATER-SOLUBLE, cream-colored, crystalline powder that is 49.6 percent mercury by weight. It was invented in the 1920s under the direction of Eli Lilly, an Indianapolis chemist whose grandfather founded the pharmaceutical company that today is one of the world's largest drugmakers. Lilly gave the solution the brand name Merthiolate and quickly discovered a burgeoning market for the new product. One of its many uses was as a preservative for the growing number of vaccines under development in the first half of the century. For decades, thimerosal was widely marketed as safe and effective. However, the preservative had been "grandfathered" onto the approved list of medical additives by the FDA, which was formed after thimerosal was invented. The product never underwent any of the rigorous safety trials now required for FDA approval.

Most thimerosal-containing vaccines are made with 0.01 percent mercury. But no one had ever bothered to add up the total sum of mercury, by weight, being injected into American infants until the job was handed to the FDA's Center for Biologics Evaluation and Research.

There was one major complication to this task. Nearly all studies of mercury toxicity in humans had investigated exposure to methylmercury, the form that is typically found in fish. Thimerosal is made with ethylmercury, a close cousin. Both are "organic" mercury compounds; that is, they are both easily absorbed by lipids, or fatty membranes. Inorganic mercury is water-soluble and more likely to be trapped by the kidneys and filtered out of the body through urination.

Organic compounds are a more dangerous form of mercury, which is among the most toxic elements found on earth. Mercury is a recognized neurotoxin that can destroy cells in key centers of the brain and nervous system. It is especially hazardous to fetuses and small infants, whose vital organs are still developing. Mercury is known to halt cell division and migration within the forming brain, and has been shown to bind to DNA, interrupting chromosomal reproduction and blocking several essential proteins.

The main chemical difference between ethylmercury and methylmercury is that the ethyl form contains an extra carbon compound on its molecule, making it larger. Some scientists contend that the extra carbon compound makes ethylmercury less likely to cross the blood-brain barrier. Methylmercury has been shown to remain in the blood longer than ethylmercury (a half-life of fifty days versus seven days for ethylmercury) and appears to accumulate more readily in the body.[38] Despite these differences, FDA researchers assumed that the two forms of mercury were equal in toxicity.

Human exposure to high levels of methylmercury had been studied in places where large-scale mercury pollution had turned up in fish (such as Japan, in the 1950s) or where seed grain treated with a mercury fungicide had been mistakenly consumed by people (as in several outbreaks in Iraq, most recently in 1971–1972). Many children born to mothers who ate the contaminated fish or grain showed some signs of developmental impairment, ranging from severe neurological disorders in the worst exposures, to problems with language, memory, or attention in milder cases.

Because mercury is excreted in part through the hair, researchers examined hair samples from mothers of the affected children. These levels were then used by three separate U.S. government agencies, the Environmental Protection Agency (EPA), the FDA, and the CDC's Agency for Toxic Substances and Disease Registry (ATSDR), to calculate what they considered to be the maximum daily "safe" level of exposure.

At the EPA, researchers looked only at the Iraqi study, and selected the lowest hair mercury level at which damage was found. They extrapolated that figure to calculate the corresponding daily exposure from food, and determined it to be 1.0 microgram (a microgram is one-millionth of a gram) of methylmercury per kilogram of body weight (a kilo equals 2.2 pounds).[39]

But the EPA took things a step further. In order to build in a "significant margin of safety," investigators divided the 1.0 microgram figure by ten. The maximum daily exposure was thus lowered to a conservative level of 0.1 micrograms per kilogram. The other agencies were less cautious. The ATSDR calculated the safety limit to be 0.3 micrograms per kilogram per day, and FDA officials set the limit at 0.4 micrograms per kilogram per day.

When FDA researchers finally did their math and converted the amount of ethylmercury in vaccines from volume percentages to actual weight, they found that most American children were being exposed to levels in excess of federal limits, especially when calculated in single-day "bolus" doses. For example, a two-month-old child weighing 5 kilograms could have been exposed to 62.5 micrograms of mercury in a single day. This would have been 125 times more than the EPA limit for that child (0.5 micrograms per day), 42 times more than the ATSDR limit (1.5 micrograms per day), and 31 times more than the FDA limit (2.0 micrograms per day).

ALBERT ENAYATI was still seething after his call with Sallie. He stormed into the kitchen, where Sima was preparing dinner. "It's ethylmercury!" he screamed, sending Payam into tears.

"It's what?" Sima said. "Albert, what on earth are you talking about?"

"Ethylmercury. That is what's in thimerosal! I just can't believe it."

"Thime . . . what? What is thimerosal?"

"Don't you remember when I called Merck last spring? They told me it was just like lemon juice? But it wasn't that at all. It was organic mercury."

Darkness fell across Sima's face. She was a chemist. She and Albert both knew about the dangers of organic mercury exposure. Both worked in pharmaceutical plants, where workers routinely handle organic mercury clad in the full protection of HazMat suits. And both had been teenagers in Iran when news of the Iraqi grain made its way across the border. They knew it had caused neurological disorders in many people.

Albert was blind with fury: at Merck, at the FDA, at America. "If I had been told that thimerosal contained mercury," he said, trembling, "if they had leveled with me back then, it would have changed everything I've done during the last six months. I would not have had all those meetings about genetics with NIH!"

"Albert, please!" Sima pleaded. "The children."

Albert softened his tone, but not his rhetoric. "If I knew they were injecting ethylmercury into my son's body when he was two days old, do you think I would've gone and helped a *gene* bank?"

Albert rushed to his office and began tapping away on the computer, hunting for safety data on ethylmercury. He found little. Most papers pertained to *ingested methylmercury* in adults. There was nothing about *injected ethylmercury* in infants. If they even existed, they were probably buried in some faraway university medical library.

Sima came into the room and sat next to Albert. She was shaking.

"You know something, Albert?"

"What is it?"

"I hope they all go to hell."

To Albert, this meant war. But one of his chief recruits, Sallie Bernard, needed more convincing. Thimerosal was a concern, to be sure, but Sallie didn't share the same sense of alarm that gripped Albert. Just because there was mercury in vaccines didn't mean the shots caused autism. Too many questions remained: Why would some kids react so horribly to the toxin while most seemed to handle it perfectly well? Besides, there was mercury in tuna, and that didn't make anyone autistic, right?

"I kind of blew him off," Sallie confessed to Tom. "There are a million other avenues we're trying to follow. This would just be one more thing to add to the plate. It's not like we don't have other things to do. Who has time to look into this mercury thing?"

But Albert was not about to give up. He kept pushing Sallie. And he kept pushing another New Jersey mother of a boy with autism, Heidi Roger, a financial director from Ridgefield Park. Her son Andrew had been diagnosed with PDD-NOS in April 1997, and Heidi—despite everything the doctors told her—felt certain she could fight the disorder and win. She had met Albert at a parent support group meeting soon after her son's diagnosis and the two became friends. Heidi, with her sharp wit and sharper Jersey accent, was a good pairing for Albert, the fighter. Heidi had joined CAN when Albert became president of the New Jersey chapter, and had spent a lot of time with him and Sallie.

Albert called Heidi after the Joint Statement was released. Like Sallie, Heidi was concerned, but not convinced. "C'mon!" Albert pleaded. "This is really bad stuff, Heidi. We're talking about organic mercury here. We have to get rid of this mercury."

"I know Albert, but . . ." She was much more interested in actual treatments than in chasing yet another wacky theory about the cause of autism.

"But nothing, Heidi. You've got to help me. I need to compile every paper on ethylmercury I can find. We have to hit the libraries. I can't do it alone."

"I don't know, Albert. I'm pretty busy these days. I'm not going to go get the freaking articles on those Iraqi children. This is bullshit."

"Oh God, no. This is not bullshit. This is important. I'm going to find out who did this to our kids, Heidi. And you're going to help."

Heidi was silent for a moment. But she knew in her heart that Albert was right. "You, my friend, are my favorite social terrorist," she said. "Sign me up."

Over the next two weeks, Albert and Heidi took turns at public libraries and medical school libraries, with pockets full of change to operate the clanky old copiers. They collected every paper on mercury poisoning they could, then ran home to e-mail each other their discoveries.

What they were finding was this: many symptoms of mercury toxicity were remarkably similar, if not identical, to the signs of autism.

Instances of mercury poisoning have been described since Roman times. The Mad Hatter in *Alice in Wonderland* was believed to be modeled on a syndrome resulting from occupational exposure to mercury vapor used in millinery, called "Mad Hatter's disease." The affliction struck a certain percentage of hatmakers in centuries past. People with Mad Hatter's disease suffered from depression, sluggishness, acute anxiety, and irrational fears. They grew nervous and timid. They blushed readily, were uncomfortable in social situations, and sought to avoid people. "Mad Hatters" were easily upset, had trouble with movement and coordination, and were prone to agitation, irritability, and aggression.

Mad Hatter's disease was just one of the wide range of bizarre disorders that mercury exposure can cause, Albert and Heidi found out. Effects can vary considerably among individuals. Age and body weight are important factors; children are far more susceptible than adults to the same dose of mercury. Other factors include the rate of exposure (chronic but low-level versus intermittent but acute exposure), the type of mercury, and the route of exposure (inhaled in vapors, rubbed onto skin, taken orally, or injected). Perhaps most important, individual sensitivity seemed to arise from predetermined genetic factors.

For these reasons, Albert and Heidi learned, there are no "typical" symptoms of mercury poisoning. Victims almost always develop some type of movement disorder, but it might range from mere clumsiness in some to severe involuntary jerking movements in others. Psychological disturbances are usually present, but these might be manifested as anxiety in certain people while presenting as aggression or irritability in others.

Albert had observed most of these signs in Payam at one time or another. "This is what happened to our freaking son," he said. Albert was as good as convinced. He fired off an e-mail to Portia Iverson at CAN.

"This is mercury," he wrote. "It is highly neurotoxic. This is important, we have to look into it." Portia never responded. Albert wrote again, and still no response came. A few days later Heidi mentioned that she had spoken with Portia, who suggested she ask Albert to halt his investigations. The national organization would look into the mercury allegation, she said. Albert should stick to fund-raising. He was good at fund-raising.[40]

But with urging from Sallie, Cure Autism Now did organize a conference call, in late August, with autism officials at the CDC. Sallie frowned as she listened in on the call. The officials offered a list of federal research projects looking into autism epidemiology. They said nothing about vaccines, mercury, or any other environmental factors. There was no sense of urgency whatsoever. When some of the parents brought up vaccines, the response was lukewarm and noncommittal, Sallie thought. "This falls so far short of what they should be doing," she told herself. "Why won't they even listen to us?"

Albert, for his part, was feeling dejected, and beginning to lose interest for lack of support. Then one day a stack of articles he had back-ordered arrived at his house. They included a recent case study of a forty-four-year-old man who, while being treated in the hospital for liver disease, received an accidental overdose of thimerosal. Within days, he lost his ability to speak. Then came the social withdrawal and, not long after that, arm flapping.[41]

Albert could not believe what he was reading. He wanted to know more. He called the university where the case study was recorded. He desperately wanted to contact the patient, to question him personally about the symptoms. But the university refused to provide any information, citing confidentiality rules. Albert tried calling the professor who wrote the article, with similar results. He wrote the school a letter. "We are looking into vaccinations, thimerosal, and autism," he pleaded. But he never heard back.

Albert was not about to quit. He called up researchers in the autism field and said, "Look at this guy in the study. He became completely autistic!" But, Albert complained to Heidi, "Nobody cares. 'Yeah, yeah,' they say. 'So what?'"

Then Albert told Heidi, "You know what? I have all these published articles. I'm going to sit down and compare the symptoms of autism and mercury poisoning. I'll write a couple of pages. Maybe eight pages. And I'll publish a paper myself."

Over the next two weeks, Albert practically lived at the New Jersey CAN office, working on his paper. The charity had an arrangement with the Bergen County District Attorney to give office work without pay to people sentenced to community service for petty crimes. One woman, caught stealing food for her family, happened to be a superb typist. Albert put her to work. In two weeks, the two of them had banged out a thirteen-page dossier on the similarities between mercury poisoning and autism.

Albert was exhausted, but he kept pushing. He had no idea how to get something like this published. He needed help, and wrote again to Portia Iverson. "I'm writing this article and I'll put your name as lead author and sponsor," he told her. "Because you have a tremendous amount of knowledge on autism, and on the scientific world. And I have very good knowledge of mercury poisoning. We could work together and you could put your name on it." Again Albert received no response from Los Angeles.

And so he turned to his friend Sallie, the marketing executive from Summit. She agreed to read the draft. Three weeks went by before Albert heard back. He was nervous with anticipation. Then the phone rang. "It's Sallie," she said. "I have reviewed the article. This is what I think."

"Yes?"

"My God, Albert. It's terrific."

WHEN LYN REDWOOD read the Joint Statement and saw that there had been "no evidence of harm" from thimerosal, she screamed out loud to no one in particular, "How could they *know* this? Nobody ever looked to see if harm had been found! Nobody researched this issue before!"

As a member of the Fayette County Board of Health, Lyn's first concern was the vaccines administered by the Health Department. Childhood immunization was one of the agency's largest undertakings, and a favorite project of Lyn, who was adamantly pro-vaccine. She called the department's head nurse.

"I need to know exactly what vaccines we are giving, what brands," Lyn said. "And I also need to know: do any of them contain thimerosal?"

"Oh right," the nurse said. "We just got a fax from the state on that. We looked and found out we were only giving one vaccine with mercury, hepatitis-B. And now that has been pushed back from birth to six months of age."

Lyn was immensely relieved. Apparently the kids in her county had largely escaped mercury exposure. But Will had not been vaccinated by the county, she remembered. Lyn had taken him to the family pediatrician for his shots. She felt nauseous. The full ramifications of the Joint Statement were beginning to hit her.

Lyn had been to nursing school, of course, where she studied the hazards of mercury. She had respect for its poisonous power. She knew it could cause brain damage, mental retardation, mental illness, and immune dysfunction. She knew that mercury is so toxic that a tiny spill, from a thermometer, can lead to the evacuation of an entire building. She went back online and looked up the MSDS (Material Safety Data Sheet) for thimerosal. "Highly toxic," it said. "Danger of cumulative effects. Avoid prolonged or repeated exposure. The chemical, physical, and toxicological properties have not been thoroughly investigated."

As Lyn read more about the symptoms of mercury toxicity, she was shocked at how similar they seemed to Will's condition. Individuals exposed to the metal, especially in the womb or during early infancy, often have difficulty speaking and understanding language. They become sensitive to loud noises, develop sensory disturbances and an aversion to touch. They become over- or underresponsive to pain. They often withdraw from social contact. They sometimes develop obsessive-compulsive disorders. They lose their ability to understand abstract ideas.

These are the hallmarks of autism, Lyn thought. This is Will.

Lyn ran to her files and pulled out the list of eleven vaccinations that Will had been given between two months and eighteen months of age. Her worst fears were realized: Will's vaccines had come from a company other than the one that supplied Fayette County. All the shots, except MMR, contained thimerosal. Lyn cried as she read the numbers and wrote them down in a little column on her pad. She had difficulty controlling the pen.

At his two-month well-baby visit, Will had received a diphtheria-tetanus shot that had 25 micrograms of ethylmercury used as a preservative. On the same visit, Will had been given an Hib shot, with another 25 micrograms, and hepatitis-B, which had 12.5 micrograms. At four months, he got the same three shots, or another 62.5 micrograms. At six months, he was given just DT and Hib, or 50 micrograms, and then he received his last hep-B at one year, which was another 12.5 micrograms. Finally, at eighteen months,

Will had received his last DT and Hib shots (plus MMR) for an additional 50 micrograms of mercury exposure.

Lyn added up her column and almost choked: Will had been injected with a total of 237 micrograms of mercury. And most of that—175 micrograms—he received in the first six months, when he weighed very little, and when the infant immune and nervous systems are still developing and more vulnerable to toxic assault, Lyn knew.

But what did Will's numbers mean in terms of the EPA limits? To find out, Lyn took Will's exposure at two months. At that age, he weighed a little over 10 pounds, or 5 kilograms. According to the EPA guideline of 0.1 microgram per kilogram per day, Will should not have been exposed to more than 0.5 micrograms of mercury on the day of his doctor visit. But he received 62.5 micrograms. Lyn did the math. She was sure she had calculated wrong. The way she figured it, Will's exposure that day exceeded the EPA limit by *125 times*.

Lyn was more shocked than angry. And she was extremely alarmed, not only for Will, but all the other kids being vaccinated at the time. "I need to let people know about this," she said to herself.

But Lyn had a difficult time processing what she was learning. She still could not believe that vaccines might be dangerous. After all, she was a committed proponent of immunization. Her nephew's wife, a chiropractor, had earlier announced to the entire family that she would not allow her kids to be vaccinated. Lyn had been horrified and disgusted. "They are making a very dangerous mistake," she told Tommy. "They need to vaccinate their kids."

Now Lyn wondered if it was she who had made the mistake. She thought back to all those babies she had held down as a nurse to give them their injections. "My God," she thought, "have I been part of the problem? All those kids that I gave shots to, am I responsible if some of them get autism?"

Guilt and internal conflict dominated her emotions. Lyn knew she would have to go public with what she had found. She would not sleep at night, knowing that so many kids were being injected with mercury in their vaccines every single day.

When Tommy got home from work that night, Lyn had him double-check her math. He arrived at the same numbers and she began sobbing again. "How could those bastards say that the exposure to mercury was so small?" she asked. "How could they say the risk is only a theoretical risk?"

Tommy had no answer. They reexamined the EPA figures and the Joint Statement. Tommy pointed out that the government had added up total mercury exposure in the first six months and then averaged it out on a per-day basis. The result showed an average daily exposure that was only slightly above EPA standards, even though on vaccination days, exposures went through the roof. (Lyn would learn that acute, high-dose exposures to mercury, called "bolus" doses, are potentially more harmful than chronic, daily low-dose exposures.)

"Think of it this way," Tommy explained, "if you take two Tylenols each day for thirty days, you'll be fine. But if you take all sixty at once, you'll probably die. It's like someone drinking a fifth of whiskey and insisting they aren't drunk, because it was the only drink they had in two months."

Lyn had to laugh at this statistical sleight of hand. "But why would the FDA, the respected FDA, issue such a watered-down report?"

"I have no idea," Tommy said. "But it doesn't look so good, does it?"

The notion that Will might have been poisoned by mercury used in vaccines horrified Lyn. But it also gave her an odd sense of relief. For the past three years, she had blamed herself for Will's decline. She had scoured her memory trying to pinpoint what had gone awry. Was it that time during pregnancy when she ate the yogurt with aspartame? Or when he had rotavirus: maybe his blood sugar fell so low it killed brain cells? Without knowing what had happened, Lyn had no way of figuring out how to fix it. Mercury was the first thing to emerge that made everything else make sense.

"If it's mercury," she told Tommy, "it can accumulate in the brain and the central nervous system. It can stay there for a long time." Mercury poisoning would be a terrible diagnosis. But what if there were ways to detoxify? What if they could reverse some of the damage? What if they could help Will and thousands of kids like him?

UP IN CHICAGO, Liz Birt read the Joint Statement one afternoon at work and was intrigued. The inquisitive attorney determined that day to scour the details of the FDA archives. She wanted to know what agency officials knew about mercury in vaccines, and when they knew it. But it was rare, in Chicago, to come across old FDA documents. A friend who ran the law library at Liz's firm was formerly law librarian at the American Medical Association. She told Liz about the *Pink Sheet*, a small-circulation pharmaceutical trade journal that covers the mazelike food and drug bureaucracy in exacting, some would say excruciating, detail.

Liz had some time available on Lexis-Nexis, the media search engine that can locate almost any printed article, anywhere. She downloaded all the *Pink Sheet*s for the past five or six years and began looking for articles on thimerosal. She found very little information. How strange, Liz said to herself. This stuff hasn't been tested. There's been no large safety trial. How is that possible?

Liz was well on her way to suspecting a vaccine connection to Matthew's illness, but for now she still had questions. Then, in September 1999, she attended a conference sponsored by CAN, where one of the main speakers was Dr. Andrew Wakefield. He had flown in from London to discuss his latest MMR findings. Liz met the young "misguided maverick," as he was being called in England, and found him to be quite rational. "He wasn't crazy, like some people had said he would be," she told her husband. "He has a deep scientific background. He's published a lot of important papers. He seems credible."

As he had done at the Orlando conference attended by Lyn Redwood, Wakefield presented results from biopsies he'd taken from inflamed lymph tissue in the GI tracts of autistic children. An independent laboratory in Ireland, run by Dr. John O'Leary, he said, had confirmed the presence of measles virus in the biopsies.

"All the kids he talked about sounded just like Matthew," Liz told her husband. The next day, she brought Matthew to the hotel, where Wakefield examined the boy right in his room. He touched his stomach and said, "I think we could help him." Liz called her husband at work and after a lengthy conversation it was decided the family would fly to London in November so that Wakefield could do a thorough review, including a colonoscopy and biopsies, on their very sick son.

Liz returned to investigating thimerosal. She was particularly interested to know what had been going on in Europe around the issue. Thimerosal, she discovered, had been removed from all childhood vaccines in Scandinavia beginning in 1992. By 1997, health officials in the European Union itself had begun looking into the preservative and its possible toxic effects. Liz learned that the Europeans, like their American counterparts, were worried about the cumulative effect of administering a string of mercury-containing vaccines to infants. Then she came across Jon Christian Ryter's warning about the Joint Statement and his account of the high-level meetings that had taken place between American and European health officials.

As Ryter noted in his Web site article, the European Agency for the Evaluation of Medicinal Products (EAEMP) had issued a white paper on June 29, 1999, announcing the conclusions of an internal study on thimerosal use in EU countries.[42] Awareness of a problem first arose in 1990, when the World Health Organization began to investigate allergic reactions to thimerosal.

"WHO was concerned that the accumulated effect of more than 200 mcg of mercury in a fetus or infant could cause moderate to severe brain damage that would result in a rise in learning impaired children," Ryter wrote. This alarmed FDA officials, who encouraged the removal of mercury from childhood shots. But in order "not to jeopardize immunization programs" it was considered advisable to eliminate it "on a gradual basis."

Liz knew something was wrong. First the FDA said that thimerosal was not harmful at the level found in vaccines. But then it admitted that no safety studies had ever been done. Then the agency said that mercury should be removed from vaccines "as soon as possible." But now Liz was reading that the FDA actually wanted to eliminate it "on a gradual basis." She frowned as she read through the contradictory documents.

"What's it going to be, guys?" she asked, looking down at the papers scattered across her desk. "Is this stuff dangerous? Or isn't it?"

Through her work with CAN, Liz had been making contacts with parents around the country. She had struck up a very close relationship with Sallie Bernard and Albert Enayati, in New Jersey. The trio began sharing lengthy e-mails on strategies for political action around research and treatment. Sallie and Albert were eager to recruit their new ally, a lawyer no less, to their fledgling mercury-autism effort. Liz had to turn them down. Matthew was so sick and there was so much else to do, including preparations for the London trip and Dr. Wakefield's evaluation. "I can't do this right now," she told them, reluctantly. "I haven't slept in two years."

THE IMPACT of the Joint Statement on Thimerosal rippled far beyond the world of autism families. It caused an uproar among right-wing, antigovernment (and anti-Clinton) alarmists, some of whom worried about jack-booted thugs in black helicopters swooping in from the heavens to whisk their children off to forced vaccination camps. Phyllis Schlafly penned a diatribe that was immediately posted on several sites.

"A scandal in mandatory mass vaccinations of infants is beginning to surface," she warned. "Vaccine-caused injuries have just forced the Clinton bureaucrats to make [some] sensational announcements that bugle temporary retreat from their plans to force all American children to submit to government-dictated medical treatment."[43]

Meanwhile, on FreeRepublic.com, the conspiracy talk waxed. On July 1, 1999, when Christian Ryter leaked the Joint Statement a full week before its release, alarmist posts appeared:

- "Guess we can give Hillary the credit for all this? I wouldn't doubt it one bit."
- "Right on, and home school if need be. I wonder if they can force this crap on you. It's very alarming. I'm upset with this type of stuff being done to America."
- "Sad to say, it all comes down to MONEY! It's hard to believe that there are those so greedy and evil that the money is more important than a human being."

- "There are enough of us here alone to start a petition to demand the government stop the inoculations until they are proven safe for the children, or we will file a class action lawsuit against them for knowingly endangering and damaging our children! It's one more way to intimidate and control us."[44]

The Joint Statement also rattled people on the front lines of public health. Some doctors launched blistering attacks against the recommendations. Instead of complaining that the statement played down the risk of thimerosal, these critics alleged that the statement was far too *alarming* and would drive fearful parents away from vaccines. Alarm over "trace mercury" in vaccines, they said, was a theoretical and unproven problem, which had been elevated to a level of importance that didn't make sense.

The controversy within medical circles was reported in a meticulously researched article in a trade journal called *Hepatitis Control Report*.[45] It quoted one unnamed "prominent Texas pediatrician," a member of the AAP, as saying, "I can't believe the Academy doesn't think it has stubbed its toe on this one."

But there was an opposing camp to the thimerosal naysayers. "Some leaders within AAP believe that the Academy did not go far enough to protect infants against mercury," the article said. "But both camps feel obligated to follow the new policies for fear of legal liability if they diverge." Bitter divisions arose between the AAP and the CDC. On October 20, 1999, the CDC's Advisory Committee on Immunization Practices (ACIP), a powerful panel of physicians and researchers whose recommendations are almost always adopted by the CDC, voted *not* to announce a general preference for thimerosal-free vaccines for use in small children. The AAP, the article said, had been urging the CDC to do just the opposite.

SALLIE BERNARD WAS IMPRESSED with Albert's work on mercury poisoning, but the mercury hypothesis still troubled her. "Intellectually I'm becoming convinced, but not emotionally, if you can imagine that," Sallie explained to her husband. "I see all this stuff in the literature making the comparisons, and everything starts to click. But then I take a step back, and say, Ah, c'mon, how could this be? Everybody gets vaccinated. How could this be the cause? After all, they must have done all the safety research. They wouldn't have given this to little kids if they didn't know it was safe."

But the more Sallie learned about the symptoms of mercury poisoning, the more convinced she became of their similarities to autism. Sallie knew that trying to convince the public, and the public health specialists, would be challenging, to put it mildly. She knew how Wakefield had been treated after publishing his MMR studies. She remembered how the CDC had rejected his ideas out of hand, before doing their own investigations. And she remembered the chilly reception the parents had received when the question of vaccines was raised on that CDC conference call back in August.

"These researchers will never give us the time of day, and no one will do anything about this," Sallie warned Albert, "unless we come out with something in their own language, that speaks to the scientific world in a way they are used to being spoken to."

The only way to do that, she figured, was to publish the paper. Her hope was to stimulate interest from the scientific community, so that they would take the hypothesis seriously and start to do research on the possible link between thimerosal and autism. "A paper will give us entrée," Sallie told her husband. Yes, the idea of a group of parents writing a medical paper seemed audacious, maybe even ridiculous. "But sometimes you get so fed up, because the researchers are supposed to be helping us find answers to our kids' problem. I know there are exceptions out there, Tom, but as a group, they just aren't doing their job."

Sallie had another motive as well: treatments. If mercury were the cause of autism, then what was the cure?

The parents would need help for such a bold undertaking, and they enlisted an autism researcher named Teresa Binstock. Teresa, in her mid-fifties, looked something like an aging mountain woman. Six feet tall and dressed in sensible shoes and a full-length skirt, her long gray-blond hair was braided into pigtails.

Teresa had amassed nearly a decade of independent research at the University of Colorado Health Sciences Center and Denver's The Children's Hospital. She had mastered several genres of medical literature and occasionally served as a consultant for physicians with difficult cases. Teresa often speaks in a quirky, formal, but offbeat manner. She can recite scientific hypotheses. Her grammar is elegant, intricate, and utterly flawless. And Teresa has Asperger's syndrome.

Teresa, an investigator in developmental and behavioral neuroanatomy, had written some papers on autism, posting several of them online. She had also worked with Portia Iverson and some of the other CAN people, adding research skills and credentials to what was largely a parents' movement.

Sallie, Albert, and Heidi continued to take turns visiting libraries, conducting online searches, and ordering back issues of medical journals. They unearthed a small mountain of evidence pointing to strikingly similar (though not always identical) traits between mercury poisoning and autistic tendencies. These included:

Minamata Disease—This syndrome was named after Minamata Bay in southwestern Japan. In the early 1950s, residents began noticing bizarre behaviors in animals living in the area, especially cats. They watched as their pets convulsed and screeched in agony as they performed tortured dances on the floor. Then cases of a previously unseen disorder began surfacing in people. It was first diagnosed in fishing communities located near a factory that had expelled heavy wastes, including mercury, into the sea. Within a year, methylmercury levels in Minamata Bay seafood were found to be extremely high. By 1957, fishing was banned in the area. But it was too late to avert the damage. Hundreds fell ill in the first year after the toxic discharge. Minamata disease caused numbness in the arms, legs, and mouth, sensory disturbance, and problems with hand-eye coordination and movement. There was a general lack of coordination, difficulty in walking, fatigue, tremors, and seizures. Victims suffered reduced or slurred speech and diminished vision and hearing. Some people went on to develop partial paralysis, jerking movements, difficulty in swallowing, convulsions, brain damage, and death. Children born to exposed mothers were the most vulnerable, as made famous in a *Life* magazine black-and-white photo of a mother cradling her severely disabled daughter in a steam room. By the time the crisis abated, some fourteen hundred residents had died and perhaps twenty thousand suffered some form of mercury poisoning.[46]

The Iraqi Grain Incident—In 1971, the Persian Gulf region suffered a catastrophic drought that wiped out wheat production in Iraq's famous "Fertile Crescent." Little seed was left for the following year's planting, so the Iraqi government imported some 178,000 tons of drought-resistant wheat seed from Mexico. The grain was treated with methylmercury (and in some cases ethylmercury) as a fungicide and dyed pink. But in much of the country, the grain arrived too late to plant as seed. Instead, villagers ground it into flour to make bread. They did not understand that the pink dye meant the seed was treated with mercury, nor did they know that the skull-and-crossbones on the grain sacks meant "poison." Thousands of Iraqis consumed bread made from the seed, apparently finding its pink color festive and attractive. Then the symptoms began. First there was burning or prickling of the skin and fuzzy eyesight. Next came loss of muscle coordination, blindness, hearing loss, coma, and sometimes death. The outbreak sent six thousand people to the hospital and 450 died. Many times that number never received medical care and went unreported. Most victims were children.[47]

"The effects on developing fetuses in mothers who ate the bread have not been fully documented," one study concluded. "But subsequent analyses indicate that the fetus may be more than 10 times as sensitive to mercury poisoning as the adult."[48] Symptoms of children exposed during pregnancy included cerebral palsy, mental retardation, weakness, seizures, visual loss, and delayed development. Older children had seizures, abnormal reflexes, and delayed development. One statement really shook Sallie, Albert, and Heidi, because it was so familiar. Children exposed to mercury in utero "appeared fairly normal at birth, with only slight abnormalities of reflexes and muscle tone, but later had seizures, long delays in learning to walk and talk, and severe clumsiness," it said.[49]

The Pig Farm Poisoning—In this bizarre case, humans did not consume mercury-treated grain directly, but rather fed upon a pig that had eaten treated grain. The family, who lived on a farm in Alamogordo, New Mexico, in the 1950s, ate from the pig for three months after slaughter. But symptoms did not arise for some time after the pig was fully consumed. Follow-up studies showed that family members suffered from quadriplegia, mental defects, and vision loss, which persisted for years. Mercury remained in their brains for years, and two of the younger children died.[50] The delayed symptoms "really drive the point home why it's so hard to correlate the mercury poisoning with autism," Heidi noted. "It's so insidious; the mercury works slowly to cause the illness."

Pink Disease—Some of the most striking parallels the parents found were accounts of a ghastly childhood disease that swept Europe, Canada, and Australia in the first half of the twentieth century. The mysterious illness, known as acrodynia, or "pink disease," began afflicting tens of thousands of children in the 1930s. Symptoms included a weepy red rash (hence the name), peeling skin, lethargy, anemia, sensitivity to light, respiratory distress, and general ill health. About 25 percent of babies with pink disease died.

Researchers now know that pink disease arose when infants with a heightened sensitivity to mercury were exposed to products containing the inorganic form, which was used as an antiseptic in teething powders, calamine lotion, and Mercurochrome. They reported that 1 in 500 exposed children developed the disease, roughly the same rate as autism in America in the late 1990s. Acrodynia, by all accounts, was a miserable condition. Descriptions of many symptoms would be instantly recognizable to parents of an autistic child. They read as if written for a textbook on autism:

> The first sign is a loss of joyfulness. The children stop playing and laughing, and may go weeks or months without smiling. Their faces reflect sadness: the forehead is wrinkled, the look melancholy or even desperate. The children appear to suffer physically and morally. At

the same time, the children stop talking. Some cry constantly. Most are cranky, complain, and moan. Affectivity is modified. Most often it is diminished or disappears completely. Some children appear unaware of their parents, don't respond to their kisses, do not seem to notice them when they come close or leave. In most children, there is some irritability, sometimes hostility. If someone comes close, they move away and cry. Some children bite or hit their mothers and siblings. Some have strange behaviors: a girl, who was very well behaved before her illness, would get up secretly and relieve herself on a rug.

Some children turn their anger against themselves. They hit themselves, bang their heads against furniture, throw themselves on the floor, pull their hair. They behave in strange ways. One little boy refused to walk and then started running away. Very often, depression follows these outbursts. The child remains completely quiet and silent and has a hostile look. Excitation and depression are often alternating. Intelligence may remain intact. But in serious cases, it appears diminished. Some children repeat the same words for hours. One child repeated constantly, "I want some coffee," with a monotonous voice.[51]

Then there was another report, the remarkable story of Heather Thiele, a perfectly normal girl who, because of her sore gums, was given a mercury-laced teething powder in the early 1950s. Years later she wrote about the experience, offering a rare glimpse of mercury poisoning from the inside. Again, her personal recollections are eerily similar to those written by higher functioning adults with autism:

Immediately, I became lethargic, sensitive to noise, light and touch, lost my appetite and consequently lost weight alarmingly. I lost muscle tone and I found it hard to hold my head up or sit, and although I was on the verge of walking, I became like a floppy doll. I would rock myself from side to side in my pram or cot, and bashed my head against the walls. Nothing seemed to pacify me, and I would go for days without sleep. I was tired all the time. I was particularly clumsy and very shy as a child. I would sit in the corner of a room, reading a book or playing, and be quite unaware of all that was going on around me.[52]

It took years before the radical theory that mercury poisoning was causing pink disease was gradually accepted, and then only against stiff resistance by industry. Once mercury was implicated in 1948, manufacturers finally began removing it. By 1954 most companies had eliminated mercury entirely from teething powders, by far the largest source of infant exposure. Removal was voluntary, but companies feared adverse publicity and potential lawsuits. Cases of the disease soon fell sharply and then disappeared entirely. Today, pink disease is virtually unheard of.

THE NEXT STEP for the New Jersey parents was to begin compiling lists of similarities between mercury poisoning and autism. They grouped the symptoms into fifteen categories and called them a "constellation" of symptoms that are common to many, but not necessarily all, cases.

They found many common impairments in sociability, for example: withdrawal, anxiety, lack of eye contact, and aggression. Common language problems included loss of speech and hearing, while sensory abnormalities included sound sensitivity and touch aversion. Similar motor disorders were also identified, such as arm flapping, uncontrolled jerking, toe walking, and poor eye-hand coordination. Cognitive impairments included poor concentration, uneven IQ test performance, and poor memory. The list continued, showing similarities in other areas: visual problems, unusual behaviors, physical disturbances, GI disorders, abnormal biochemistry, immune dysfunction, central nervous system structural pathology, and neurochemistry abnormalities.[53]

With the able guidance and contributions of Teresa Binstock, the New Jersey parents worked together for several months. "And before I knew it, that primitive little ten-page paper I had written had evolved into an elegant sixty-page treatise," Albert marveled. "Sallie was so knowledgeable about autism. She read all the articles. She knew all the symptoms."

Sallie insisted on crafting the report in the most professional and scientific manner possible. She was serious about getting it published in a peer-reviewed journal, and harbored no illusions about the scrutiny that would be brought to bear on their work. "Unless you can publish what you write," she told her friends, "you're only talking to yourself, talking to the wind." And even if they did manage to publish, she added, "Nobody is going to pay any attention if we don't speak in their language. Scientists aren't going to read anything unless it's written in scientific jargon."

Sallie also knew that resistance would come from within the autism community itself. She knew that some parents were openly scoffing at the Jersey group's ambitions. More than a few skeptics called them crazy. One night, when everyone was gathered in Sallie's office reviewing another draft of the paper, she warned Heidi and Albert about what they were up against. "Given the topic, the other side is going to treat us just like they treated Wakefield," she said. "And we're just a few off-the-wall parents, to be looked down upon by scientists and clinicians."

Albert rolled his eyes. "I don't give a damn about those guys," he said. "They are the ones who did this to our kids."

"I know," Sallie said, "but we are writing about vaccines, the sacred cow of public health. We are putting vaccines in the same context as toxicology. They will come after us. We must be prepared."

Public ignorance was another barrier. "How are we going to let everybody in the world know that most of their diseases are caused by environmental influences?" Sallie asked. "Bad diet, drug taking, lead in thirty-year-old houses, environmental toxins. None of that is sinking in. When we cry 'mercury,' people are going to look at us and go, 'Huh?' "

The same was true for challenging the genetic theory of autism, she said. It was accepted as gospel by leading researchers. "Not only do they say that autism is genetic," she added, "they say it's prenatal, it manifests in utero. But we are talking about something that happens after birth. What we have here," she finished with a sigh, "are several big strikes against us."

LYN REDWOOD was now convinced that mercury had played a role in her son's disease. She was upset to learn that Will's exposure had not just come in vaccine form. Lyn remembered the Rho(D) immunoglobulin injections she had received while pregnant. She looked up the brand of Rho(D) she received and felt sick to her stomach. Each injection had contained a whopping 65 micrograms of ethylmercury, more than twice the level in any vaccine, and each was administered prenatally.[54]

Lyn was furious that the Joint Statement of the FDA, the American Academy of Pediatrics, and the Public Health Service claimed there was "no need" to test children for mercury exposure. If Will had mercury poisoning, Lyn wanted to know about it. And she wanted to know what, if anything, she could do to make it better. She called a toxicology lab for information about mercury testing, but was disconsolate to learn that heavy metals are detectable in the blood only if the exposure was recent (within fifty to seventy days) or if it was ongoing. Will was now five and a half years old. The lab workers said there was no way to determine his exposure levels during infancy.

Lyn hung up and pondered this newly blocked road of inquiry. Then she remembered that hair is often tested to determine heavy metal exposure. But so what? She had recently read that hair tests were only accurate for about one year after exposure. A sample taken now wouldn't provide any evidence on Will's levels during his first year of life. Lyn was about to give up.

A few weeks later, while rummaging through some old belongings in a closet, Lyn stumbled upon Will's baby book. She had put it away long ago, when Will stopped having milestones to record in its pages. Inside was a hair sample from his very first haircut at twenty months. Will should have been excreting vaccine mercury at this time. A hair analysis would indicate if his mercury "burden" had reached dangerous levels.

Lyn knew the beautiful lock of baby hair would be destroyed. It was the only one she had, the only physical relic of a much happier time. She plucked the lock from its box and stared at it a moment. This was going to be hard. You know what? she thought. It's worth it to get an answer. She dropped the hair in a baggie and sent it to the lab.

While waiting for the hair results to come back, Lyn prepared for her second major autism conference, this one scheduled for early October 1999 in Cherry Hill, New Jersey. It was sponsored by another emerging influential organization, Defeat Autism Now! DAN! had sprung from a small group of forward-thinking physicians and scientists who joined forces to exchange information and ideas in order to "defeat" autism as quickly as possible. The DAN! doctors had first come together in January 1995 under the auspices of Bernie Rimland's Autism Research Institute. A top priority was to issue a guideline for physicians in the clinical assessment of autistic patients and the creation of appropriate treatments. A year later they issued a consensus document on "state-of-the-art" diagnostics and treatments, known as the "DAN Protocol." Lyn wanted to find out all she could about the new approach. Tommy agreed to go to New Jersey with her.

Despite her excitement over DAN! Lyn was preoccupied with Will's hair test. On the morning that she and Tommy were leaving for the airport, Lyn couldn't resist the urge to call the lab. She knew it would be days before they returned, and the results were to come in by fax. To her surprise, the test was complete. The fax would be sent right over. Lyn ran upstairs to her office and waited nervously, not wanting to miss her flight, but not willing to leave until she had those numbers. The phone rang and the fax paper slowly crept from the machine. Lyn's eyes followed the chart as the results appeared line by line. She immediately noticed that two metals were far out of the normal reference range: mercury and aluminum. Lyn tore the fax paper from its spool and ran to meet Tommy in the car. She looked at the paper again. Lyn knew from the EPA Web site that hair levels of mercury above 1 part per million (ppm) were considered cause for action. A reading of 5 ppm means mercury poisoning.[55] At twenty months of age, Will's hair had contained 4.8 ppm.

"I have no idea what these levels mean in terms of damage to kids," she said to Tommy. "Do you?" Tommy looked at the fax. "All I know," he replied sourly, "is that they are too damn high."

Lyn nodded. She was unhappy, but also oddly relieved. "But you know something, Tom?" she said. "This is the closest thing to an answer we've ever gotten. This is the only test result to come back with a detectable biochemical abnormality." And, she added, "Will never eats fish, and he doesn't have any fillings. There is no other possible source for the mercury in his hair than thimerosal."

THE DEFEAT AUTISM NOW! conference was an absorbing two-day gathering of parents and some of the world's most innovative autism experts. The consensus seemed to be that there was still no decisive proof of autism's origin. But the DAN! doctors had developed a series of interventions that, based on their success rate, did seem to indicate that autism was a combination of ailments—including immune dysfunction, GI problems, poor nutrient absorption, gut inflammation, and viral infection—possibly sparked by some environmental trigger of a genetic predisposition.

Among the triggers discussed were vaccines, pesticides, diet, infectious diseases, and environmental pressures from pollution and other sources. There was some, but not much, talk of heavy metal exposure. Dr. Kenneth Bock, for example, said that toxic metals can suppress immune responses and pave the way for a host of serious ailments. A "down-regulated" immune system becomes so dysfunctional it begins to reverse the normal immune response, which is generally divided into two categories, called TH1 and TH2. TH1 enhances immunity by promoting the growth of certain immune cells that attack infection, whereas TH2 induces immunity through antibody production. When the ratio of TH1 to TH2 is reversed (producing more TH2 than TH1), the antibody response can overtake the system.

Near the meeting's close there was a roundtable session that offered parents a rare opportunity for a back-and-forth discussion with researchers and doctors. It seemed like an eternity before Lyn got to ask her question.

"My name is Lyn Redwood, the mother of a little boy, Will, who is really struggling with PDD-NOS," she began nervously. Lyn clutched the report from the toxicology lab and brandished it in the air. "I have to announce that I've just discovered that Will received one hundred and twenty-five times his allowable exposure to mercury from vaccines in a single day. And I found out his mercury hair levels were five times the allowable EPA levels. What should I do?"

The room was silent. No one knew what to say. "I only hope," Lyn said, looking each doctor straight in the eye, "that this question of mercury in vaccines will be pursued with all the vigor it deserves." Lyn sat down, her face red with excitement, knowing she had unleashed something important. A tearful woman approached the Redwoods and told them that her autistic son had also been found to have very high mercury levels.

"Really?" Lyn asked anxiously. "And what are you doing for him?"

"We just started chelation on him," the woman explained. "It's where you give the kids this agent, a sulfur compound, which binds with the mercury so that it can be cleared from the system. We've already noticed a difference; you should try it."

Lyn knew what chelation was. Once back in Atlanta, she could not wait to find out more about chelation and mercury. The word (pronounced key-LAY-shun) is derived from the Greek word *chele,* or claw, because the technique in a sense "scrapes" metals from cells. Developed by the U.S. Navy to treat lead poisoning in sailors in the 1940s,[56] its use had been expanded, unofficially, by some doctors, for the treatment of autism. The process is complex, and has not been clinically proven to successfully treat mercury toxicity (though there is ample anecdotal evidence). Simply put, heavy metals bind to certain sulfur-based amino acids, which are then eliminated normally from the body. Theoretically, once the metals are removed and their toxic effects eliminated, it might be possible to begin reversing some of the damage.

Chelation therapy has two steps. First the loosely bound body mercury must be eliminated, usually with dimercaptosuccinic acid (DMSA). This is typically given orally, in a one-week-on, one-week-off pattern, with dosages administered every four hours. Excreted mercury levels are measured in the urine. Once urine levels have come down and stabilized, some doctors then chelate the mercury that is tightly bound within the cells. This is typically done using a substance called lipoic acid.

Chelation can be dangerous. Side effects, while not common, may include mineral depletion, skin reactions, nausea, headache, dizziness, hypoglycemia, fever, leg cramps, or loose bowel movements. Some of the more serious complications reported have included kidney damage, decreased clotting ability, anemia, bone marrow damage, insulin shock, and embolism. The entire process must be done under strict doctor supervision and with proper nutritional support. Regular monitoring of blood counts, kidney and liver function, and mineral levels is essential.

Several products are currently in use as chelators. Many doctors consider DMSA to be the best and safest. The FDA, while not approving DMSA for autism, has approved it to remove lead from the body. It has been tested in children and found to be effective, but only when properly used. Chelation for autism remains highly controversial. The overwhelming opinion in traditional medicine is that it's an unproven therapy probably best avoided.

Lyn decided she was going to try it. She was given the name of a doctor who had treated several autistic kids with oral DMSA. She contacted him and he walked her through the protocol. Tommy wrote a prescription for DMSA, and within days, they chelated their son.

The Redwoods were already treating Will with an experimental substance called secretin, a hormone derived from pig blood. Secretin is also found in humans, in the pancreas, liver, upper intestinal tract, and brain. But it seems to be deficient in many children with autism. One of its functions is to stimulate the pancreas to secrete a fluid with a high concentration of bicarbonate. This assists in neutralizing stomach acids, permitting a variety of important enzymes to break down and help absorb nutrients, which may in turn help bring proper nourishment to the brain, something that apparently was not happening in children with autism. Another theory is that secretin combats low serotonin levels in the brain, also a common problem in autism. Serotonin is known to regulate several brain functions affected by autism, including learning and attention.

Secretin was highly controversial, and it never panned out as an effective treatment for autism (though many parents swore that it had helped their children's cognitive function and GI health). But the Redwoods noticed some improvement after several treatments. Will's speech had grown clearer, his vocabulary improved, and so did his gut problems. But the benefits of secretin wore off after a few weeks. The Redwoods would watch helplessly as their son began to slip away again.

Once they added chelation to the regimen, Lyn noticed that the benefits of secretin were more sustained. The progress, Lyn believed, was augmented by a battery of diet and nutritional supplements she was giving to Will, based on the DAN Protocol.

On the first administration of DMSA, Lyn expected mercury to come pouring out in Will's urine like tea from a teapot. It didn't happen. The doctor had said it might take five or six cycles before the mercury was removed from his tissues and measurable amounts eliminated through his urine. But after several more rounds, they still did not see appreciable levels of mercury being excreted.

Despite the lack of mercury he excreted, Will made significant improvements after each round of chelation. His vocabulary continued to grow. And even though he still mostly parroted the words he heard on Bugs Bunny and other cartoons, he seemed to know what he was saying. One day when Lyn picked Will up from school, she saw him walking on his tiptoes, cradling an imaginary rifle in his arms like Elmer Fudd.

"Will?" she asked. "What are you doing?"

"Shhhhh!" he said, putting a finger to his lips. "Hunting wabbits." Lyn had to smile and laugh, just a little.

After a few months, the Redwoods dropped the secretin altogether. Will's condition continued to improve. He ate more and gained weight. He seemed more aware of his surroundings. His speech became clearer and more complex.

Before treatment, Will would say something simple, like "Juice," when he wanted a drink. Soon this utterance had expanded to "Want juice." A few weeks after that, it became "Want juice please Mommy." To Lyn and Tommy, even these basic words were exquisite.

ONE DAY, not long before Thanksgiving 1999, when the sky was heavy with rain, Lyn was doing her daily Web search when she found the issue of *Hepatitis Control Report* that detailed the bureaucratic hand-wringing over the Joint Statement on Thimerosal. She was struck by the comments of Dr. Neal Halsey, director of the Institute for Vaccine Safety at Johns Hopkins University School of Medicine, and the undisputed vaccine authority. At the time, Halsey was completing a four-year term as chair of the AAP Committee on Infectious Diseases.

Halsey had been convinced that the government's findings on thimerosal were "worthy of alarm," the article said. He and his colleagues at the AAP had argued that doctors "should be told soon about the amount of mercury in vaccines and the conflict with a federal guideline."[57]

But CDC officials argued against precipitous action. "They pointed out that no child was known to be harmed from thimerosal, and they were loath to undermine confidence in existing vaccines by labeling some vaccines 'bad' (thimerosal-containing) and some 'good' (thimerosal-free)."

Halsey and others at the AAP held fast, stating that pediatricians who failed to reduce mercury exposures in infants might "face a flurry of lawsuits, perhaps claiming that children had acquired learning disabilities from mercury exposure."

The fight quickly devolved into an argument over postponing all vaccines from the first six months to a later time "when infants' bodies were larger and better able to tolerate mercury," the article said. But delaying DTP and Hib could expose infants to serious infections. It became evident that the "delayed" vaccine would have to be hepatitis-B.

CDC staff resisted even this minor change. They worried that delaying the birth dose "would cause hepatitis-B vaccination rates to slide," the article said. "Once the policy was changed it could be difficult to switch back." The CDC worked "furiously" against delaying the shot. "Negotiations continued with AAP nearly around the clock. Everyone was becoming exhausted. As the groups continued negotiations over days, worries increased that the story would leak to the press in an uncontrolled way, triggering a general vaccination scare. After a week of late-night meetings, the exhausted group struck a compromise." Halsey acknowledged that many colleagues were "angry with him and miffed about the way the issue was handled," the report said.

Lyn was impressed. Halsey sounded like a powerful potential ally, especially when she read the last sentence of the article. "No one knows what dose of mercury, if any, from vaccines is safe," Halsey said. "We can say there is no evidence of harm, but the truth is no one has looked."[58]

Lyn Redwood knew she had found a sympathetic ear. Halsey had composed an editorial about the Joint Statement in the prestigious *Journal of the American Medical Association* (JAMA), which Tommy received at home. Halsey argued that *all* vaccines given before the age of six months should preferably *not* contain thimerosal. When mercury-free vaccines were unavailable, "exposure to no more than one thimerosal-containing vaccine at each visit would reduce exposures while ensuring that infants are fully protected."[59]

Halsey also noted that bolus doses of mercury "may pose more risk than small daily doses." Moreover, he speculated that the toxicity of ethylmercury in vaccines could be having an "additive" effect on top of methylmercury exposure from fish, incurred by mothers while pregnant. The EPA had recently estimated that 7 percent of U.S. women of childbearing age consume 0.1 microgram per kilogram or more of mercury per day from fish; 1 percent are exposed to nearly 0.4 micrograms per kilogram per day or more. Large predator fish with long life spans are the most contaminated. The average can of tuna contains 17 micrograms of methylmercury. A single ounce of swordfish can have 30 micrograms or more.[60]

"Mercury accumulated in these women is transferred to their children prenatally and in breast milk," Halsey wrote. Subsequent exposures from other sources, "including biologic products, are presumed to be additive to their baseline body loads."

On November 22, 1999, Lyn faxed a letter to Dr. Halsey. Tommy, the M.D., signed it for good measure. "You were correct in your opinion that CBER's findings were worthy of alarm," Lyn wrote. "But what is disturbing to me is that in many of the recent articles I have reviewed, there is a consistent theme that there is, 'No evidence of harm having occurred from thimerosal vaccine administration.' No evidence of harm does not equate with no harm having occurred."

Lyn also criticized the method used to factor high bolus doses of mercury into much lower average daily amounts. "Intermittent large exposures (which our children have received with immunizations) may pose more risk than small daily doses," she wrote. "This only serves to falsely minimize this toxic exposure. If you look at the mercury from a daily dose perspective, then no one vaccine containing thimerosal would be able to meet EPA's limit.

"Almost an entire decade of children have been exposed to levels of mercury in vaccines that exceeded Federal Guidelines," Lyn continued. "These numbers will only continue to increase until all thimerosal is withdrawn. The CDC's decision not to give preference for thimerosal-free vaccines is a grave injustice to the health of our children that borders on medical negligence. It appears that the Vaccine Program itself has taken priority over the children that it is responsible for protecting. Who will be responsible for investigating reports of neurotoxicity from thimerosal? Who will be responsible for uncovering the truth that no one has investigated? I look forward to your response."

The letter was copied to the U.S. Surgeon General, the U.S. Public Health Service, the American Academy of Pediatrics, the American Academy of Family Medicine, the National Immunization Program, the Agency for Toxic Substances and Disease Registry, the Autism Society of America, and Cure Autism Now.

The next morning, Lyn's phone rang. It was Dr. Halsey. He was interested in what she had to say and asked her to mail a clean hard copy of the letter to him that he could share with colleagues. Lyn cried when she hung up. Someone had listened.

Lyn's letter found its way on to the FEAT list and several other autism sites, along with her e-mail address. Within hours, her inbox began filling with messages from parents around the country. Their kids also showed dangerously high levels of mercury, far in excess of EPA standards.

Lyn decided to launch a Web site of her own with free space she received as part of her Internet account with Mindspring.com. Soon she was getting hundreds of hits a day. Lyn included a link where parents could send in reports on their autistic children. She was looking for accounts of children who had been tested for mercury and undergone chelation therapy. She wanted to see how much mercury they had received, how much they had excreted, and if chelation made any difference in the child's condition.

Information from parents of affected children began flooding in, and Lyn was overwhelmed with data. One letter was from a general practitioner named Woody McGinnis, who had been a specialist in Tucson treating children with autism and ADHD. He had two adopted kids with attention deficit disorder. Woody had sold his practice to an HMO and now spent his early retirement researching neurodevelopmental disorders.

Woody asked Lyn if he could help, and she jumped at the offer. Woody was working with a doctor in Arizona, treating adults and children (some of them autistic) who had mercury poisoning. In some cases, patients had excreted up to 80 micrograms of mercury in their urine after chelation. Many of them, he added, reported remarkable improvement in clinical symptoms after the procedure. Lyn asked him to collect case studies from his clinic.

Woody was delighted to comply. Eventually Lyn and Woody compiled a dossier of cases, beginning with twenty profiles. Lyn posted each case study on her Web site.

On Thanksgiving morning, 1999, the Redwoods' kitchen was filled with the cozy smells of a warm holiday meal already fragrant in the oven. The guys were watching football and Hanna helped out at the stove, chatting amiably with her mom about school and boys and the upcoming Christmas vacation. The phone rang and Hanna answered.

"It's for you, Mom," she said. Lyn wiped her hands and walked to the phone.

"Mrs. Redwood?" It was a man's voice, a man with an accent. "Hello, Happy Thanksgiving. I'm sorry to bother you but it's very important. It's about thimerosal. I saw your letter to Dr. Halsey."

Lyn was busy, but this sounded like a good call. "Yes, go on," she said.

"I'm now sure that mercury caused my son to develop autism," the man said. "I've been working on a paper comparing autism to mercury poisoning. The symptoms are indistinguishable. I'd like to find out about your work, especially the case studies."

"Sure," Lyn replied. "I'd be happy to! May I ask who's calling?"

"I'm calling from New Jersey," the man said. "My name is Albert."

ON NOVEMBER 29, Liz Birt and her husband drove to O'Hare Airport and boarded a flight to the UK, bringing along Matthew and a guarded sense of hope. During the four-day visit, they stayed with friends, British parents of an autistic boy who lived in London near Royal Free Hospital, on Pond Street.

Liz will never forget the first time they walked to the hospital. It was a raw and dim afternoon and the weak autumn sun hung low in the chilly English sky. Liz turned the corner and saw an aging high-rise built in the 1960s, very institutional looking and depressing. Inside, the halls were filled with the cries of suffering children and the biting smell of rubbing alcohol. Liz had never taken Matthew to a public hospital before. She was a little shaken.

Matthew's crib was enclosed in railings. "It looks like something out of Bosnia," Liz thought. But the nurses were friendly and the rooms clean. The hospital employed a top gastroenterology group and one of the foremost pediatric GI specialists in the UK, Liz was told, Dr. John Walker-Smith. After they settled in, Dr. Walker-Smith and a squad of seven GI specialists led by Dr. Simon Murch, an expert on pathologies of the infant gut, entered the room. Liz was amazed to see such a large team. Dr. Murch began palpitating Matthew's abdomen and peppering the parents with questions. Did he have allergies as a child? "No," Liz said. What were his sleeping and eating patterns like? "Rotten as hell," she replied.

"And how is his bowel? Is everything working properly?"

Liz laughed. "Not exactly. He has endless, horrible diarrhea. It's just awful."

Dr. Murch thought otherwise. He believed that Matthew was "impacted," the medical term for severely constipated. Liz said that couldn't be possible. Every expert back home, not to mention their own travails, indicated chronic diarrhea.

"What happens in many of these cases," the doctor explained, "is they get so blocked up that whatever they manage to squeeze out, it looks like string. Because they're forcing it around the blockage. It's terrifically agonizing."

Could that really be the case? Matthew was unquestionably in pain. Dr. Murch ordered an X-ray that same day, and it confirmed his suspicions. Matthew's colon "contained a fecal mass the size of a grapefruit," the doctor told the couple. What appeared to be diarrhea was, in fact, overflow from persistent constipation. It took two days of laxatives and thirty diapers until Matthew was completely cleaned out.

On the third day, Matthew was finally ready for his endoscopy and colonoscopy. Several biopsies were also planned from the inflamed lymph nodes the doctors expected to find in his gut. The tests were difficult, and Matthew had to be sedated. "He's just a little boy, he's only five!" Liz cried. She wandered into the waiting room alone. "What am I doing here?" Liz asked herself. "How did I end up in London in this depressing old hospital?"

The following day, Dr. Wakefield, Dr. Murch, and the team went over the results with the anxious parents. "Matthew's esophagus is inflamed," Andy informed them solemnly. "There are visible variations throughout his intestines, a loss of vascular pattern that indicates inflammation." The two parents nodded, unsurprised, as Andy continued, "His lymph tissue is swollen and the pathologic analysis from his biopsies shows chronic active panproctocolitis, or inflammation of the entire colon and rectum, including inflammation of the intestinal lining, as well as cysts in the intestinal lining." This was a sign of ongoing inflammatory bowel disease, most likely related to some type of autoimmune disorder.

Wakefield came to dinner that night. He told Liz he had been asked to testify in the spring of 2000 at a hearing of the House Government Reform Committee, whose chairman was the conservative Republican Dan Burton of Indiana. Liz was thrilled. The lawyer in her saw a fresh opportunity to bring the vaccine debate directly to Washington. Surely in the marbled halls of American power, she thought, there would be sympathetic ears eager to learn of the damage that had been inflicted.

"That's great, Andy," she said, smiling for perhaps the first time in weeks. "When you tell Congress you've found measles virus in our kids, well, *somebody's* got to look into it! It's going to change things. Let me know what I can do to help from over there." Years later, Liz would laugh at her naïveté. "I thought people would instantly say, 'Oh! This is a big problem. We have to do something.' That hasn't been the case at all."

THE BUSY WEEKS squeezed between Thanksgiving and the end of 1999 seemed indistinguishable to Sallie, Albert, Heidi, and their new ally, the mother from Georgia, Lyn Redwood. Lyn was recruited to add some of her case studies to their paper, "Autism: A Novel Form of Mercury Poisoning," which was growing larger by the day.

Meanwhile, Teresa Binstock, the researcher with a high-functioning case of Asperger's, came to stay with the Enayatis, sleeping in the guest room for the next six weeks. Albert had been laid off from Pfizer and had ample time on his hands. The two began work early in Albert's home office (he was still unemployed), often staying up until far past midnight, poring through more studies and honing the scientific style of the paper under Teresa's skilled hand. One question was the all-important conclusion: what would be the most salient points to make in that single final paragraph? The parents chose to focus on pink disease, and its parallels to autism.

"The history of acrodynia illustrates that a severe disorder, afflicting a small but significant percentage of children, can arise from a seemingly benign application of low doses of mercury," the parents wrote. "This review establishes the likelihood that Hg [mercury] may likewise be significant in Autism Spectrum Disorder, with the mercury derived from thimerosal in vaccines rather than teething powders. Due to the extensive parallels between autism and mercury poisoning, the likelihood of a causal relationship is great.

"Given this possibility," the paper concluded, "thimerosal should be removed from all childhood vaccines, and the mechanisms of mercury toxicity in autism should be thoroughly investigated. With perhaps 1-in-150 children now diagnosed with ASD, development of mercury poisoning–related treatments, such as chelation, would prove beneficial for this large and seemingly growing population."[61]

Six months had passed since the Joint Statement on Thimerosal was issued. The time had come for the parents to bring their mercury-autism findings to the health establishment and to the public at large. The pressure on Sallie was daunting. She knew that intense scrutiny would be brought to bear on her work, which detractors were sure to vilify. It was an audacious premise, one that essentially accused the American health establishment of poisoning an entire generation of children, however inadvertently. "Please be critical," Sallie pleaded when sending the final draft to her associates. "Better my friends to point out inconsistencies or error than the wolves that lurk beyond."

Down in Atlanta, Lyn continued collecting reports from parents eager to share the medical histories of their children. In nearly every case, it was the same story: A normal birth and infancy followed by usually rapid regression beginning around eighteen months to two years (when the MMR shot is typically given), followed by loss of speech, social withdrawal, and GI distress. And when "challenged" with chelation, many children yielded extraordinary levels of mercury, often followed by significant mental and physical improvement.

BY THIS POINT Lyn had stopped working altogether in order to devote more time to Will. Like many parents of autistic kids, she learned how destructive the disease can become for the entire family. Will demanded her attention nearly 100 percent of the time.

But Lyn had two other children and a husband, and there were never enough hours in a day to take care of everyone properly. Hanna was now fifteen years old. A typical teenager, she had recently become a high-maintenance child. It was a time when she depended on her mother for advice, support, and answers to questions that arise in a confusing, grown-up world. Hanna needed emotional support, and Lyn felt torn between her needs and Will's.

One afternoon Hanna came into Lyn's office, wanting to talk about problems at school. She was fighting with her girlfriends and needed some motherly advice. Lyn put down her work and gave her undivided attention to Hanna. It was gratifying to be part of her daughter's life, to be involved. Just as Lyn was about to impart her wisdom, though, a hellish wail rose from downstairs. It was Will.

Lyn rushed to the living room, where she'd left Will in front of the TV. Something on the screen had alarmed him. As she tried to calm Will, Drew burst into the room. "Mom! I'm late for practice!" he cried. "And you didn't wash my clothes!" Lyn looked at the pile of dirty laundry in the washroom. Her eyes panned around the house, to the dinner that was still uncooked, the bills piled up by the phone, the unfed dogs outside.

Lyn had not slept an entire night in weeks. She was exhausted, guilty, and overwhelmed. Her house, her home, her whole family seemed to be fraying at the edges. She was so bankrupt of energy, it was nearly impossible to hold it all together. For a second, she considered walking out the door, never to return, then quickly put escape out of her rattled mind. Lyn needed to be the strong one. She needed to be the mom.

On the rare occasion when Lyn could get away, she often found herself up in Atlanta, at the relatively peaceful Emory University medical library, of all places. One day she found a study of the toxic effects of mercury on monkeys, how exposure made the poor apes lose affect and withdraw into morose pools of inattention.

Lyn went to make copies of the report, flipping through the pages. There were photos in it and one showed a monkey, obviously depressed, with eyes as lost and faraway as Will's. It was the saddest picture of the saddest monkey she'd ever seen. Lyn cried while pressing the book to the copier. When she got home, she pinned the photo to her bulletin board, where it remained for years. Lyn called him the "Mercury Monkey."

SHORTLY AFTER NEW YEAR'S DAY, 2000, with their paper almost finished, the New Jersey parents began thinking about what they were going to *do* with the thing. Of course they planned on sending it out to peer-reviewed journals. But they also had loftier plans.

Albert was determined to get the paper into the hands of every top-level official at the FDA, the CDC, the AAP, the NIH, and whatever other alphabet soup agency he could think of. Not sure where to begin, he placed a cold call to Dr. Neal Halsey at Johns Hopkins for advice. He knew the doctor had responded well to Lyn, and Albert prayed he would get equal treatment. Halsey took the call and suggested that Albert contact Dr. William Egan, acting head of the FDA's Center for Biologics Evaluation and Research (CBER), who had sent out the letters to the drug companies the previous July, asking for their plans to either remove thimerosal from vaccines or explain their reasons for not doing so.

Bill Egan is a nondescript-looking bureaucrat with graying hair and wire-rimmed glasses. He had worked in government vaccine programs nearly his whole career and was a top-level official at the FDA when it came to regulating the nation's vaccination supply. It took a while, but Albert finally got Egan on the phone.

"Thank you for speaking with me, Doctor," he began. "I know you're busy."

"What can I do for you?" Egan asked, politely enough.

"It's about the mercury in vaccines. We're a group of parents of autistic kids, and it's come to our attention that the symptoms displayed by our children are very similar to those caused by mercury poisoning."

There was silence on the other end of the line. Albert kept talking.

"We are writing an article. And when we finish the article we are going to send it to you. This really concerns us. We expect you to look into it."

"Mr. Enayati," Dr. Egan said, "we are reviewing this as well."

This was unexpected. "You are? And what have you found?"

"There is some concern here at FDA. But we do not believe that thimerosal in vaccines could cause autism. The amount of mercury involved is very low." Everything that needed to be done on the matter, he said, was being done. "The government has changed the immunization schedule," Egan said. "We don't give hepatitis-B vaccinations to newborn children. And the mercury is coming out of the shots anyway. I'm not sure what more there is to discuss."[62]

Looking back on that conversation, Albert still smolders. He didn't know it at the time, but federal health officials were indeed paying far closer attention to thimerosal and developmental disorders than anyone imagined. More than a year later, in 2000, Albert and the other parents would learn that health officials had looked at closely guarded government data on the connection between thimerosal and autism. The officials, their detractors would allege, knew there was a potentially serious problem, but they chose to remain silent. Instead, they sought refuge behind the impenetrable walls of bureaucracy, away from the prying eyes of the inquisitive public, especially those overwrought, emotional parents screaming about vaccines. "The FDA knew what was going on," Albert said years later.

"They knew when I spoke with Egan. They just didn't say anything. They must have thought, 'These people will never figure this out.' I'm sure that's what they thought. But they were wrong."

4. Red Flags on the Hill

THERE ARE FEW PROPONENTS of childhood vaccination in the United States more ardent than Dr. Paul Offit, chief of the Division of Infectious Diseases at the Children's Hospital of Philadelphia and an authority on immunology and virology. In early 2000 Dr. Offit, a personable and articulate physician with salt-and-pepper hair and professorial wire-framed glasses, was making the rounds on radio and cable television to promote his new book, *Vaccines: What Every Parent Should Know* (with Louis Bell, M.D.). What every parent "should know," Offit said, was that the vast benefits of vaccines far outweighed any risk of harm, most of which was theoretical anyway.

Offit tried to reassure parents who were growing nervous about the long list of shots their kids were getting. But not everyone was buying his message.

"Do not be misled, it's not the objective scientific book I was hoping for," one reader said in a review posted on Amazon.com. "It's no better than the worst of the reactionary anti-vaccine books, riddled with errors that exaggerate safety."

Another reader/reviewer wrote that "the sole purpose of this book is to convince parents to vaccinate their babies when and how the medical establishment/drug industry wants them to." The writer said her pediatrician had lent her the book because it presented both sides of the issue. But the doctor had mistakenly left a form letter inside, provided by Merck Vaccine Division, telling pediatricians they "highly recommend the book for parents to 'dispel all of the misinformation,' out there," the reviewer said. "Everyone should proceed with caution when a multi-billion dollar conglomerate gives their stamp of approval on a book." In fact, the conglomerate in question had purchased twenty thousand copies of the book for distribution to doctors' offices around the country.[63]

But Merck was more than Offit's book distributor. The corporation was also, effectively, his business partner. Offit was a consultant for the drug giant, working on the development of a new Merck vaccine against rotavirus, the infection that had made Will Redwood so sick. Offit's partner had received at least $350,000 in grant money from the company to help develop the vaccine, for which the two doctors shared the patent.[64]

And there was an added bonus, from Merck's perspective at least. Dr. Offit happened to sit on the CDC's Advisory Committee for Immunization Practices. The advisory committee is an influential body of physicians and researchers whose charge is to promote and oversee vaccine use in the United States. Among their chief tasks is to recommend which vaccines should be included on the national childhood immunization schedule. In most states, those shots are mandatory for children to attend school. For the vaccine companies, it guarantees them a built-in annual market.

In 1998 the advisory committee voted to recommend adding a new vaccine against rotavirus, Rotashield, made by Merck's competitor Wyeth Lederle, to the schedule.[65] Rotavirus is a serious illness that can cause acute diarrhea in kids under five. It sends some fifty thousand American children to the hospital each year, at a cost of $264 million in medical care, and $1 billion in societal costs, according to the CDC.[66] Dr. Offit voted on three separate occasions to support the Wyeth vaccine, including the final vote to recommend it to the schedule. He said he faced no conflict of interest, because Wyeth and Merck were competitors; however, recommending one new vaccine brand opens the door for others to be approved, regulatory experts say.

But there was a problem with the Wyeth vaccine. At least ten children developed a deadly bowel obstruction called intussusception in the first two weeks after vaccination.[67] In October 1999, the panel withdrew its recommendation. This time, however, Offit abstained from the voting. "I'm not conflicted with Wyeth," he explained, "but because I consult with Merck on the development of rotavirus vaccine, I would still prefer to abstain because it creates a perception of conflict."[68]

Weeks later, Wyeth voluntarily pulled its product from the market.[69] To vaccine critics, it was just another sign of the public health establishment's overzealous drive to vaccinate every child against every potential illness quickly and without regard to possible side effects. In 2004, interestingly, Merck submitted its own rotavirus vaccine for approval by federal regulators.

LYN WAS SPENDING another long evening upstairs in her office. She clicked through Web pages as the computer screen flickered green in her bloodshot eyes. Pausing for a moment, she looked up at the Mercury Monkey, whose photo was tacked to her wall. The monkey looked sadder than ever, she thought.

On this particular night in January 2000, Lyn was researching the growing reported incidence of autism cases in the United States. Caseloads began to rise slowly in the 1970s and continued upward through the 1980s, she learned. But then, in the early 1990s, the numbers spiked dramatically and never came back down. What on earth, Lyn wondered, had changed during 1990–1992 that could account for such an abrupt upsurge?

One possible explanation was that in 1992 the system that offers services to (and counts) children with learning disabilities—the Department of Education's IDEA program—was overhauled and expanded. Perhaps many parents simply failed to report diagnoses like autism until their school systems actually offered the services to address their kids' never-ending needs.

But Lyn believed there was another, equally plausible (or additional) explanation. She retraced the history of the childhood immunization schedule. As a nurse, Lyn recalled that a new, reformulated Hib vaccine was added to the childhood schedule in 1988, calling for four shots in the first year, beginning at age two months. Some, but not all, brands of Hib vaccine contained 25 micrograms of ethylmercury—each.

Then, in 1991, hepatitis-B was added to the list. At the time, all hep-B shots contained 12.5 micrograms of mercury. The schedule was three injections in the first year, beginning with the now-controversial "birth dose."

Lyn did the math. The CDC's immunization advisory committee, by voting to add four Hib and three hep-B shots to the schedule, had saddled some kids with an additional 137.5 micrograms of ethylmercury during their first, most vulnerable year. Prior to 1988, only the DTP shot had mercury (four shots with 25 micrograms each). In just three years, total potential exposure leapt from 100 micrograms to 237.5 micrograms. And these figures did not account for additional maternal exposures from Rho(D) and the flu shot.

A few nights later, back online, Lyn found the site of the Institute for Vaccine Safety, run by Dr. Neal Halsey, who never wavered in his support of childhood immunizations. (Though he did not believe in a link between thimerosal and autism, he did think there could be an association with less severe neurological disorders.) Halsey had made very compelling observations in an FDA-sponsored workshop in August 1999, including the following information taken from his slides:[70]

- "All children are not created equal with regard to their risk from exposure to mercury," Halsey said. One needed to consider the type of exposure (chronic versus bolus), age, weight, metabolism, excretion rates, and "genetic predisposition."

- The smallest newborns weigh half as much as the largest babies. Relatively speaking, they were exposed to twice as much mercury per kilogram.

- Exposure at two months poses a greater potential risk than the same dose at six months, not only because children weigh less, but because the brain "is more vulnerable early in life."

- Some studies of methylmercury exposure in pregnant women showed that larger, intermittent bolus doses might be more detrimental to fetuses than chronic low doses.

- Adverse effects in these studies, while minor, were noted primarily in boys, although "the biologic explanation for increased susceptibility to mercury of the male fetal brain has not been determined."

- Given the EPA daily guideline of 0.1 microgram per kilogram, many children at two months of age received almost 90 times the daily limit in a single doctor's visit. And the smallest babies were given approximately *eight months'* worth of daily exposures (240 times the daily limit) in a single day.

- Ethylmercury exposure from vaccines came *on top of* maternal exposure of methylmercury in fish. Some children were born with mercury exposures *already* above federal guidelines, even before getting their first shot. "Although safety factors have been built into these guidelines," Halsey said, "we do not know what the effects of additional mercury will be on the developing brain."

- Thimerosal is an imperfect preservative. Some vials of DTP, for example, were contaminated with streptococcus bacteria.

Lyn was thunderstruck by Halsey's revelations. She immediately sent copies of his presentation to the New Jersey parents. She also linked it to her own Web site, which was now having so many hits per day she was getting warnings from Mindspring.com threatening to close the address if it continued receiving such abnormally heavy traffic.

Around this time, Lyn began to hear talk of a long-forgotten FDA memo, published in the early 1980s in the *Federal Register,* referring to thimerosal's safety problems. There were references to the report online, but it was hard to find an old copy of the *Federal Register.* One spring morning in 1999, Lyn headed to the library at Georgia State University, in Atlanta. There she looked up the government journal on the school's microfiche system. It took a while to search through the film, but she found what she came for.

In 1982 an independent panel convened by the FDA had called for removing all mercury-based preservatives including thimerosal from over-the-counter topical products such as Mercurochrome, skin bleaching agents, eardrops, eyedrops, and nasal sprays. The panel ruled that such products should be reclassified as "not generally recognized as safe and effective."[71]

Moreover, mercury was an unreliable preservative, the memo said. It was more bacteriostatic than bactericidal—it slowed the growth of new bacteria but did not kill them altogether. Thimerosal was singled out as being "no better than water in protecting mice from fatal streptococcal infection." It was more deadly to healthy cells than it was to harmful bacteria. It was 35.3 times more toxic for embryonic chick heart tissue, for instance, than for *Staphylococcus aureus.*

In prior studies thimerosal was found to be among the most toxic of some twenty mercury compounds the panel looked at. It was also highly allergenic. (Interestingly, symptoms did not usually appear until well after exposure.) One guinea pig study showed that 50 percent of the animals developed "delayed hypersensitivity" to thimerosal, the document said. "And it is reasonable to expect it will act similarly in humans." In fact, published trials in Sweden and the United States had shown hypersensitivity to thimerosal in 8 to 26 percent of patients.

"The panel concludes that thimerosal is not safe for over-the-counter use because of its potential for cell damage if applied to broken skin and its allergy potential," the memo concluded.

Lyn was starting to lose it.

"They knew in 1982 that this stuff was too toxic to rub on your skin," she thought. "But it's perfectly okay to inject into newborn babies."

In 1982 the FDA had called for a period of public comment and solicited evidence on the safety of mercury compounds. Nothing was sent in. Years later, in 1998, when the FDA finally published its decision to reclassify thimerosal as "not generally recognized as safe and effective," not a single company had stepped forward to furnish any safety data whatsoever.

"These manufacturers have known for some time that if adequate data were not submitted to support safety and effectiveness, cessation of marketing of the current products would be required," the FDA said. All OTC products with "active" mercury ingredients would be pulled from the shelves in six months "regardless of whether further testing is undertaken to justify future use." Violators would be subject to "regulatory action."[72]

This gave Lyn an idea. If the FDA could recall thimerosal from over-the-counter products, why couldn't it do the same for vaccines? Yes, the preservative was being phased out voluntarily and gradually, but why couldn't it be yanked from the shelves?

Lyn was also curious about other ingredients that were brewed into the vaccines Will received. To a layperson, they sounded like something from a poison factory manual (though, as any toxicologist will attest, it's the dose that makes the poison.) The following are just some of the components used to make a variety of vaccines sold in the United States: formaldehyde, aluminum hydroxide, aluminum phosphate, ammonium sulfate, calf serum, fetal rhesus monkey lung cells, monkey kidney cells, chick embryo, fetal bovine serum, washed sheep red blood cells, casein from pig pancreas, phenoxyethanol (antifreeze), neomycin and streptomycin (antibiotics), and, incredibly, diploid cells originating from *aborted human fetal tissue*.[73]

Nauseating as the list was, it was the presence of aluminum that caught Lyn's eye. The metal is used in many vaccines as an "adjuvant," meaning that it helps the immune system induce a healthy antibody response against the "antigens" (usually viral proteins) found in most vaccines. Lyn remembered that Will's baby hair showed very high levels of aluminum, which she knew to be neurotoxic in high doses. Lyn also remembered from her nursing school days that when mercury and lead are combined, the compound becomes much more lethal than either metal alone: they act synergistically. Might it stand to reason that aluminum had a similar effect on mercury?

Six months before, Lyn never dreamed she would be up nights pondering the finer points of metallurgy. Now she couldn't stop thinking about it. Mercury is a "heavy" metal, she knew. It sinks like a bullet in water. She wondered if it was possible that, instead of remaining suspended in solution, some mercury particles might clump together and settle to the bottom of the vial. Could there be more thimerosal in the last dose drawn from a ten-dose vial than the first? Many parents Lyn interviewed said they saw the nurse toss away a multidose vial after vaccinating their children, meaning that they got the final shot. Vaccines come with instructions to shake vigorously before each injection. But Lyn knew that this precaution, especially in busy clinics, was not always followed religiously.

AFTER HER TRIP to London, Liz Birt vowed not to rest until she solved the mystery of Matthew's regression and chronically inflamed gut. She also offered to do whatever was necessary to further the research of Andy Wakefield. Because of the doctor, Matthew was on antiinflammatory drugs to calm his swelling colon and daily laxatives to prevent any "grapefruit" from recurring. Eventually Matthew began sleeping on a regular basis, and so did Liz. He no longer screamed inconsolably. He didn't lie on the sofa rubbing his stomach or wail into the long dark night. And he stopped his terrible toe walking.

The psychiatrists had told Liz that such bizarre conduct was common in autistic children. They had called it "self-stimulating" behavior. They said it was mostly harmless, if difficult to watch. But having seen Matthew writhe for so long in agony, Liz knew it had nothing to do with "stimulation." It was a frenzied response to pain.

Home life for Liz was increasingly troubled. Matthew's gut problems suddenly got worse all over again. He had become even more hyperactive, if that were possible. He tore through the house knocking over vases, jumping on beds, ripping apart books. He adopted a nonverbal mantra that he repeated incessantly. "Agghhheeee! Agghhheee!" he screamed. The racket drove Liz crazy, which only made her feel more guilty. Matthew frequently managed to escape from the house. Sometimes it took hours of searching before they found him, often walking alone down by Lake Michigan, or in the middle of a busy street.

Liz had taken Matthew off dairy and wheat products, and this seemed to help. Matt became more focused, she thought. He didn't seem doped up all the time anymore. But like many autistic kids, Matthew had become addicted to the casein and glutein proteins, and there was nothing that would keep him away from cookies, crackers, milk, or cheese. More than once, Liz walked into the kitchen to find that Matthew had broken the locks on the cupboard and helped himself to copious amounts of wheat products. She would find him on the floor, in a total stupor, like a heroin addict after a fix.

By early 2000, Liz had founded Medical Interventions for Autism (MIA), a nonprofit charity dedicated to raising funds for Wakefield's MMR research. And she was in constant communication with some New Jersey activists she had met through Cure Autism Now: Sallie Bernard, Albert Enayati, and Heidi Roger. In February, the results of Matthew's biopsies were faxed from across the Atlantic. The samples had been sent to the laboratory of John O'Leary, a professor of cellular biology at Trinity College in Dublin and a close associate of Andy Wakefield.

One morning, driving to work, Liz got a call from Wakefield on her cell phone. Dr. O'Leary, he told her, had found exactly what Liz had expected and dreaded in equal measure: measles virus had invaded Matthew's bowels and nervous system.

By the time she got to work, Liz was a blubbering mess. She crawled into the office and closed the door. A coworker, who was also a good friend, came in to give her comfort. She understood what Liz was going through, and Liz was extremely grateful to have her there that morning.

Liz was not certain if the measles virus had caused Matt's autism, or whether his autistic condition left him more vulnerable to viral infection. But she was certain the two were connected. Liz shared the sad news with her New Jersey friends. Sallie, Heidi, and Albert were sympathetic, but they wrote back saying they had to beg off the MMR crusade, at least for now. Their immediate goal was to get their mercury paper published.

Liz was disappointed, but she understood, and continued searching for additional allies to pursue the MMR connection. Somebody she almost instinctively turned to was Beth Card Clay, a Republican staff member of the House Committee on Government Reform, chaired by the colorful and controversial congressman Dan Burton. Burton was serving his ninth term from central Indiana's Fifth District, one of the most conservative in the country. Liz had met Beth in 1999 at the same New Jersey DAN! conference that Lyn and Tommy Redwood had attended (though she and the Redwoods didn't cross paths at the time). Beth eagerly asked Liz to send in Matthew's biopsy results.

As it turned out, Liz had a second connection to Dan Burton. She had been in e-mail contact with the congressman's daughter, Danielle Burton Sarkine. Danielle's own son, Christian, had declined practically overnight into full-blown autism in 1997, after receiving nine vaccines in a single visit to the doctor. Seven of them contained thimerosal. Within two days, the normal two-year-old was running amok and banging his head against the walls. He started flapping his hands like a wounded sparrow. He developed constant constipation and diarrhea. He no longer met the gaze of his mother. Then he stopped talking. It was not the first time that vaccines had seemed to harm a Burton kid. In 1993 Danielle's daughter, Alexandra, became so sick the day of her hepatitis-B vaccination she almost died. Neither child's case, of course, could be definitely linked to vaccines, but they were awfully suspicious, Dan and Danielle Burton thought.

CONGRESSMAN BURTON'S measured speech and poker-faced expression served him well in his capacity as chairman of the powerful Committee on

Government Reform. Armed with subpoena power and an inquisitive mind that liked to dig around in places that his opponents would rather keep in the dark, Burton had looked into everything from Janet Reno's handling of the Waco disaster (he called for her resignation), to Vice President Al Gore's missing White House e-mails on campaign fund-raising (Burton called for an Office of Special Counsel investigation). Burton committee hearings were sometimes packed with curious Capitol Hill staffers eager to catch the fireworks.

To the Clinton camp and most Democrats, Burton was a constant political thorn, with a reputation for being unduly drawn to conspiracy theories. He was perhaps best known for pumping gunshot into a watermelon to prove his personal theory that Clinton aide Vince Foster did not commit suicide, and must have been murdered, presumably by Clinton henchmen. During the Lewinsky affair, Burton famously called Clinton a "scumbag," even though he was forced to admit that he himself had fathered an illegitimate child.

Burton took his grandchild's illness hard. Soon after Christian's quick decline, he began looking into vaccine safety. In August 1999 he presided over a hearing called "Vaccines: Finding the Balance between Public Safety and Personal Choice." The star witness was Clinton-era surgeon general David Satcher, who defended the national vaccine program with fervor. Burton had also invited a panel of parents, including Barbara Loe Fisher, to talk about their suspicions that vaccines had irreparably damaged their children, and a panel of doctors and academics eager to tout the safety of vaccines. The testimony centered around the vaccines themselves, with no mention of thimerosal.

Beth Clay, who specializes in health care reform and alternative medicine, was appointed by Burton as staff director of what was becoming a sprawling investigation into autism and vaccines.

LYN REDWOOD'S WEB SITE was now getting hundreds of hits a day. Without asking for it, she was becoming the Dear Abby of autism. The traffic overwhelmed her, but it was also exciting. Lyn spent so many hours answering parents' queries—how to test for mercury poisoning, how to diagnose symptoms, how to locate doctors willing to do chelation—that her fingers throbbed from overuse.

Lyn also kept in close contact with the New Jersey group. She was already thinking ahead, anticipating the months after the paper's release. She proposed three steps for dealing with its aftermath: demand the immediate removal of thimerosal from U.S. vaccines and biologics; establish a national parents' advocacy and research group focused on mercury and autism; make the government and/or industry compensate injured families for the misery and costly therapy they faced.

Lyn found a ready ally in Albert. "We should go public with our hypothesis ASAP," he told Lyn. "Then we'll get thousands of parents to join us. And we must take this to the CDC. We have to talk to them about our concerns, about removing mercury from vaccines, and finding a way to fix what's wrong with our kids."

"But how?" Lyn asked.

"We tell them that thimerosal is a national emergency," Albert said. "They need to start spending money on *independent* researchers to verify our hypothesis now. Otherwise more kids will be exposed, and no kids will be treated."

Noble as the goal was, Lyn wondered if high-level bureaucrats would deign to grant an audience to a loose gaggle of pissed-off parents, let alone take their ideas under consideration. On the other hand, the group had approached independent doctors and researchers to draft a paper, and none of them wanted to touch the subject. Most of them told the parents they were crazy, or simply stopped responding to their entreaties. Still, *somebody* had to get on the government's back about this, Lyn thought.

"Please think about what I say," Albert pleaded. "If we don't demand anything from government agencies, I promise you, they won't do anything. We have to confront them, Lyn. It's the only way these kids are going to get any attention. And you have to help me convince Sallie and Heidi to go along."

Lyn was moved. "Count me in," she said. "But we've got to make sure this gets brought up at the next Burton hearings. Congress needs to know that a federal agency allowed our kids to get excessive levels of a known toxin. And in a vaccine! Something meant to protect them, not harm them."

"Ironic," Albert said. "Isn't it?"

Lyn laughed. "I think *panic* is a more fitting word," she said. "FDA, CDC, I don't care who it is, Albert, we're going to make them face up to the fact that they messed up. They have to help fix this generation of autistic children that they created."

Lyn was on a sleep-deprived adrenaline roll. The next day, as promised, she wrote to Heidi and Sallie. "I'm going to my State Senator and my Congressman to see if we can get FDA to do something about the damage they have allowed to occur to our children," she announced. "They should take the fall for this. I would just be happy if someone would face the music on this and say, 'We screwed up,' and then pay for my son's therapy, which is costing well over $1,000 a month."

Lyn's powers of persuasion were eroding Sallie's resistance. In an e-mail back to Lyn, she revealed her growing contempt for the experts. "Just a cynical question," she wrote. "If these guys know so much and spent their whole lives looking at mercury, why wasn't this paper written by one of them fifteen years ago, before my son was shot up with thimerosal? Or even five years ago, so he could have been detoxed as a child?"

Sallie noted that one article on pink disease, from 1953, "specifically points at vaccines as contributory causes, because they not only contain thimerosal, but also set off an immune reaction to it.[74] Why didn't all these mercury pros jump all over this, especially since parents have been complaining about vaccines since the 1960s? Sorry to vent! I'm so ticked off that no one figured this out in 1982 when the Feds said take thimerosal out. It's déjà vu all over again. Makes you sick."

LYN CONTINUED making friends and winning Internet allies. One key player who entered her electronic circle was Rick Rollens, the father of an autistic boy in California. Rick was a well-placed political operative in Sacramento with very close ties to Governor Gray Davis. Rick lived with his wife, Janna, in a large custom-built home in Granite Bay, an attractive bedroom community outside Sacramento tucked into the gentle folds of the Sierra Nevada foothills. The Rollens had two sons, Matthew, who was thirteen, and Russell, their autistic boy, who was eight. Rick is a hulking man with the subdued demeanor of one who has witnessed the violent suffering of a loved one.

Rick had served a long and distinguished career in Democratic politics. In 1973, while working as an aide to California congressman Jerome Waldie, he helped draft the articles of impeachment against Richard Nixon. His stint in the House was followed by twenty-three years in the California State Senate. He worked his way up through the ranks and eventually became secretary of the upper house, where his ties to Governor Davis proved valuable. In 1996 Rick resigned to dedicate his career and life to finding a cure for Russell's disability. He also became a lobbyist and consultant. He and Janna intensified their search for effective treatments, or perhaps even a cure, for the boy they loved so dearly.

Like many autistic kids, Russell began life healthy and robust. But at seven months, after his third DPT and first Hib shot, he began to slip. A year later, after his MMR, he lost his remaining cognitive skills within days. He couldn't sleep. He had chronic GI problems. His bad behavior became worse, his pain more acute, his screams more harrowing. Six months later, he was diagnosed with autism.

Rick had helped establish Families for Early Autism Treatment (FEAT) along with other Sacramento area families. He was also a key player in creating the MIND Institute (Medical Investigation of Neurodevelopmental Disorders) at UC Davis with three other area fathers. The state-of-the-art complex brings together parents, educators, physicians, and scientists in an integrated collaboration on research, treatment, and education. Studies cover fields as diverse as molecular genetics, cognitive therapy, and clinical pediatrics. In less than a year, the fathers were able to raise more than six million dollars to help build the institute and convince the UC Davis School of Medicine and Medical Center to sponsor and house the program. Subsequently, Rick Rollens was responsible for securing an additional eighty million dollars in state and private contributions for the MIND Institute and other autism causes.

Rick also convinced the legislature and Governor Davis to produce the first-ever comprehensive epidemiological report on the increase of autism cases in California.[75] The report, which found a 273 percent increase in eleven years, is what made the alarming news in the state in April 1999. At the time, Rick estimated that six new cases of autism were entering the California system every day, seven days a week—or one new child *every four hours*. Each of those kids would end up costing taxpayers at least two million dollars, he said. Unlike children with cancer or AIDS, autistic kids don't die from their disease. They require a lifetime of care.

Rick returned to the legislature in 1999 and secured one million dollars to fund a study to examine factors that could be responsible for the increase in reported cases of autism. This effort resulted in a report that, among other things, sustained the finding that the increase was real and could not be attributed to other factors such as people moving to California to avail themselves of services or shifts in diagnostic criteria.[76]

Rick knew his way around Washington as well as Sacramento, and Burton had asked him to testify at the August 1999 hearing on vaccines. Rick had evoked tears from many inside the hearing room that day eight months earlier. It was the first time that anyone had brought the autism-vaccine issue to the attention of Congress. Rick depicted the appalling symptoms that wrecked Russell's life. He discussed the frightening numbers coming out of California, and compared them to those from another alarming study, in Brick Township, New Jersey, where the CDC had identified an inexplicable "cluster" of autism cases in the gritty, working-class borough. Of the town's roughly 6,000 children, 40 had been diagnosed with full-blown autism. This figure, 1 in 150 kids, was *twelve times higher* than that found in any previously published federal study.[77] It was unclear whether the New Jersey numbers were part of a nationwide trend or just a freak "cluster" produced by reasons yet unknown. Rick told the committee that, given the numbers coming out of California, a national trend was probably at work.

"I reside in a community approximately three thousand miles from Brick Township, a community that is almost in every way as different from Brick as two communities in our country can be," he said. "The prevalence of autism in our elementary school district of less than three thousand students is 1 in 132 children. Brick Township and Granite Bay are not clusters of autism, but snapshots of what is occurring in your districts and throughout this country. Seek and you shall find."[78]

One thing was certain, Rick told the hearing room, these breathtaking statistics could not be explained away as simply the result of better reporting and awareness of a genetic disorder. Autism was epidemic in America. "Surely any intelligent person cannot with a straight face suggest that it's all genetics, or better recognition of one of the most recognizable of all childhood disorders," Rick said. "Any of you who spend five minutes with an autistic child will thereafter be able to recognize autism from across an airport."

Rick also warned the room about letting government and industry guard the immunization henhouse. "Is it appropriate to continue to entrust the CDC, the public health community, and the indemnified vaccine manufacturers with the responsibility of guaranteeing the parents of this country that this potent class of poisons we know as vaccines will NOT cause autism?" he asked. Those same groups had vested interests as "the most aggressive promoters of vaccines," Rick said. He likened the situation to asking Big Tobacco for an independent study "to ascertain if there is any relationship between cancer and smoking."

LYN AND RICK ROLLENS had become good friends even though they hadn't actually met. Now they would get their chance. Dan Burton had scheduled another autism hearing, on April 6, 2000, and Rick was planning to attend. He was not going to testify this time. But he helped organize a special forum at the National Institutes of Health for the day after the hearing. It was a rare chance for parents converging on Washington to question and confront government scientists about their apparent reluctance to investigate thimerosal and vaccines.

Rick had also helped set up a press conference prior to the hearing. Dan Burton, Barbara Loe Fisher, Bernie Rimland, Andy Wakefield, and other proponents of the autism-vaccine theory, including Burton's daughter Danielle, were scheduled to speak.

Lyn wanted Rick to exert his considerable influence to get thimerosal placed on the agenda of the hearing itself. But even this seasoned player was unable to pull those strings. Besides, Andy Wakefield and his MMR theory were still making the headlines, Rick said. He had been in touch with Wakefield and his colleagues. They did not want anyone mucking up the waters with talk of ethylmercury, lest it detract from the dramatic news of measles virus in autistic kids.

Lyn pressed Rick to get Andy to reconsider. Why should mercury compete with MMR for attention, she asked, when attention needed to be paid to both? "I don't know, Lyn," Rick said one day before the hearings. "I've been feeding the mercury stuff to Andy. But he is pretty convinced it's MMR."

Lyn reminded Rick that his son Russell, just like Will, showed signs of regression *before* the MMR shot. "And anyway, why would some autistic kids get colitis, but not others, if they all received MMR?" Those were good questions that needed to be posed to Wakefield. Meanwhile, Lyn should try to work on Danielle Sarkine, Rick suggested. It was worth seeing what kind of influence Danielle might be able to exert over her father. Maybe she could convince him to open the discussion to thimerosal.

ANOTHER KEY ALLY who turned up on Lyn's e-mail in the spring of 2000 was Shelley Reynolds, an outspoken Baton Rouge, Louisiana, mother of a four-year-old autistic son, Liam. Shelley and another Louisiana mother, Jeana Smith, had helped start a parents' activist and support group called Unlocking Autism (UA).

UA was organizing a rally dubbed "Hear Their Silence" for the Washington Mall, two days after the Burton hearings. Shelley recruited Lyn to spread the word through her emerging electronic network. Shelley and Jeana were also scheduled to testify at the congressional hearing. Lyn helped the women with their testimony and told them how to calculate the total mercury levels their children had received in vaccines. Yet again, it was the same, sad old story.

Liam had been a normally developing boy until the age of seventeen months, when he received his MMR and Hib vaccines. Soon after, according to Shelley, he became obsessed with removing his shoes and putting them back on, in a repetitive ritual that he alone understood. He screamed if his parents dressed or undressed him. He would stare for hours at television and not move if someone blocked the view. He no longer wanted to sing his favorite songs, but simply covered his ears and screamed "No!" at the sound of music. Next came the stinging acidic diarrhea that burst from his gut ten times a day. Within a year, Liam no longer said "Mamma" or "Daddy" or "Love you."

One day, Lyn asked Shelley, "Do you think vaccines played a role?"

"*Think?*" Shelley laughed bitterly. "I *know*. I'm dead certain of it." And Shelley was not alone. Her group had gathered thousands of photos of autistic children to be displayed at the Washington Mall rally. They had surveyed these parents and found that nearly half believed their kids' autism was linked to vaccines.

In the final days leading up to the Burton hearing, the NIH forum, and the rally, Lyn and Albert did not relent in their push to get thimerosal into the hearing. Albert called Danielle Sarkine to deliver a personal appeal. "Your father must give us the opportunity," he pleaded. "I'm hoping and praying that he will open his heart and see how hard we've worked on this issue."

Danielle was moved by Albert's dedication. She would see what she could do. Danielle was also in touch with Lyn, whom she had found through her Web site. Lyn had already sent copies of her case studies to Burton, and Danielle offered to make sure her father read them. "Get all the mercury stuff to me directly," she said, "and I will get it to Dad when we have lunch this weekend. Then I can really pound it into him and say, 'Guess what, Dad? The day Christian was injured was the day he had 62.5 micrograms of mercury injected into him.' That should get his attention!"

ON WEDNESDAY, April 4, 2000, hundreds of parents from around the country began to converge on Washington. The next three days would be packed with a press conference, a congressional hearing, an NIH debriefing, and a major rally on the Mall, all in the name of autism. It was an exciting time. The mainstream media had stepped up coverage of the vaccine-autism movement, and Burton's hearing was sure to draw some marquis-name journalists.

Sallie, Albert, and Heidi could not get to Washington until the day of the rally. Lyn flew up from Atlanta the night before the hearing. She and Albert had failed to secure a thimerosal slot during the testimony, or even at the press conference. But the parents were still keen to disseminate their message as widely as possible. They needed something simple they could hand out, a one-page flyer, but all they had was their long, cumbersome report. Sallie managed to boil the entire mercury paper down to a leaflet, with bullet points outlining the common signs of mercury poisoning and autism. The flyer also issued a call to arms for parents to demand the removal of thimerosal from vaccines.

"There are still 30 vaccine products on the market with thimerosal in them, poisoning our children every day," the flyer warned. "Yet the FDA has only 'encouraged' the manufacturers to take it out, and the CDC remains quiet, despite knowing that children are receiving more mercury from vaccines than government mandate allows. If you don't think this is right, call . . .

Dr. William Egan, head of the vaccine division at FDA (301) 827-0655

Dr. Walter Orenstein, head of immunization programs at CDC (404) 639-8200

Dr. Marie Bristol-Power, the autism coordinator at NIH (301) 496-1383."

Lyn had arranged to stay at the same hotel as Rick Rollens and a small army of other parents. Rick was traveling on the nonprofit dime of the MIND Institute; any frill was one frill too many. They ended up in a dingy motel across the Potomac in Virginia.

Lyn arrived alone on a stormy evening (Tommy was on ER duty) and gagged when she saw the shabby lobby. Tiles were chipped from the dusky walls and a pink plastic bucket collected rainwater dripping from the peeling ceiling. Her room was no better.

It took two hours for Lyn to steel her nerves and leave the room. She walked through the rain to the nearby Pizza Hut. It was getting late and only a few stragglers were there eating. Lyn ordered a pizza and a much needed beer. She settled in for a lonely meal. Then she heard a male voice.

"Are you Lyn Redwood?"

Lyn looked up to see a large man with a friendly, confident smile.

"Yes. How did you know?"

"You look like the person who is most out of place here. I'm Rick Rollens."

From that moment on, the trip improved greatly. Lyn and Rick talked for what seemed like hours. Back at the motel, Rick introduced her to a dozen parents in town for the events. Lyn felt like crying again, not from self-pity but from the quiet joy that comes from entering a warm huddle of kindred spirits. Out of a hodgepodge of desperate and sad people was emerging a community of brave souls united in grief and hope. Lyn had found a whole new family that extended well beyond her own.

THE EARLY MORNING LIGHT broke with startling clarity. Lyn saw that the rain had moved on, leaving a tender April dawn in its wake. Everyone had breakfast together and shared a van ride across the Potomac and into the capital for the 9:00 A.M. press conference in the Rayburn Office Building, home of the Government Reform Committee.

Lyn looked around and saw a Who's Who of the autism world. There was Dan Burton, of course, tall and straight in his charcoal gray suit and red power tie. And there was his daughter Danielle, looking pretty but also a little nervous about speaking at the crowded event. Lyn was introduced to so many people she almost forgot to hand out Sallie's flyer. She met Andy Wakefield, in from London, and Barbara Loe Fisher, of the National Vaccine Information Center. There was jovial Bernie Rimland, founder of the Autism Research Institute; Dr. Walter Spitzer, Professor Emeritus of Epidemiology at McGill University in Montreal and one of the world's premier statistical analysts; Vijendra Singh (now at Utah State University), who had identified the problem with brain autoantibodies and MMR; and Ray Gallup, a New Jersey father and founder of the Autism Autoimmunity Project.

And, of course, Lyn finally met Shelley Reynolds and Jeana Smith, the two Louisiana moms from Unlocking Autism who had organized the rally on Saturday. The three women hugged and carried on like long lost girlfriends.

The press conference went by quickly. Burton discussed how his committee had come to investigate vaccine safety and the path he intended to follow in exploring the connection between vaccines and immune dysfunction in children. He introduced Danielle, who gave an emotional account of what had happened to Christian. Everyone was careful to stress that they were not questioning the benefits that vaccines had conferred on society. But they called on the government to accelerate its research into the issue.

"This is a historic day," Barbara Loe Fisher said. "It marks the first time that researchers stood publicly with parents of vaccine-injured children and issued a united call. We can't wait for one more generation to be born before we commit the will and resources to answer outstanding questions that beg to be answered."[79]

Lyn was giddy. She had never heard so many people speak so eloquently about vaccines and autism under one roof. She followed the crowd from the press conference and down the hall to the committee hearing room.

The place was packed. An overflow audience had lined up early to get into the hearing. There were so many people that two adjacent rooms with closed-circuit screens were opened to accommodate them. There were parents and doctors, Capitol Hill staffers, Washington reporters, and well-paid lawyers in expensive suits.

Some of the men waiting in line looked as if they had slept on the street. Lyn asked Barbara Loe Fisher who they were. "Place savers," she said. "The drug executives offer money to these guys to wait in line for them. They don't want to wait themselves, so they pay someone else to do it."

The event was at turns exhilarating, exhausting, tearful, and tense. It was, as the *New York Times* reported, "A long and contentious hearing."[80] Dan Burton convoked the session with all the usual formalities and delivered his opening statement.

"We have received hundreds of letters from parents across the country," he said, holding up several thick binders. "Here are some notebooks, and each one of the pages represents a parent who has a problem with a child with autism. They have shared with us their pain and their challenges. My staff tells me that some of them cried when they read some of these letters. And I have a pretty hard-nosed staff."[81]

Burton was alarmed at the growing number and frequency of childhood vaccines, he said. And he questioned the use of certain vaccine ingredients. "Why is it," he asked, pausing for dramatic effect, "that the FDA licenses vaccines that contain neurotoxins like mercury and aluminum?" Lyn sat up in her chair. Finally, she thought, mercury in vaccines had reached the halls of Congress. Research into these additives needed to become a top priority, Burton said. "We cannot stick our heads in the sand and ignore this possibility. If we do not take action now, ten years from now, it may be too late, not only for this generation of children, but for our taxpayer-funded health and education systems, which could collapse from trying to care for all of these children."

Following custom, the Ranking Minority Member, Henry Waxman, spoke next. The California Democrat had built his twenty-five-year career around health care and health care reform, especially on children's issues. Waxman is an ardent proponent of vaccination. Long skeptical of a link between vaccines and autism, he has never publicly ruled it out, either.

"We know there is a genetic component to autism," Waxman said. "We've seen some dramatic discoveries recently in the genetics of autism like the discovery of the Fragile X gene and the gene that causes Rett syndrome.

"I also understand that this hearing was called to consider a theory that certain vaccines cause autism," Waxman continued. "From my discussions with medical experts, scientists, and the autism community, it is clear that this is only a theory." The AMA, no less, had recently concluded that "scientific data does not support a causal association" between vaccination and autism. "I believe that we need to increase our efforts to understand the causes of autism," Waxman said. "In this search, no possible cause, including vaccines, should be off the table." Lyn knew there was a "but" coming.

"But," Waxman said, "in medicine the best answers come from research that can withstand the rigors of the scientific method." It was a hard statement to argue with.

Burton called the first panel to the table. The group, the first of three panels (nineteen witnesses were scheduled for the long day), was composed of parents, including Shelley Reynolds. The Louisiana mother spoke slowly and looked at Waxman directly.

"We have no doubt that our son developed his autism as a direct result of an adverse vaccine reaction," Shelley declared. She had not wished to believe this theory. It was too painful to think that this disaster could have been averted, that it wasn't preordained by mangled genes. "If I could strike that belief that I held him down on the table for his shots and go back to the Russian roulette of genetics, I would take it in a heartbeat," she said. "The pain of knowing that I inadvertently caused him harm due to blind trust in the medical community is nearly unbearable."

The room was silent, save for the sniffling of the choked-up attendees. Even some of the seen-it-all camera crews were getting misty-eyed.

Shelley stepped up her assault. "How can pharmaceutical companies concoct substances with mercury, formaldehyde, antifreeze, lead, aluminum, aborted fetal tissue, and live viruses," she demanded to know, "and not expect that, as they continue to pour these highly toxic and reactive substances into children—increasing dose after dose, all on the same day—it will not alter their minds and bodies? I need someone to explain to me why it is acceptable to have products on the market that exposed my son to 37.5 micrograms of mercury in one day, at a time when he should not have been exposed to more than 0.59 micrograms, given his body weight."

Autism, Shelley told the committee, was no genetic mishap that occurred in the womb. "We have talked with thousands and thousands of parents from across the country," she said. "And their story is the same: Child is normal; child gets vaccine; child disappears within days or weeks into the abyss of autism." Shelley looked up from her statement and scanned the faces of the committee members. "I know my children," she said. "And I know what happened to my son. As far as I am concerned, the needle that silently slipped into my baby's leg that day became the shot heard around the world."

The room exploded in deafening applause. It was electric. Sadly, for Lyn, these words were the last mention made of mercury for the rest of the day.

But the show had to go on. And what a show it was. Lyn was particularly moved by the next parent, a father from Durham, North Carolina, named Scott Bono. Scott, it turned out, had met Beth Clay, Burton's senior staffer, when her South Carolina high school marching band traveled to march in President Carter's inaugural parade and she stayed in Scott's best friend's home in Falls Church, Virginia. After the first vaccine hearing, Beth got dozens of calls from parents who saw it on CSPAN, including one from Scott Bono. Returning his call would reconnect the two after more than twenty years. Because the Bonos' story was so striking, and they had substantial medical documentation, Beth asked Scott to tell the story of his autistic son, Jackson, to Congress. Scott leapt at the chance.

Scott's wife, Laura—a petite southern charmer who is dwarfed by her large husband—was originally from South Carolina and had become a prominent and vocal autism activist in the Raleigh-Durham area who had made several lobbying trips to Washington. Scott is a gentle giant of a man with dark brown eyes, brown hair messed on his head, bookish glasses, and, often, a grin across his face that even Scott would describe as "goofy." He is a prankster, given to sharing ribald jokes with buddies. But on this day, in the hearing room packed with people and the national media, Scott was deadly serious.

"We had a perfectly normal pregnancy and birth of our son," Scott began. "In the first sixteen months of life, he learned language, played with toys, appropriately began pretending skills, initiated contact with his twin sisters, and could light up a room with his wonderful personality. He was brighter than most, and he could even tell the difference between a Concorde jet and a 727 at such an early age."[82]

But then, in August 1990, Jackson departed on "a journey into silence, bewilderment, and a medical enigma," Scott said. "That was when he received his MMR immunization. Jackson would not sleep that night. He developed unexplained rashes and horrible constipation and diarrhea. After eating, he experienced projectile vomiting. Over the next weeks he would slip away, unable to listen or speak. He retreated into autism.

"What was the reason for this change?" Scott asked, looking up from his text. "It is my sincerest belief that it was that shot."

The Bonos were left struggling with the pain, heartbreak, and overwhelming costs of caring for an autistic child. "Hundreds of thousands of dollars over the past eight years," Scott said. "After going through all of our savings and retirement, we continue to accumulate debt to meet his educational and therapeutic needs and his medical needs."

But there were other incalculable costs, Scott added, his voice slow and soft with pain. "How do I put a cost on not sleeping for six years? How do I put a cost on attention not paid to my daughters, because I am seeing to the needs of my son? How do I put a cost on locking every door and window at all times for fear of him wandering from the house?" Scott's voice broke with emotion. Many people were again reduced to tears.

Not all the parents were in the vaccine-autism theory camp, however. One father invited by Waxman was flatly unconvinced that vaccines caused his child's autism. His name was Dr. Wayne Dankner and he had traveled to Washington with his thirteen-year-old autistic daughter, Natalie, who sat quietly in the hearing room. Dankner was a pediatric infectious disease specialist from San Diego, and his words must have come as a welcome breath of balance to the pro-vaccine camp.

"Other parents on this panel may feel otherwise, in fact, definitively feel otherwise, but I have seen no sound evidence linking autism to the MMR or any other vaccine," he said.

Waxman pounced at the opening. "How can you say that, when the other parents have given us evidence that, in their view, their children developed autism after the vaccine? Isn't that sound evidence?" he asked, with what Lyn felt was overcooked sarcasm.

"As a *scientist*," Waxman added, smiling, "how do *you* think we should consider it, and what do we need to prove that there is a connection, if there is one?"

"My reading of what has been correlated to date does not appear to indicate a causal link," Dankner said. "I think that debate has not been settled and probably needs to be." But, he added, "I have seen children who have been harmed by vaccine-preventable diseases." This had made him cautious, "because if vaccine rates fall in the United States, I can almost guarantee, from my own personal experience, that there will be individuals who will suffer."

Waxman picked up the lead: "Are you saying to us, in other words, that we should not be alarmed about vaccinations and have parents refrain from having their kids vaccinated because of this theory, which, at this point, you do not think has gone through a scientific evaluation to be established as scientific fact?"

"I think an alarmist view is always of concern," the doctor said. "I'm a cautious individual, and I think we just need to be cautious in how we approach this issue."

The second panel, as expected, proved to be more contentious. Seated in a row along the witness table were Andrew Wakefield, John O'Leary, and Vijendra K. Singh, proponents of the MMR-autism hypothesis. Next to them were witnesses from the "other side." (Many vaccine defenders do not like to think of themselves as members of one camp pitted against another, but at this hearing, that was how the battle lines were being drawn.) The group included Dr. Brent Taylor, a colleague and critic of Wakefield from London's Royal Free and University College Medical School, Coleen Boyle and Dr. Ben Schwartz, officials from the CDC, and Dr. Paul Offit, the Philadelphia pediatrician.

Wakefield walked the committee through his MMR research. He announced that other labs had replicated his own discovery of measles viral proteins in the guts and nervous systems of kids with regressive autism and bowel disease.

O'Leary, the Irish microbiologist who had examined the biopsy from Liz Birt's son, defended his lab and his reputation against the barrage of attacks he had recently been subjected to. Critics had carped that O'Leary used inferior equipment and failed to maintain a sterile working environment. O'Leary insisted his team went to "desperate lengths" and used "revolutionary" technology to ensure the most accurate sampling possible. The detection of measles RNA in the children's biopsies, he maintained, could not have come from another source like lab contamination, as some critics asserted.

Chief among those critics was Dr. Brent Taylor, the professor of community and child health at Royal Free and University College School of Medicine. "The belief that MMR is the cause of autism is a false hope," Taylor said, "Mr. Wakefield and Professor O'Leary's testimony notwithstanding." He went through the many high-profile studies that had roundly refuted Wakefield's hypothesis. And he cautioned that false speculation about MMR threatened public health. In the UK, vaccination rates had dropped from about 90 percent in 1995 to 75 percent in 1999. "There is almost an exact parallel fall [in] confidence in the safety of MMR vaccine," he said, blaming "two papers produced by Mr. Wakefield and colleagues."

The final panel did not get under way until late in the long afternoon. The crowds were thinning and most of the media had left to cover other news. They should have stayed. The reporters would have witnessed a sound bite–rich exchange between Burton and Dr. Deborah Hirtz, a researcher from the National Institute of Neurological Disorders and Stroke. Burton pursued the doctor until she finally admitted that a vaccine-autism hypothesis was, at the very least, plausible:

> MR. BURTON: A number of people testified from the health agencies that there's no scientific evidence that autism is related to vaccines. How do they know that?
>
> DR. HIRTZ: They do not.
>
> MR. BURTON: How do you know that? There is an increase from 1 in 10,000 to 1 in 400 or 500, so we have an epidemic on our hands. And yet the health agencies of this country are telling us there is no connection between these vaccinations and autism. How do you know?
>
> DR. HIRTZ: I do not know that there is no connection. What I know is that the evidence that has been reviewed by the British Medical Research Council and the epidemiologic evidence does not support a large-scale causation. But I think . . .
>
> MR. BURTON: How do you *know* that?
>
> DR. HIRTZ: . . . But I still think that there are . . . there may be certain children who are susceptible, and that is what we have to go after. It is very important that we look for why children develop autism and whether there might be a small minority of children who have some susceptibility, and we are not ruling that out.

At the end of the seemingly endless day, Waxman went on the offensive. He suggested that Burton was looking for cheap publicity. The chairman was playing to the media and playing to fear. "What we have in this hearing is a sensationalization by the chairman in order to get all these cameras to report to the American people that there is this connection because he believes it, and many other people believe it, and therefore a lot of others who watch this will think, 'I will not immunize my children.' "

Still, Waxman did offer an olive branch of sorts across the political aisle. He had drafted a letter to Health and Human Services Secretary Donna Shalala, urging her to convene a panel of experts from the NIH, the CDC, and the FDA to review any possible association between vaccines and autism.

"Given the grave possibility that immunizations against life-threatening childhood diseases may decline as a result of unsubstantiated allegations of vaccine-induced autism," he wrote, "I would want you to act as expeditiously as possible." He invited Burton to cosign the letter.

But Burton worried that drug company money flowing to independent "experts" that advise the government had corrupted their ability to conduct an objective review of the data. Burton wanted to ensure that the experts were "not controlled by the health agencies of this country that may have some people who have some possible conflicts of interest." He insisted that "we have some people who are totally unbiased."

Waxman seemed annoyed. "Well," he said, " 'Independent' means no conflict of interest. I would not want a panel that had people with a conflict of interest. But I do want a panel of experts, and I think that the NIH and the CDC and the FDA can give us a panel that can do this evaluation."

Derisive laughter crackled through the room. Many parents who stayed until the end were getting a little punch-drunk. To them, "government independence" on autism was a comic oxymoron.

"I do not know why some people find that amusing," Waxman defended himself. "But I think—" He was interrupted by Burton, eager to wrap things up. Burton said he could live with federal bureaucrats looking into the vaccine connection, as long as "there is no conflict of interest . . . we would not have any problem with that."

WHEN THE HEARING ENDED, Liz Birt walked over to Andy Wakefield and gave him a hug. She was glad to see the doctor again, especially on Capitol Hill. Liz was planning a major fund-raising dinner for Wakefield back in Chicago the following night. She needed to fly out soon to oversee last-minute details of the sit-down dinner for four hundred, including guest speaker Dan Burton. But nothing could have kept her away from this hearing.

Unlocking Autism was throwing a post-hearing reception for Dan Burton in an ornate salon on the House side of the Capitol building. Liz and Wakefield joined the stream of parents filing out of Rayburn and into the soft afternoon, welcome relief after a day under the harsh glare of fluorescent lights. They strolled up to the Capitol, whose graceful marble dome glowed pink with the first rays of twilight. Everyone appeared a little ragged, but they were smiling.

When Liz arrived at the reception, she was introduced to an activist mother from Georgia named Lyn Redwood. Liz wanted to socialize, but she had arranged a meeting between Wakefield and Congressman Dave Weldon, a conservative Republican from central Florida. Weldon was sympathetic when it came to the vaccine-autism hypothesis; he was a respected M.D. and friendly with Dr. Jeffrey Bradstreet, also from Florida, the doctor who spoke at the Orlando conference in 1999.

Dave Weldon was an articulate, ambitious politician in his mid-forties, tall, dark, and soft spoken. He received Liz and Wakefield warmly in his office, alongside key aide Stuart Burns, a young southern conservative. Weldon offered his help to make sure the health authorities complied with the Waxman-Burton request for a review of all data on vaccines and autism. Liz knew that the doctor-congressman was going to make an outstanding ally.

It was not the only alliance forged that day. Back at the reception, Lyn Redwood had recognized Scott Bono from his turn at the witness table. She approached Scott and Laura, who were chatting with Scott's old school chum, Beth Clay. Lyn had been thrilled with his testimony. She remarked how familiar Jackson's story sounded compared with Will's. She told the Bonos how she had added up the mercury he received, and how horrified she was to find it was 125 times over the EPA limit.

The Bonos regarded Lyn with alarm. They had heard Shelley Reynolds testify about mercury, but it didn't really sink in. Lyn handed them one of her flyers, which Laura scanned, growing more ashen as her eyes moved down the page. A slight tremble shot through her arm and she set down her drink. "Scott, you've got to look at this," she said. "This is it. This is what happened to Jackson."

Scott read the paper and responded in much the same fashion. "My God," he said, turning to Laura with a look of someone just diagnosed with cancer. "You're right. It's the mercury. It messed up his immune system. It let the MMR virus take over."

They fell silent. The chit-chat of other guests filled the uneasy pause. Lyn knew what the Bonos were going through. It was a dreadful second of clarity when all that seemed so senseless began to make terrible sense indeed.

"Those motherfuckers," Scott said.

Lyn told the Bonos about her plans to form a parents' group, to get the warning out about mercury in vaccines, and to fund research into mercury toxicity and promising new treatments like chelation. The Bonos found Lyn's passion infectious. They agreed on the spot to join forces. It was the beginning of a special friendship and an inseparable alliance between the two southern families.

Just when Lyn thought that things were really looking up, they got even better. Someone had offered to share a hotel room with her at the Omni Shoreham, in the upscale Woodley Park section of the Capitol, where Unlocking Autism had booked a block of rooms for parents attending the rally. When Lyn arrived, she saw a check-in table set up for rally arrivals. She walked over and gave her name. "I know you!" cried the young mother checking people in. "You're the Mercury Mom!"

Lyn was startled and delighted. Obviously word was getting out. Once you acquired a nickname, you knew you were on the right track.

ON FRIDAY, Lyn Redwood, Rick Rollens, Scott and Laura Bono, Shelley Reynolds, Jeana Smith, and about fifty other parents headed out to Bethesda, Maryland, not far over the Washington, D.C. line. There in the Thatcher Auditorium at the National Institutes of Health, they had a morning meeting with top NIH researchers. Armed with questions and shielded by their numbers, they were feeling confident.

It was quite a meeting. The staid NIH campus had seen nothing like it since the angry-mob days of ACT UP a decade before, when the AIDS group plagued government facilities with cacophonous theatrical demonstrations.

One of the parents, Karyn Seroussi, a longtime autism activist and author of the book *Unraveling the Mystery of Autism*, posted her perception of the rambunctious meeting a few days later on the FEAT site. "Unfortunately their agenda was, 'Sit quietly while we tell you all about autism,' " she complained.[83]

Dr. Marie Bristol-Power, NIH chief of autism research, outlined the agency's research under way and spoke glowingly of a new twenty-year longitudinal study that, she said, was the "best bet for collecting data on normal brains, looking at environmental factors, and so forth."

Twenty years? This was not what the parents had come to hear. In twenty years they might be dead. Who would look after their kids then? Murmurs of dissent rumbled through the auditorium.

Rick Rollens was agitated. He stood up and interrupted the doctor. "There is revolutionary research that needs to be done, and right away!" he admonished her. "We have started some of that work out in UC Davis, at the MIND Institute. I urge you and your agencies to cooperate with us in this effort."

The parents went wild with applause. Rick had started a trend, to the mortification of the NIH staff, who must have thought they were coming to deliver a nice talk on autism to a group of appreciative parents. Karyn Seroussi rose to her feet. "Many of us here are not just parents, but researchers as well," she said. "We have come up with great ideas for controlled studies to look at immune panels, food allergies, nutritional deficiencies, gastrointestinal problems, and so on. Why aren't you looking at these areas, instead of the traditional brain-and-genetics stuff?"

At this point the parents were asked, more or less, to shut up. Dr. Stephen Foote, chief of neuroscience at the National Institute of Mental Health, began speaking about how brain imaging would prove to be an invaluable tool. He spoke "as if we were in kindergarten," Seroussi recalled. "Dr. Foote said, 'We have sophisticated technology for looking at the brain. It is called *M-R-I.*'" This condescension, she said, had the parents "hopping mad." Catcalls echoed through the gallery.

The next victim was Dr. Deborah Hirtz, who had testified the day before and had stumbled a bit when Burton pressed her on vaccine safety. "What is autism?" she asked to plaintive groans from the audience. "Autism is a rare disorder. It is believed to be genetic and neurological." Eyeballs rolled in collective disbelief. The audience knew what autism was, and they were tired of being told it was genetic. This was getting ridiculous.

Hirtz went on with her Autism 101 lesson. Seroussi was writhing in her seat. It all became too much for Michael Goldberg, a pediatrician from UCLA. "Why are you wasting our time with 20-year-old information?" he yelled. "You people need to have a major paradigm shift in your perception of autism! These kids are not behaviorally challenged, they are physically ill. Until you recognize this, you are going to waste another twenty years looking at the wrong issues."

Dr. Hirtz looked crushed, as if she'd never been interrupted in her entire career. Goldberg continued, "We are looking at a terrible, tragic epidemic that will sacrifice an entire generation of children unless you can do something remarkable. You need to listen to our findings as parents and pediatricians. We know that autism is immunological. Why don't *you* know this? We already have studies looking at treatment through correcting the immune dysfunction. Why aren't you interested in these studies?"

Goldberg kept talking a few minutes until the moderator interrupted. "OK, this is how this meeting is going to go," the scientist told the unruly parents. "We will finish our presentations. You will be allowed to ask questions. *Afterward!*"

Karyn Seroussi could bear no more. "How *dare* you patronize us with this kind of information?" she protested. "We are not stupid! We are educated, informed parents who have done thousands of hours of research in autism. We did not come here to be lectured to. We came to be listened to."

Visibly shaken, she turned to address her comrades. "My child had chronic ear infections and allergies but developed typically. After his MMR vaccine, he had seizures and a high fever, and within three weeks lost all social and language skills and developed chronic gastrointestinal problems. To how many people does this sound familiar?"

Everyone's hand in the audience shot up.

The government moderator was flummoxed. "Fine," he announced, trying to appear collected but coming off as snippy. "I guess we'll just fast-forward through our presentations and let *you* people do all the talking."

"Unfortunately for him," Seroussi wrote, "the next presentation was from a guy from NIH Infectious Diseases and the slides said things like, 'Why Vaccines Are Safe And Effective.' I really started hollering then. 'Look at that nonsense! Did you actually think you were going to convince us that we don't have a problem? Listen to me: WE ARE NO LONGER SUSCEPTIBLE TO YOUR PROPAGANDA!'"

The meeting was half over. "If the NIH is going to continue wasting time," Karyn Seroussi huffed, "Then I am leaving to go have lunch. Would anyone like to join me?"

A good twenty people marched toward the door before Barbara Loe Fisher, of the National Vaccine Information Center, moved to stem the flow. "Hang on!" she cried. Things calmed down. She asked the scientists to finish talking, but added, "We would like a chance to speak when you're done." Even Karyn Seroussi sat down.

When the parents were finally allowed to pose their questions, Lyn Redwood got up to ask, calmly and politely, why her son was given ethylmercury in his vaccines in amounts that were well in excess of federal guidelines. The parents clapped enthusiastically, but none of the scientists had a satisfactory answer.

When it was over, Rick Rollens urged the NIH staff to consider holding more meetings, Seroussi wrote, "and Hirtz was glaring at him with an 'over-my-dead-body' expression on her face." Seroussi approached Marie Bristol-Powell, shook her hand, and thanked her. Toward the end of the session, Dr. Bristol-Powell had softened her tone a bit. She had even referred to autism as being "epidemic" at several points.

"I told her she was the only person on that stage who was actually listening to us," Seroussi said. "She had the strangest expression on her face. I looked into her eyes and I thought, 'Oh God, she believes us and she can't say anything.' I hope I'm right, but I don't know what good it'll do."

A month or so later, Karyn Seroussi would come to regret the confrontation. "In many ways I regret that I wrote the e-mail, and that it even took place." The meeting went badly for the hosts, to be sure, but it also went badly for the audience. The last thing she wanted was to further polarize the parents and professionals who so needed and wanted to work together on this problem. "To publicly humiliate those in power felt good," she confided, "but it was stupid and non-productive, and I am ashamed of my outburst."

Seroussi refused to believe that any of the scientists on that stage "were anything but painfully ignorant, living in their ivory research towers with a pre-existing autism paradigm," she said later. "I do not believe that any of them even suspected that their policies were poisoning our children. I guessed that Bristol-Powers was beginning to understand that environmental factors had to be involved, and that we were facing an epidemic, but I doubt she was even subconsciously considering that the vaccines were implicated."[84]

SATURDAY DAWNED into another lovely spring day. Lyn peered down from her new hotel room to the flowering trees and tulips below. The hard part was over, she thought. Now to the fun stuff: the rally. It was also the day she would at long last get to meet her fellow fighters from New Jersey.

After breakfast a small band of parents boarded the Metro and headed for the Mall. Thousands were expected and a huge staging area was set up with a large platform for speeches and live music. There was also a stretch of grass where families (many people brought their kids, even their dogs) could relax and picnic. On one side, dozens of booths were set up for autism organizations from around the country.

Among the day's speakers were some of the parents who testified at the Burton hearing. Maya Angelou spoke and read a poem. Dan Burton delivered a blistering speech about getting to the bottom of the autism mystery, even if that meant taking on the vaccine industry. Lyn couldn't help herself. Caught up in the moment, the lifelong Democrat grabbed a poster and scrawled "BURTON FOR PRESIDENT!" on the back. Hundreds more took up the call, chanting for several minutes. Burton stood onstage and beamed.

Lyn wandered around the sun-splashed scene. Families were picnicking on the grass. People tossed Frisbees. Children ran and cavorted beneath colorful banners and flags fluttering in the April breeze. Lyn was not able to bring Will to Washington so she carried a large color photo with his name at the bottom.

A man recognized her. He came up and threw his arms around her in a bear hug.

"At last! I am so happy to find you!" the man said. It was Albert, walking around with Payam. Grinning, Albert led Lyn to the CAN booth, where Sallie and Heidi were selling T-shirts, signing up parents for volunteer work, and distributing their flyer.

Everyone took turns staffing the booth or grabbing fistfuls of leaflets and heading out through the crowd. People seemed very receptive. Lyn noticed them reading the flyer intently. Many were shaking their heads in disbelief.

It was an uplifting time for all of them. Lyn was thrilled to finally meet the people she had been working so closely with. "Misery loves company," she told the others. "And we've all had the same misery in our lives."

5. Hidden Agendas

ALLIE, Lyn, Heidi, and Albert returned home from Washington recharged. They were ready for the next steps in a long march to proving their unpopular theory. Top priority was to present the mercury paper personally to the public health bigwigs. It was a powerful tool, they believed, for demanding the removal of all mercury from vaccines.

The long document still had not been readied for publication. But Sallie had been asked to submit a shortened version of the paper to a Scottish journal called *Medical Hypotheses,* published by Elsevier, a global multimedia publisher of scientific and medical information, including the *Lancet.*

The journal wholly admits to taking a "deliberately different approach to peer review," and according to its Web site will "publish radical ideas, so long as they are coherent and clearly expressed." The editor's role is that of a " 'chooser', not a 'changer.' "[85] The *New England Journal of Medicine* it is not. Many critics of the parents' mercury paper still point to where it was first published as evidence of its questionable integrity.

Sallie shortened the paper and sent it off anyway. After all, this *was* a peer-reviewed journal. Sallie was listed as lead author, followed by Albert, Teresa, Heidi, Lyn, and Woody. To this day, the controversial paper is often referenced as *Bernard et al.*

In April, Sallie got the word from Scotland: *Medical Hypotheses* had accepted the manuscript. "Now that we know we'll be published, it's really time to get vocal," she said. She sent copies right away to Bill Egan at the FDA, Marie Bristol-Power at the NIH, and Dr. Walter Orenstein at the CDC's National Immunization Program.

"Our review of the available medical literature," Sallie wrote in her cover letter to Egan, "found that the symptoms and abnormalities which characterize autism are identical to those found in past cases of mercury poisoning."

"Due to the high likelihood that many if not most cases of autism are caused by the mercury in childhood vaccines containing thimerosal, and due to the fact that every child today can be fully vaccinated using a thimerosal-free product, I am asking you to join me in urging the FDA to call for an immediate ban on thimerosal-containing childhood vaccines."

THE HEAT was being turned up on Dan Burton. The congressman had been taking fire for what critics considered to be his unseemly grandstanding on the subject of vaccines and autism. Henry Waxman, for one, was not at all happy with the chairman's performance at the last hearing. On April 17, Waxman blasted Burton on the op-ed page of the *Los Angeles Times* in an essay titled "Bad Information Can Be Deadly."[86]

The April autism hearing offered "heart-rending testimony from parents of autistic children, who sincerely believe that vaccines caused their children's condition," Waxman wrote. "And a few hand-picked researchers lent a scientific veneer by testifying that they believe vaccines may cause autism." But Waxman claimed to see through the veneer. "Virtually every medical expert around the world" had come to an entirely different conclusion. "The scientific evidence does not support a causal association between vaccines and autism," he said, taking special aim at Wakefield. "Wakefield has made similar announcements in the past, only to have them invalidated when his findings could not be duplicated."

A week later Burton fired back in a letter to the *Los Angeles Times*.[87] "Mr. Waxman apparently believes that having a dialogue about the possible links between autism and vaccines is dangerous," he wrote. "He suggests that the Committee ignore the near-epidemic rise in autism, and hide the discussion from the public eye so that parents will continue to vaccinate their children without awareness of the growing concern about adverse events."

Insisting that he was not antivaccine, Burton still urged parents to inspect the package insert of their kids' vaccines. "Some of the ingredients may shock them," he said: "aluminum, MSG, formaldehyde, and mercury."

In the first six months of life, he added, "the amount of mercury that is injected into children through vaccines exceeds federal safety guidelines. The FDA knows that mercury can cause neurodevelopmental delays, yet has licensed these mercury-containing vaccines anyway. Why are we injecting known toxic substances into our children? Instead of hiding our heads in the sand to protect the status quo, it is time to admit that the U.S. Government failed the American public by not funding adequate studies to determine the long-term effects of vaccines on our children."

DOWN IN ATLANTA, Lyn Redwood persisted in her mission to land the big meetings with government health officials. She called every office that had received a copy of the mercury-autism paper. She badgered staffers until they gave her a response. The first answer came too quickly, from the office of Marie Bristol-Power at NIH. There would be no meeting.

Lyn wasn't making much progress with the FDA or CDC, either. She was fed up, frankly. "It's time to go to the media with this," she told Sallie one night. "I've been patient enough. I have written letters without response. We've been told that removal has been 'requested,' so there's nothing more to do. That was almost a year ago."

Teresa Binstock counseled patience before running to reporters. The mercury paper had not yet been printed, and premature attention might be counterproductive. "Publication will earn us more allies and will be an important step in giving credibility to the concept," she said. "So my vote is no."

Albert refused to give up on meeting with the NIH, CDC, and FDA, despite Lyn's lack of progress. Albert was relentless and charming in his quest, and he became an authority on the cold call. "He's really our ambassador of goodwill," Sallie marveled to her husband. "He just picks up the phone and very emphatically says, 'We're a bunch of parents, and we really need to meet with you. We have something very important to discuss. And we need to know, please, on what date can we do that?'" Before long, Albert had somehow charmed his way into back-to-back meetings with officials at the NIH and FDA. The CDC, however, was still dragging its feet.

Encouraged by his own success, Albert began working his charisma on another target: Dan Burton. Albert lobbied Beth Clay relentlessly for her boss to hold a hearing exclusively on thimerosal. On May 3, 2000, Albert got the great news: Burton had agreed. The hearing was scheduled for July. Even better, the parents would be invited to testify on behalf of their new hypothesis. Burton and his staff wanted to meet with everybody on May 16, when they came to town for their twin meetings at the NIH and FDA.

. . .

EVERYONE ARRIVED in the parking lot of the NIH that warm May morning practically in unison. Lyn had come up from Atlanta, Woody McGinnis flew in from Arizona, and Sallie, Heidi, and Teresa drove down from New Jersey with Albert. There was a newcomer on the team that day, too, another parent of an autistic child, and an M.D.: Dr. David Baskin, professor of neurosurgery at Baylor College of Medicine in Houston. He knew Albert and Sallie from CAN, and they invited him to come.

David Baskin implored the group to formulate a concise strategy before the meeting. They filed into a café on the campus for some impromptu caucusing. Woody was eager to broach the subject of chelation. Some kids had excreted up to 80 micrograms of mercury, he said. Such a high level was an unmistakable implication of thimerosal. But David Baskin urged caution. There was little if any scientific evidence to support chelation treatment. "Our credibility will suffer if we even bring it up," he said.

The parents ambled over to the meeting hall, where they were met by smiling staffers who led them into a small conference room on the second floor. Then a fire alarm went off. Everyone headed back downstairs to the parking lot, where they waited forty-five minutes until the all-clear was given.

When things finally got under way, a dozen NIH staff people were sitting at the table, including directors from two of the agency's institutes: Stephen Foote, director of the Neuroscience Center at the National Institute of Mental Health (NIMH), and Duane Alexander, director of the National Institute for Child Health and Human Development (NICHD).[88] Sallie wasted no time. She presented her case in concise PowerPoint slides on the wall—perfect for her businesslike demeanor. She meticulously went over each category of symptoms for autism and mercury toxicity.

Then Teresa and Woody began a wide discussion of experiments being conducted outside the federal bureaucracy. They mentioned several epidemiology studies, some animal models, and, David Baskin's concerns aside, clinical trials for chelation therapy.

Teresa said urgency was key. "Clearly some of the studies NIH is talking about will take a long time here, we're talking years," she said. "That's why studies like chelation are so very important to initiate as soon as possible. Many children are showing very positive responses to chelation. Waiting for long-range strategies is not in the best interests of children whose neurotypicalities may have a mercury component."

Teresa inquired about applying for NIH grants to study the mercury-autism hypothesis. Chelation, she added, could be a useful tool in diagnosing mercury toxicity, as measured by the amount of metal excreted through urine. It could also play a major role in treating the disorder itself. But the parents had more than chelation on their wish list. Lyn read from a laundry list of studies. Most already existed in proposal form, written by researchers around the country. Now they needed NIH funding. They included:

- Electromagnetic imaging to detect if mercury is present in the brains of autistic children versus controls.
- Animal studies where mice or monkeys are injected with bolus doses of thimerosal. These animals would include subsets of "high responding" and autoimmune-prone specimens.
- An epidemiological study of vaccinated versus nonvaccinated groups of children to determine the rate of autism cases in each. Nonvaccinated groups might be found in the Amish or Christian Scientist communities, where parents obtained a religious exemption.
- An immune assay of autistic kids versus controls to see if lymphocyte imbalances in the sick children were significantly greater than in normal kids.
- A comparison of typical EEG patterns from past mercury poisoning cases with those of autistic subjects.
- A study to measure the amount of thimerosal actually in vaccines, and the variability in amounts withdrawn in any given batch.

When Teresa asked if chelation case histories could be used as the basis for a research proposal, Dr. Alexander said that they could. He also showed unusual interest in pink disease. Sallie mentioned the disorder and his ears perked up. "So, you believe that autism is very similar to what happened in acrodynia?" he asked Sallie.

"I think it's the same thing. It's the same type of cause," she replied. "And once we get rid of the thimerosal, we'll see it go away, like we saw with acrodynia."

"Well, that is interesting," Dr. Alexander mused. "I remember acrodynia from my early days as a physician, and it does seem similar."

Teresa walked away from the meeting enormously encouraged. "Bottom line," she wrote in an e-mail to people in the autism community, "these folks appear to be taking very seriously thimerosal's possible (even probable) link with many cases of autism. They seem to care. The preponderance of evidence suggests the link is causal!"

The parents filed out of the room and out to their cars. They drove through the flowering Maryland suburbs and over to Rockville, home of the

FDA, where they were to meet with William Egan and other members of the CBER team.

Sallie, Albert, and Lyn were far less sanguine than Teresa. They were dismayed at the blasé reception they were given at the NIH. "They sat there very stone faced the whole time," Lyn told Tommy back home in Atlanta. It seemed as if the scientists were going through the motions but not really interested, she said. "They listened politely to what we had to say, took a few notes, and then basically announced, 'Okay thanks. Good-bye.' "

LYN HAD ALWAYS THOUGHT of the FDA as a gleaming bastion of hygiene and health. She imagined its headquarters as sleek and modern, like something from a Stanley Kubrick film. But the parents pulled up to an old, undistinguished brick building instead. They were met by staff and escorted downstairs into a musty subbasement jammed with filing cabinets and lined with thick steel doors. Fluorescent lights buzzed and flickered overhead. They were led into a small, windowless conference room and seated around an old table on metal chairs. Lyn regarded her surroundings. "This is the FDA?" she muttered to Sallie. "It looks like a stuffy old elementary school. Are they strapped for funds? Is that why they can't do vaccine safety studies?"

Sallie laughed and told Lyn to be sure to ask the feds the same question.

Several officials entered the room, including Dr. Egan, Dr. Kathryn Carbone, from CBER's Division of Viral Products, and Dr. Leslie Ball, who had calculated vaccine mercury exposure prior to release of the Joint Statement in 1999.[89] Lyn was keyed up to confront Dr. Ball in person. At long last, she could finally ask the doctor the question that had burned inside her for so long: Why had she chosen to average out mercury exposures into small daily doses?

When everyone introduced themselves around the table, and Lyn's turn came, she pounced. "Dr. Ball," she said, staring straight at the doctor, "your calculations on mercury exposures have bothered me now for a long time."

"Oh?" said Dr. Ball, in a manner seemingly defensive to the parents. "In what way?"

"Well, every toxicologist I have spoken to, outside of government, that is, tells me you cannot legitimately average these types of bolus dose exposures, which occurred only on three days, over a six-months period of time."

Dr. Ball was silent. So was everyone else. "Mercury has a long half-life, as I'm sure you know," Lyn persisted. "These bolus injections build on each other. So what I am asking is, Why on earth did you average it out this way?"

Ball seemed nervous, Lyn thought. She spoke haltingly. "I—I don't know," she said, looking around apprehensively at her superiors. "I am not a toxicologist. I am a pediatrician. I just did what they told me to do."

Lyn was staggered. Holy cow, she thought. This is a young female pediatrician who couldn't have been at the FDA for very long. If the FDA had something this concerning, they needed to put senior people on it, not some new pediatrician who didn't have the experience or background.

Lyn looked Dr. Ball in the eyes and continued thinking. The FDA must have, what, fifty or a hundred toxicologists on staff? Why did they shuffle this off on her? Why did they tell her to do the modeling this way?

It was time for Sallie to move on to her mercury-autism presentation, much like the one she had given at the NIH. It was received with even less enthusiasm here.

The discussion then turned not to research, but to regulation, the bailiwick of the massive administration. The parents formally requested that thimerosal be immediately banned, or at least temporarily withdrawn from the market pending further evaluation.

"Children are being harmed, right now as we sit here talking about it!" Albert said forcefully. He looked at Dr. Egan. "What the hell, Doctor, are you going to do about it? We are not leaving here without an answer." But Dr. Egan offered no answer. He looked pale and distracted. It seemed he would rather be anywhere else in the world than in this oppressive little room brimming with hostile parents.

"Dr. Egan?" Albert persisted. But Egan just dropped his head and stared at the table.

David Baskin broke the silence with an unrelated question. Egan looked relieved at the change of subject. He sat up in his chair, ready to answer. But Egan was interrupted.

"No! Wait!" It was Kathryn Carbone, from CBER's Viral Products Division. "I, for one, would really like to hear Dr. Egan's answer to the question. Dr. Egan?"

Lyn was amazed. Clearly there was a lot of politics going on beneath the surface. Maybe the parents had more allies at the FDA than they realized. You can tell when someone is conning you and toeing the company line, Lyn thought. Kathryn Carbone was not one of those people. For months, Lyn had been keeping track of good people and bad, on a writing pad she called her "Little Black Book of Players." She got it out and wrote Dr. Carbone's name on her "Good Guy" list.

Everyone was still staring at Egan, waiting for an answer. Slowly, he shook his head and then looked up. "We can't do a recall," he said. "There is no evidence to support such a decision on the part of FDA. And acting without supporting evidence could potentially open up the agency to litigation."

"Litigation?" Lyn whispered to Sallie. "That's great. The FDA is afraid of being sued by the industry it is supposed to regulate. There is something very wrong here."

By the time it ended, rush hour had descended and the group was already two hours late for their meeting with Dan Burton on Capitol Hill.

Lyn had to catch a flight back to Atlanta. As she headed for the parking lot, Leslie Ball approached her and walked Lyn to her car. "She seemed very interested in what we had said at the meeting," Lyn told Tommy that night. "She said a member of her extended family was affected. She seemed genuinely sympathetic in a way that she hadn't been during the meeting." Lyn decided that Dr. Ball would be a good person to work on in the coming months, an insider ally, perhaps. But she wasn't ready to enter the doctor onto her "Good Guy" list.

LANDING A TÊTE-À-TÊTE at the CDC was proving to be elusive, Albert's charm notwithstanding. The parents did not know it, but CDC vaccine officials were busy at the time. They were preoccupied with an internal review of data on the effects of thimerosal in childhood vaccines.

Starting in the summer of 1999, researchers at the National Immunization Program had quietly commenced a major analysis of data on hundreds of thousands of children who received varying amounts of thimerosal in vaccines during the 1990s. The records were part of a government monitoring program, launched in 1990, called the Vaccine Safety Datalink (VSD). The Datalink draws together large databases from several health maintenance organizations. In sum, the HMOs have received some twenty-five million dollars in federal taxpayers' money for participating.[90] The database, according to the CDC Web site, "makes it possible to do large epidemiologic studies of vaccine adverse events, captures information on less commonly occurring types of adverse events, and helps determine whether an event is linked with a vaccine or with some other cause."[91]

CDC officials had looked at the records of some four hundred thousand children enrolled in four HMOs on the West Coast. In May 2000, they presented their findings at a joint meeting of the American Academy of Pediatrics and the Pediatric Academic Societies, in Boston.

It didn't take long for Lyn to get a copy of the abstract. The study was called "Infant Exposure to Thimerosal-Containing Vaccines and Risk for Subsequent Neurologic and Renal [Kidney] Disease."[92] The lead author was Robert L. Davis, associate professor of pediatrics and epidemiology at the University of Washington and senior adviser for vaccine safety to the Vaccine

Safety Datalink. Other authors included CDC staff members Thomas Verstraeten, Frank DeStefano, and VSD chief Robert T. Chen.

The team had calculated the total ethylmercury exposure each child had received at one and three months. Using average birth weights, they compared these amounts to the EPA's daily exposure limit for methylmercury of 0.1 microgram per kilogram. Over half the kids, they found, had exceeded the EPA limit.

Next they looked at the number of adverse "outcomes" reported among the children, including those with degenerative disorders (286 cases), developmental disorders (3,702), kidney disease (310), autism (153), ADD (346), and "developmental delay" (2,568). Among these adverse outcomes, they found no significant difference between children who fell below the EPA exposure limit and those who had exceeded it.

"Among children followed up to six years of age," Davis et al. concluded, "ethylmercury exposure at one and three months of age is not associated with adverse neurodevelopmental or renal outcomes."

Lyn was shocked to read that the government was sitting on thimerosal safety data. Why hadn't anyone told them about it? Surely officials at the NIH and FDA must have known about the Datalink. Surely they were aware that their CDC counterparts were examining data for potential problems associated with thimerosal.

Either way, Lyn was unimpressed with the study. She dismissed it as a rudimentary and meaningless analysis, one that could not accurately predict the risk of autism based on what she considered to be such crude calculations.

Lyn had several questions. Why did the team only look at exposures at one and three months? Why didn't they extend their analysis out to include exposures at six months, or even the total cumulative exposure during the first eighteen months? And why had they simply divided the children into those who fell above and below EPA levels? At each visit, the kids had received varying amounts of mercury, ranging from 0 to 62.5 micrograms or more, depending on which brands they got.

Lyn thought the researchers should have broken the data down into different levels of exposure. They should have compared outcomes between kids who, at three months, received no thimerosal, and those who received a low level (12.5 micrograms), a moderate amount (37.5 micrograms), or at the highest end, 62.5 micrograms or more. This would have painted a more accurate picture of the risk of injury at each level of exposure.

Lyn also noticed that prenatal exposure from Rho(D) was not factored in.

Lyn posted the Davis abstract on the mercury-autism Web site alongside her own editorial comments. "Interesting how you can design a study to support your own hypothesis," she said.

Sallie was appalled as well. "What a piece of junk," she wrote to Teresa. "If CDC does not agree to reanalyze the data, then we know they're not dealing honestly with us."

Teresa concurred. "Acting to defuse Davis in its current form, and to have them improve their model, *or* offer alternative models, is important ASAP," she wrote. "This is a good example of how an inaccurate model can skew data and conclusions." Caught up in the moment, she called the study "a whitewash for [the CDC's] Chen and other ethylmercury injectors."

Later that night Sallie called Lyn about the Datalink study. "I think the only way we're going to know what went on at CDC is to access the raw data ourselves," she said. "We need to have an independent analysis done. We need to look at the autism outcomes at each level of exposure, not just those above and below EPA."

Of course Lyn agreed. "I think I could find a statistician to do it," she offered. "There must be someone out there not on the government or drug company payroll."

"Great," Sallie said. "But first, let's get our hands on that database."

"WE NEED A LAWYER," Lyn said one May afternoon to Rick Rollens. "I don't think we're equipped to launch major legal action against two huge bureaucracies on our own."

The looming legal battles they faced were exhausting to even think about. How on earth, Lyn wondered, were they going to force the FDA to remove mercury from vaccines while simultaneously pressuring the CDC over access to the Datalink? "We need someone good who will do this for free. Know any parents who are attorneys?"

Rick had just the person in mind. "I do know someone, in Chicago," he said. "Her name is Liz Birt. You met her briefly at the reception in the Capitol building."

Lyn called Liz the next day. "Tell me, what do you know about FDA?" she asked.

"Well, they keep drug companies in line, make sure drugs are safe and effective."

"We want to get rid of all the vaccines that still have thimerosal in them," Lyn said. "Do you know anything about FDA recalls?"

"Very little, but I can find out. I can go look at the regs," Liz said.

Lyn was pleased. "That would be great. We've been banging down doors trying to get these people to listen to us. We met with FDA, but our demands fell on deaf ears."

Liz promised to try to help. Time was always at a premium, of course, especially with a sick son and her work for Wakefield's MMR crusade. But she would try. Before hanging up, Lyn asked one more question: "What do you know about the CDC?"

"Not much. Why?"

"We found out they've got safety data on thimerosal. They just announced that it played no role in neurological disorders. We think that's crap. We want to get the data ourselves. Do you have any idea how to go about doing that?"

"Well," Liz said, "I could send them a letter. We could just ask."

"And if they say no? I'm pretty sure they'll say no."

"I guess we'd have to file a FOIA request then."

"A what?"

"Freedom of Information Act. In theory, when it works, it provides public access to unreleased government documents."

"You know how to do that?"

"Sure," Liz said. "Piece of cake."

After the phone call, Liz dialed up an old pal, Jim Moody, an attorney who lived in Washington. Jim and Liz had known each other since high school days in Kansas City and remained very close over the years.

Jim Moody is a seasoned D.C. attorney with close ties to power brokers of most every political stripe. An uncompromising libertarian who is deeply distrustful of big government, Jim is equally cynical about big business. He founded the Washington-based Advocates for a Competitive Economy, which represents small producers of commodities like milk, hops, and apples against powerful (he would say "extortionist") trade boards that demand contributions for national campaigns, such as the "Got Milk?" series.

Jim disliked both major parties. He had no more respect for George Bush than for Bill Clinton. He did, however, enjoy the company of some rather notorious conservatives. He was Linda Tripp's attorney during the Lewinsky scandal. Jim delivered Tripp's phone tapes to Ken Starr and almost brought down a president. He counted among his friends Matt Drudge, the Internet muckraker, and Anne Coulter, author and scourge of the left.

When Liz called Jim to tell him about the thimerosal controversy, he didn't think it sounded crazy at all. It sounded like a fine scandal. He wanted to help Liz and her son Matthew, and he was salivating at the prospect of sticking it to the feds for what he would come to call the deliberate poisoning of a generation of American kids.

"The first thing you've got to do," he told Liz, "is get organized. If you want to be an effective presence in Washington you've got to come up with an official-sounding group. No one will listen to a bunch of parents. You need a name. You need a board of directors and a mission statement and all that. You need to become a kind of lobbying organization if you want to make any changes at FDA or anywhere else."

But, he cautioned, the chances of a recall were slim. "The FDA could have recalled this crap a long time ago if they wanted to," he said. "They had plenty of regulatory power to do so. But they didn't."

"Why the hell not?" Liz asked.

"You know why not," Jim said. "A lot of those researchers are squarely in the pocket of the drug companies. They won't do anything to upset their benefactors. And their second priority is not to lose face. It sounds to me like they really fucked up on this one," he added. "The FDA should have caught this a long time ago. You wait and see. They will go to unbelievable lengths to avoid owning up to what they let happen."

BETH CLAY had big news for the parents, and she was eager to share it. Burton's staff had a just-released copy of a government-commissioned report on mercury poisoning in humans. Its significance for the thimerosal investigation, she said, was considerable.

The report, *Toxicological Effects of Methylmercury*, was sponsored by the EPA and prepared by the National Research Council of the National Academy of Sciences. The National Academy of Sciences is a private institute with which Congress and governmental agencies contract to provide independent analysis of science and technology issues.

Beth sent a copy of the groundbreaking report to Lyn. The day it arrived, Lyn took a highlighter pen and devoured its contents in a single sitting. The paper's main objective was to revisit the EPA maximum daily exposure limit and determine whether it was scientifically justifiable. The report concluded that the 0.1 figure indeed was the appropriate one. But it also suggested that this level might still be *too high* for certain sensitive subpopulations, especially children. It left open the possibility that the limit might need to be readjusted to ensure that it was broad enough to protect all individuals.[93]

"Due to inter-individual variation, there is no single correct value," it said. "Failure to consider inter-individual [toxic] variability can result in [a limit] that is not protective of a substantial portion of the population. We need to better understand how this chemical affects brain development in fetuses and children."

What this meant, Lyn knew, was that the EPA levels were established to provide sufficient protection for the average adult individual. But they did not take into account infants and children, who might also have exceptional sensitivity to mercury. What was the "safe" level of exposure for them? Was there even a safe level at all?

"Although we believe EPA's guideline on methylmercury is generally adequate to protect most people," the press release issued with the report said, "more must be done to gain a better understanding of various risk factors for the U.S. population."

One of those risk factors lurked in the human mouth. The major source of "elemental" mercury exposure was found to be vapor from fillings. (Some 3,000 metric tons of mercury were used in 1999 by American dentists for fillings.) In one study, two-thirds of college students with dental fillings excreted mercury in their urine that "appeared to be derived from vapor released from the amalgams," the report said. "The vapor enters tissue, including the brain, where it is oxidized into inorganic mercury."

As for environmental "organic" mercury exposure, it varied among Americans depending on where they lived and how much fish they ate. Lyn was not surprised to read that fish was the main culprit. But how did the heavy metal get into fish? The answer was coal-burning power plants, which generate significant amounts of mercury. Inorganic mercury emitted from power plants returns to earth in rainfall, where it washes into lakes and rivers, and eventually winds up in the ocean, the report said. Once in the water, the inorganic mercury is converted to organic methylmercury by aquatic organisms. It then enters the food chain and eventually lands on the dinner table in the form of, say, a tuna casserole. A full 90 percent of the methylmercury will be absorbed into the GI tract of anyone who eats the food, the report said.

Pregnant women who ingest methylmercury can easily pass it on to unborn children. The placenta provides little protection. "Fetuses are particularly vulnerable to methylmercury because of their rapid brain development," the report said. In fact some unborn children "may currently be receiving exposures at levels that cause observable adverse neurological effects." The committee estimated that each year sixty thousand U.S. children may be born "with neurological problems that could lead to poor school performance because of exposure to methylmercury in-utero."

Although there was no mention of thimerosal or ethylmercury, Lyn found the whole report fascinating, but also upsetting.

Let me get this straight, she thought. Mercury goes from a power plant into the air, back down into the water, into fish, into pregnant women, and then into unborn kids who go on to develop neurological problems. That convoluted route is dangerous. But injecting mercury into little babies is perfectly okay? How stupid do they think we *are*?

IN EARLY JUNE 2000, CDC vaccine officials finally relented and at last granted a meeting with "Bernard et al." The parents couldn't help but wonder if the sudden change of heart had anything to do with the fact that Dan Burton had recently announced two hearings on vaccines and autism.

The meeting, actually a video teleconference, was slated for June 15, the same day as the Government Reform Committee hearings on CDC and FDA conflicts of interest. Some participants were to gather at CDC headquarters in Atlanta, where Lyn would head up one delegation, and everyone else would meet at a CDC office in Washington.

Before the meeting, Lyn drove to the airport to retrieve two recently acquired allies, flying in from New Orleans for the occasion. One was Dr. Jane El-Dahr, chief of Pediatric Allergy, Immunology, and Rheumatology at Tulane University Medical Center. The other was a graduate student, Susan Owens, who was studying the role of sulfur in human biochemistry. Susan explained to Lyn that, in healthy people, certain sulfur-based proteins bind with mercury and other heavy metals, helping to eliminate them from the body. It was, in a way, an internal natural chelation mechanism. Autistic children, however, were found to be dangerously deficient in these sulfur proteins. The result was an acute inability to shed the toxins. This would explain why so many autistic children were excreting high levels of mercury after chelation therapy. Lyn was amazed.

They arrived at the Atlanta site, a CDC facility in a nondescript office park miles from the main CDC campus. The women were led down a corridor to a windowless conference room already jammed with twenty or so staff members, mostly from the National Immunization Program. Technicians were busy setting up the cameras, monitors, and microphones for the Washington hookup.

The CDC staff listened politely as the parents made their case.[94] Sallie, in Washington, began with the now-familiar mercury-autism presentation based on the parents' paper. In Atlanta, Jane El-Dahr discussed the autoimmune damage caused by mercury exposure, and Susan Owens talked about low "sulfation" in autistic kids.

When Lyn's turn came, she challenged the assertion of many researchers that ethylmercury was not as harmful to the brain, nerves, and other tissues as methylmercury. She pointed to several reports suggesting that ethylmercury was toxic in its own right, even if methylmercury was "more" toxic. One study from China in 1984 showed that people who ingested a single ethylmercury dose of 0.5 micrograms per kilogram from tainted grain suffered "significant impairment," much like the Iraqis exposed to methylmercury. It would appear that the two forms were more or less equal in the damage they could do.

Another study, conducted in Japan in 1971, showed that human intoxication with ethylmercury salts often produced symptoms similar to methylmercury poisoning. This team found that ethylmercury, once it passes through the blood-brain barrier, is converted to inorganic mercury at a higher rate than the methyl form. Inorganic mercury remains in the brain and central nervous system longer than organic mercury.

Finally, Lyn told the CDC staff about a 1985 study from a team headed by Dr. Laszlo Magos, a respected toxicologist from the UK's Medical Research Council Laboratories. His team exposed groups of rats to equal amounts of ethyl and methyl mercury. They found higher mercury levels in the brains of the methyl-exposed rats. In the ethyl-exposed cases, however, there were higher concentrations of mercury in key brain centers that govern motor and sensory functions, speech, and communication.

The CDC workers sat stone-faced, seemingly unimpressed. Lyn moved on to the case studies. She discussed the encouraging results obtained through chelation. She put up slides of the lab reports from children who underwent chelation therapy. Most of the metals excreted were well within the normal ranges, as represented by short black horizontal bars. The markers for mercury, however, looked like single long strands of spaghetti, often extending to the edge of the page. One child had dumped out 87 micrograms of mercury after a single round of chelation.

"These children underwent repeated psychological evaluations by entirely independent therapists," Lyn said. "Nearly all the kids who underwent chelation therapy showed significant improvements in behavior and health over a short period of time."

When Lyn finished, Sallie asked the CDC folks for their questions and comments. She was looking forward to a lively debate, a spirited exchange of ideas. But not a single question was asked. The stone faces sat in silence. This meeting was clearly ending.

"You may be aware," said Dr. Martin Myers, one of the directors at the meeting, "that the CDC has looked into the question of thimerosal exposure and developmental disorders. Among children followed up to six years of age, ethylmercury exposure at one and three months was not associated with adverse neurodevelopmental or renal outcomes."

And with that, CDC staffers distributed a one-page handout to the parents as they got up to leave from their respective conference rooms.

"What's this?" Lyn asked one of them.

"We've looked into this," he said. "There's nothing there. But if you want to know more, we will be presenting data on the study at our next public meeting."

"Really? And when is that?"

"Next Wednesday. Right here in Atlanta."

Lyn glanced at the handout. It was the same Davis et al. abstract they had seen posted on the Internet. Only in this version, on the back of the page, the analysts had in fact broken down the various mercury exposure levels, to 0, 12.5, 25, 37.5, 50, and 62.5 micrograms. They then compared the risk of developing autism or other adverse outcomes associated with each exposure level. As before, they found no statistically significant difference in outcomes among the exposure categories.

"My God," Lyn thought. "Maybe we *are* crazy. Maybe we are completely wrong, and they are right."

What Lyn and the other parents did not know, and would not learn for another year, was that the CDC had found preliminary evidence of an association between thimerosal and adverse outcomes. But the agency, whose mission is to protect the public health, did not share this information with those most affected by it.

DAN BURTON looked stern as usual that June morning as he presided over the June 15, 2000, Government Reform Committee hearing on conflicts of interest in the vaccine approval process. "We've been focusing on two important advisory committees," he intoned. "The FDA and the CDC rely on these advisory committees to help them make vaccine policies that affect every child in this country. We've looked very carefully at conflicts of interest. We've taken a good hard look at whether the pharmaceutical industry has too much influence over these committees. From the evidence we found, I think they do."[95]

The FDA panel, called the Vaccines and Related Biological Products Advisory Committee (VRBPAC), makes recommendations on whether new vaccines should be approved and licensed. The CDC's Advisory Committee on Immunization Practices (ACIP) recommends which vaccines to add to the childhood schedule.

Burton learned that many advisory panel members had received research grants from drug companies, either for themselves or their academic institutions. Others got plum speaking honoraria, travel funds, or other benefits. Incredibly, some of these "independent" experts owned stock in the companies whose products were under review. Some, like Paul Offit, even shared the patents on certain vaccines. And even though they were required to recuse themselves from voting on products in which they held a direct financial stake, the advisers could lobby colleagues in closed-door meetings.

Burton was eager to air some dirty regulatory laundry. He believed the conflicts might have played a role in why so many new vaccines were added in quick succession to the schedule, including the ill-fated Rotashield.

"Was there evidence to indicate that the vaccine was not safe?" he asked.

"If so, why was it licensed in the first place? How good a job did the advisory committees do? We've identified a number of problems that need to be brought to light and discussed."

Burton asked that the financial reports of the advisory committee members be included in the public record. Henry Waxman strenuously opposed that. "There's a right way and a wrong way to investigate conflicts of interest," Waxman scolded the chairman. "The right way is to investigate first, and then reach conclusions later. The wrong way is to accuse first and then investigate later. Unfortunately, our Chairman has a propensity to investigate in the wrong way, not just in this issue, but in other issues. He has made unsubstantiated allegations that smear people's reputations but turn out to have no basis in fact."

Burton continued his line of attack. He said that an "old boys' network" of vaccine advisers was rotating between the CDC and FDA, at times serving simultaneously. "How confident in the safety and need for specific vaccines would doctors and parents be," he asked, "if they learned that:

- Members of the FDA and CDC advisory committees who make these decisions own stock in drug companies that make vaccines.
- Individuals on both advisory committees own patents for vaccines under consideration or affected by the decisions of the committee.
- Three out of five of the members of the FDA's advisory committee who voted for the rotavirus vaccine had conflicts of interest that were waived.
- Seven of the 15 members on the FDA committee were not present at the meeting, two others were excluded from the vote, and the remaining five were joined by five temporary voting members who all voted to license the product.
- The CDC grants conflict-of-interest waivers to every member of their advisory committee a year at a time, and allows full participation in the discussions leading up to a vote by every member, whether they have a financial stake in the decision or not.
- CDC's advisory committee has no public members—no parents have a vote in whether or not a vaccine belongs on the childhood immunization schedule. The FDA's committee only has one public member.

"The entire process has been polluted and the public trust has been violated," Burton charged. "No individual who stands to gain financially from the decisions regarding vaccines that may be mandated for use should be participating in the discussion or policy making for vaccines."

Waxman jumped to defend the advisers and went on the attack against Burton. "My fear is that the Chairman has reached a predetermined conclusion that vaccines are dangerous," the Democrat said. "It is difficult for him to persuade others to agree with his conclusion because it is so far out of the scientific and medical mainstream. But rather than accept the fact that he may be wrong, the Chairman decided that those who disagree with him must be part of a drug company conspiracy."

Waxman doubted that Burton would be able to demonstrate that "vaccine decisions have been tainted by scandal." Burton countered that he found it hard to believe the government could not find "leading experts" without financial interests in the drug industry. "The problem with the bureaucracy is, you keep saying, 'Well, we can't do this because we might not be able to attract people to these advisory committees,'" he said. "Look, there are 700,000 doctors. There must be somebody else out there in that vast mass of humanity that has the expertise to be able to be on these advisory boards."

JUST DAYS after their meeting at the CDC, Lyn was hitting the books once again, this time at the medical library of Atlanta's Emory University, where fatigued med students crashed on the couches in the main lounge. Lyn was doing research on blood and hair levels of mercury in exposed patients, when she found an article that she could have used as ammunition against the CDC in Atlanta.

The study appeared back in 1995 in the journal *Environmental Health Perspectives,* published by the National Institute of Environmental Health Sciences, a division of the NIH. The article was titled "Neurobehavioral Effects of Developmental Methylmercury Exposure," and was authored by Steven G. Gilbert and Kimberly S. Grant-Webster, researchers at the University of Washington's School of Public Health.

Because infants and fetuses were more sensitive to the adverse effects of methylmercury, the article warned, federal standards for daily exposure should be lowered radically in order to protect the most sensitive segments of the population. "Based on results from human and animal studies on the developmental neurotoxic effects of methylmercury," it concluded, "the accepted reference dose should be lowered to between 0.025 and 0.06 mcg/kg/day. Continued research on the neurotoxic effects associated with low level developmental exposure is needed."[96]

Lyn's face froze. Here was an article in a government-sponsored publication arguing that the lowest current maximum exposure level, 0.1 microgram per kilogram, was still too high. Lyn got out her calculator again. If the maximum level had been established at 0.025 as recommended, then Will's exposure of 62.5 micrograms at two months of age would have been *500 times* over the limit, rather than 125 times, as she had calculated previously.

"My God," Lyn thought. "If Davis had applied this standard to his study, almost all the kids with autism would have fallen above the EPA limit." Lyn was so angry she could not sit still. She felt the need to pick up the phone and talk to someone. She needed to vent. She thought of Bob Davis out there at the University of Washington. Why not? She picked up the phone and quickly punched in the numbers.

"Dr. Davis, this is Lyn Redwood," she began, "the mother of a boy with autism from Atlanta."

"Yes." His voice was cordial, but not warm. "How can I help you?"

"It's about your VSD study."

"What about it?"

"I don't think you did this right."

Lyn could tell that Davis would ignore this. Instead, she found the doctor showering her with sympathy. It was the last thing she wanted. "I'm sorry about your son," he said. "I can't imagine what it must be like."

"Thank you, I appreciate that. But I'm going to say it again, Doctor." Biting her lip in resolve, she said, "I think you got it wrong. You didn't look at cumulative exposure. You only looked at the first three months of life. And you did not factor in prenatal exposure from Rho(D) globulin."

Davis said he would consult with colleagues and thanked her for "pointing out that potential source of exposure."[97]

ON JUNE 21, 2000, the CDC's Advisory Committee on Immunization Practices held a regularly scheduled meeting in Atlanta. The Vaccine Datalink thimerosal study was included on the agenda, and there was no way that Lyn was going to miss it.

The Mercury Moms fully expected the CDC to announce that it had found zero associations between thimerosal use and neurological disorders, as they had been told at the CDC teleconference. They assumed that the Davis study would be presented, and that would be that. The mercury case would be closed and the controversy would fade away.

Lyn braced for a battle. She had collected letters from Sallie, Heidi, Albert, and Teresa, all of them attacking Davis and his colleagues for what they said was a shoddily constructed report. Lyn herself prepared a critique of the analysis that she planned to deliver during the public comment session. She also had the parents' mercury-autism paper in hand, to be entered into the record.

But halfway into the meeting, Lyn returned the speech to her briefcase.

The CDC team, it turned out, had performed another round of analyses on the data, and produced decidedly different results.[98] This time the team, led by Dr. Thomas Verstraeten, looked at some 110,000 children enrolled in just two

of the HMOs: Northern California Kaiser (NCK) and Group Health Cooperative (GHC). The two were chosen because they had computerized records of all
patient data, making complex analyses possible, explained Verstraeten, a thin,
pleasant-looking man with curly dark-blond hair, wire-frame glasses, and a
slightly guttural Flemish accent, a product of his native Belgium.

This was certainly news to Lyn. Still, she expected that this new version
would reveal the same lack of association between thimerosal and neurological outcomes found in the Davis study.

She was unprepared for what was to come next.

"It is difficult to interpret the crude results," Verstraeten began, somewhat hesitantly. Lyn expected to hear vague reassurances from the European
statistician, but instead he announced: "Researchers found statistically significant associations between thimerosal and neurodevelopmental disorders."

Lyn thought she had surely misheard. Was it possible the government was
admitting that thimerosal had harmed kids? Her head buzzed.

The team had calculated the "relative risk" for a number of outcomes,
based on various exposure levels among the children, Verstraeten said. In
other words, they determined the odds of there being a neurological outcome
with each incremental increase in exposure (0, 12.5, 25, 37.5, 50, and 62.5
micrograms or more).

"What these estimates suggest," Verstraeten said, "is that there seems to
be an increasing trend, an increasing risk for any of these outcomes, any of
these neurological developmental outcomes, with increasing thimerosal exposure among kids who received the highest exposures, compared with children who received little or no mercury at all."

The researchers first combined a number of outcomes into a general umbrella category called "neurological developmental disorders," which included
autism, and found "an increased risk with increased cumulative exposure at
one month, three months, and six months of age," Verstraeten said.

Lyn was horrified and fascinated at once.

When the general NDD category was broken down into individual outcomes, the team also found a "statistically significant relationship for tics and
exposure at three months," Verstraeten announced. For ADD, a relationship
was found for exposures at six months; for language and speech delays, relationships were found for exposures at one, three, and six months; and for
"unspecified delays," relationships were found for exposures at two and
three months.

Most of the increased risks were only moderately elevated, but the trends
were unmistakable, and many results were statistically significant. For instance, the increased risk for a "neurological developmental disorder" with
every microgram of exposure at three months was calculated at 1.007, or a

FIGURE 1. Relative risk +95% CI of *developmental neurological disorders* after different exposure levels of thimerosal at 3 months of age, NCK & CHC, Cycle 7.

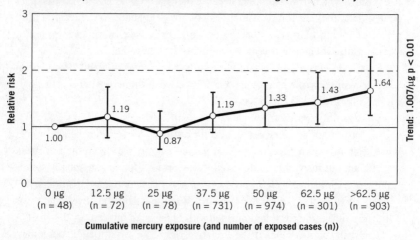

Cumulative mercury exposure (and number of exposed cases (n))

Source: Dr. Thomas Verstraeten, from Graph 2, "Minutes from the Meeting of the Advisory Committee on Immunization Practices," CDC, Atlanta, July 19, 2000.

"trend" of a 0.7 percent increased risk per microgram. As Verstraeten explained it: "If you go from 12.5 to 62.5 micrograms of cumulative mercury exposure in the first three months of life, that would be an increase of over 50 micrograms. We have to multiply this number (1.007, or 0.7 percent) by 50, and that would mean a relative risk of 1.35 for this category." In other words, children exposed to 62.5 micrograms were 35 percent more likely to have a neurological developmental disorder than children exposed to 12.5 micrograms.

The relative risk of 1.64 was considered statistically significant because the margin of error (the 95 percent confidence interval) remained above a risk of 1.0.

When the team broke down the umbrella NDD category into individual outcomes, they found the following.

For attention deficit disorder, they found a statistically significant, dose-dependent response for exposure at six months of age. The increased relative risk for each microgram of ethylmercury was 1.006—or 0.6 percent. Therefore, a child who received 62.5 micrograms by six months of age was 30 percent more likely (RR 1:30) to develop ADD than a child who received 12.5 micrograms (because 0.6 percent multiplied by 50 mcg = 0.30).

In the same way, statistically significant increased risks for language disorder were found at one month (RR 1.019, or a trend of 1.9 percent per microgram), three months (RR 1.021, or 2.1 percent per microgram), and six months of age (RR 1.06, or 0.6 percent per microgram). The results at three

FIGURE 2. Relative risk +95% CI of *developmental language disorder* after different exposure levels of thimerosal at 3 months of age, NCK & GHC, Cycle 7.

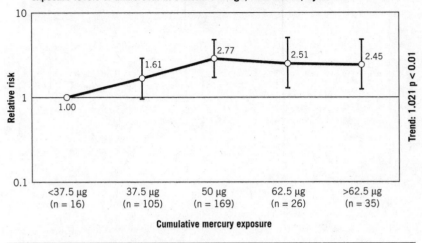

Source: Dr. Thomas Verstraeten, Graph 12, from "Minutes from the Meeting of the Advisory Committee on Immunization Practices," CDC, Atlanta, July 19, 2000.

months of exposure were especially alarming. Using the same example of a 50-microgram differentiation, children who received 62.5 micrograms of ethylmercury by three months of age, compared with children who received 12.5 micrograms, had an elevated risk of 2.10—they were 110 percent more likely to develop a language disorder.

Increased risks per microgram of exposure were also found for speech delay: one month (RR 1.011), three months (RR 1.008), and six months (RR 1.002); unspecified delays: two months (RR 1.005) and three months (RR 1.007); and tics: three months (RR 1.021).

"Some of these are borderline statistically significant," Verstraeten said. "Some of them are highly statistically significant."

As for autism, the relative risk at three months of age in the highest exposure group was calculated at 1.69, meaning that these children were 69 percent more likely to develop autism than baseline, which in this case was "less than 37.5 mcg." The findings, however, were not statistically significant because the margin of error (95 percent confidence interval) fell below a risk of 1.0, meaning that the results could be due to chance alone.

It was not the only big news of the day. The CDC team had conducted a Phase II segment of the study. They had acquired data from a third HMO outside of the Vaccine Safety Datalink system, Harvard Pilgrim, in Massachusetts. The investigators wanted to see if their findings in the first two HMOs could be replicated in the third. But, Verstraeten said, "Analyses of these data using

FIGURE 3. Relative risk +95% CI of *autism* after different exposure levels of thimerosal at 3 months of age, NCK & GHC, Cycle 7.

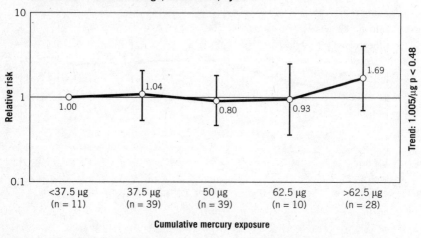

Source: Dr. Thomas Verstraeten, Graph 4, from "Minutes from the Meeting of the Advisory Committee on Immunization Practices," CDC, Atlanta, July 19, 2000.

the same methods as the first study did not confirm results seen in the first phase."

Even if the CDC had not replicated the findings in the Harvard Pilgrim HMO, and even if they could not show a definitive link with autism, the fact that they had associated thimerosal with other neurological disorders was unprecedented. Lyn turned to the well-dressed men sitting on either side of her.

"Can you *believe* this?" she asked them, practically giddy. "They're confessing! They are admitting that thimerosal causes harm! This is amazing."

The two men sat expressionless. They were neither impressed nor amused. Lyn surmised that they were pharmaceutical reps, and she let it go.

There was yet one more surprise in store for Lyn. Dr. Paul Stehr-Green, an associate professor of epidemiology at the University of Washington, announced that the CDC had convened an invitation-only meeting two weeks before, at the Simpsonwood Retreat north of Atlanta, where government, academic, and drug industry officials had reviewed and commented on the Verstraeten report.

"The group expressed unanimous feelings that the findings supported a statistically significant, although weak association, but that the implications for obvious reasons are profound," Stehr-Green said. He said that new studies should be pursued "with a degree of urgency," not only for the sake of U.S. public health policy, "but for public health policy around the world."

Dr. Stehr-Green then projected a slide describing the conclusion of the consultants at Simpsonwood: "Although the findings of the VSD screening analyses were insufficient to support a causal relationship between exposure to thimerosal-containing vaccines and selected neurological disorders, [this] should be vigorously pursued along several lines of investigation." The jury, in other words, was still very much out.

Lyn whipped out her cell phone and called Sallie. "What do I do?" she asked. "I came here ready to trash the Davis study, but now they are saying there are statistically significant associations between thimerosal and neurological outcomes. Help!"

"Lyn," Sallie replied, "you know how to handle this. They just gave you an opening, so run with it. You'll have to wing it. I know you can."

When it came time for public comment, Lyn was one of the first to line up at the mike. "My son was one of the children that received the highest possible amount of exposure. I feel strongly that mercury toxicity from excessive exposure to thimerosal played a significant role in the development of his disease," she informed the panel. "I have been researching mercury toxicity and I have found the parallels between mercury toxicity and those of pervasive developmental disorder uncanny, so uncanny that I can't think it could possibly be a chance occurrence," she continued.

"I have worked for the last six months with a number of other parents and have compiled a document that I would like to present to the Committee today that identifies a lot of the parallels between autism and pervasive developmental disorder and mercury toxicity," she said. "I would just like to say, please don't compromise our children. Don't let the vaccine programs take priority over their safety."

When it was over and Lyn was driving home, she shuddered at the thought of what Verstraeten had admitted. She traveled down the Interstate toward Tyrone, barely able to grip the wheel. She felt as if she knew a terrible secret, one that could spark mass panic. She wanted to shout from her car, warn everybody on the highway about the dangers of thimerosal. How many more kids would be injured? Lyn felt like a different creature from the people in the other cars going about their lives. She knew, but who would listen?

"My God," she muttered, "this really *did* happen. Our worst fears really were true." Until now, this had been the parents' offbeat hypothesis and theirs alone. They had no one in power to support them. Now they had the first bit of official evidence to back up what they had been saying.

"I guess," Lyn told herself, "we're not so crazy after all."

6. Safe Minds

IT'S GOING TO BE a scorcher," Lyn muttered as she set out on a muggy morning stroll through the still-sleepy streets of Capitol Hill, the rising sun just a dull glow in the eastern haze. It was July 11, 2000, and the summertime tourists and congressional staffers were still a few hours away from their descent upon the marble halls of power. Lyn had found a moment to steel her wits for the day ahead: another Government Reform Committee hearing chaired by Dan Burton, and this time the Mercury Moms were slated to testify.

She wandered back to her hotel, a "boutique" B&B in the shadow of the Capitol, where she was rooming with Liz Birt, in from Chicago. They had coffee and croissants on dainty twin sofas in the lobby's intimate anteroom, as Lyn nervously speculated on how the hearing would go. "There are some pretty big guns on the other side," she said.

"I know," Liz said, her face tight and set for battle. "FDA. CDC. NIH. They're all going to say our theory is bunk."

"I just hope we're ready for the attack," Lyn said.

"We're ready, Lyn. We've been preparing for months, we have the science."

"But *still*. They're going to try to make us look like a bunch of hysterical mothers. Like we think we know more than they do."

"Maybe," Liz suggested, "we do."

The women walked outside into the pea-soup morning and crossed the west lawn of the Capitol to the Rayburn Building. Sallie and Albert were already there, enjoying the fresh blast of chilled air in the small anteroom reserved for witnesses and staff. Beth Clay was conferring with committee staff when Lyn and Liz walked in.

The hearing would be divided into two panels. The parents, there to make the mercury connection case, would speak for two hours before lunch. The government panel of vaccine experts would then testify for two hours after lunch.

In addition to the three Mercury Moms and Albert Enayati, two other mothers had traveled to Washington to testify. Sharon Hunniston, a physician from Virginia, was a noted vaccine expert and former CDC employee. Also on hand was Stephanie Cave, a physician from Baton Rouge, who claimed to have had remarkable success giving chelation therapy to ASD kids. Lyn admired the sharp-talking, strong-willed Cave, who with her tall and square frame, short-cropped hair, and southern accent cut a commanding presence.

The doors swung open and committee staff led the parents into the cavernous wood-paneled hearing room, its oversized windows laced with bronze Art-Deco grills. There were views out to Independence Avenue and the Capitol gardens beyond. Various Hill staffers had wandered in. But there were no media.

The parents took their front-row seats. Liz jabbed a gentle elbow into Lyn, motioning her to look toward the back of the room, where three men in dark suits surveyed the crowd. One of them spoke into a cell phone.

"Security?" Lyn wondered aloud. "Secret Service?"

Beth, who was sitting nearby, had a more sinister theory. "Pharmaceutical guys," she said. "Here to report to headquarters about everything that's said today." Lyn turned around to gaze at the men. She tried to make eye contact, but they only stared at the ceiling, or out the window into the languid haze.

Committee members entered the chambers and took their seats along the elevated podium. Meanwhile the back of the room had filled up with busloads of tourists, filing through to see their government in action. Lyn, for one, was somewhat unnerved by the unexpected audience of camera-toting families in Bermuda shorts.

Dan Burton's opening statement began somewhat defensively, not surprisingly, given all the criticism he had taken for his pursuit of the autism-vaccine question.

"For the last year," he began, "the Government Reform Committee has been looking at issues regarding vaccine safety, research, and policy. A few people have tried to portray this investigation as anti-vaccine. Nothing could be further from the truth."

Was it irresponsible to hold hearings? "Of course not," Burton answered his own question. "If someone holds hearings on mismanagement at the Department of Education, that doesn't mean they're anti-education."

Then he shifted to combat mode. "The FDA continues to allow mercury-containing vaccines to remain on the market," he said. "Today, over eight thousand children in America may be given a toxic dose of mercury in their vaccines. No area is so sacrosanct that the world will come to an end if we ask some sensible questions and expect to get some sensible answers."[99]

The attack drew an equally heated counterattack by Democrat Henry Waxman.

"The purpose of this hearing appears to be to publicize the theory that thimerosal is causing autism," Waxman said. "The evidence to support this theory is virtually nonexistent. I fear that once again we are pursuing an anti-vaccine agenda in disregard for the scientific and medical consensus on the safety of vaccines."

Waxman complained that Rep. Dave Weldon, the Republican from Florida who had met with Liz and Andy Wakefield in the spring, had been invited to sit with the committee during the hearing, even though he was not a member of that panel.

Waxman continued: "The Chairman has promoted allegations that MMR vaccines cause autism. And he has alleged that parents should be skeptical about vaccines because our government is beholden to the drug industry."

Though Burton had to squirm to contain his anger, he remained silent, if somewhat smug, a wooden gavel always at hand. "This," said Waxman, looking directly at the chairman, "is a backward attitude to take."

Burton ignored the Democrat. With the obvious advantage of his power, he allowed his nemesis to finish. He did not answer the challenge. In fact, Liz thought she saw him yawn and check his watch. After a respectful interval, Burton called the first panel, the parents, to the witness table.

Lyn went first. Dressed in a simple black business suit, with scant makeup and no jewelry, she was trembling and obviously nervous. But she minced no words. "Millions of children have been needlessly exposed to toxic agents from federally-sponsored vaccine programs and have suffered neurological damage," she said, looking up at the panel to gauge their reaction. The Republicans seemed supportive, with encouraging little nods and smiles. The Democrats, Lyn thought, were impassive at best.

"Since last fall when I discovered my son's mercury toxicity, I have spent every free moment further investigating this issue," Lyn continued, her voice shaking from the enormity of the moment, from the pressure of having tourists watch her testimony, and from the sheer emotion that packed every word. "I did research, I made phone calls, I wrote letters and actually went in person to meet with FDA and CDC officials to voice my concerns."

By now, Lyn was fighting back tears. It had been an exhausting few months, and this was the most draining moment of all. "All of my efforts," she said with deep sadness in her voice, "seemed to fall on deaf ears. The statement that there is 'no evidence of harm' does not equate to *no* harm having occurred. The truth is that we have not adequately looked, or we just refuse to see."

There were rumblings of approval among many in the audience. It heartened Lyn, gave her more confidence. Her voice steadied as she drove home the speech. "It is time," she demanded, "for someone to step forward and acknowledge these facts and provide the science to fully investigate what has happened to our children and what can be done to help them. Some may say we don't have a smoking gun, but the truth is there are bullets all over the floor!"

Several tourists gasped audibly, a rare occurrence in a congressional hearing. The committee looked stunned, the parents content. Lyn felt dizzy.

Sallie went next. Dressed in a white suit with black piping and matching scarf, her light blond hair clipped short, she cut a handsome figure at the witness table.

"I have some slides," she said in typically unruffled fashion. Sallie projected her charts onto a screen that Burton's staff set up in the hearing room, which had fallen into silence. "Research conducted by me and others has shown that the characteristics of autism itself are identical to those arising from mercury exposure."

Audible gasps rippled though the room. Many tourists shook their heads and shuffled their feet uncomfortably. By the time Sallie got to pink disease, she and the other parents could tell: people were becoming convinced. She told the panel that acrodynia was an example of how a severe disorder, afflicting a small but significant percentage of children, can arise from a benign application of low doses of mercury.

Then Sallie turned to the Vaccine Safety Datalink. "A recent CDC study has found a statistically significant association between thimerosal and vaccines specifically, and attention deficit disorders, speech delay, motor tics, and neurodevelopmental disorders in general," she said. "Given this possibility, thimerosal should be removed from all childhood vaccines, and the mechanisms of mercury toxicity in autism should be thoroughly investigated."

When Stephanie Cave's turn came, she began by reminding the congressmembers that, contrary to what they might have heard, autism in America "is truly an epidemic. If you have the idea that it is not, I invite you to sit in my office for two hours." Her clinic was treating over three hundred autistic children, she said, with an additional hundred and fifty waiting to get in.

Cave said she was convinced that mercury had caused the autistic symptoms, because the vaccines corresponded to "critical periods of neuronal development" in infants, when the blood-brain barrier is not fully developed and bile production is minimal, "making it more difficult for metals to be cleared from the body."

Cave's clinic had studied the body's detoxification process and found it to be "woefully inadequate in developmentally delayed children." Ethylmercury, she insisted, enters the brain and is converted to inorganic mercury, which cannot cross back over the blood-brain barrier. This inorganic form, she said, was more likely "to cause autoimmune antibodies to brain tissue, and this is what we are seeing in these children."

And, Cave added, mercury exposure was causing problems beyond autism. "I fear that we've underestimated the devastation by concentrating only on the autistic children," she said. She had found elevated mercury levels in children with milder difficulties, like learning disabilities, ADHD, and Asperger's syndrome.

As a rule, Dr. Cave tested every developmentally delayed child patient for the presence of heavy metals. "Hair is screened, followed by a determination in urine after a challenge of an oral chelator," she said. "It's rare that we find a child with developmental problems who does not have increased levels of mercury in the urine after a chelation."

The children were responding well to oral chelators and supplements to remove metals, she said. "The changes in the children are remarkable with each dose of a chelator. The chance for recovery is evident on a daily basis. Changes in neurological functioning are remarkable with each day of treatment."

Liz was next to take the microphone. Dressed in a dark red jacket, with no-nonsense reading glasses framing her unflinching face, she looked more like an angry librarian than a skilled attorney. She outlined her son's misery in depressing detail. "Matthew has physical problems, including antibodies to myelin basic protein, abnormal EEG, inflammatory bowel disease, and live measles virus in his terminal ileum," she said. "His immunologist believes that the thimerosal contained in the vaccines contributed to the development of these medical conditions and they have led to his contraction of the live measles virus by priming his immune system for an adverse reaction.

"My son was injured for the greater good," Liz went on. Committee members leaned forward in their plush leather chairs. "But these children have voices. They have the voices of their parents, many of whom are in this room." Liz continued, her voice rising, "And those voices will be heard, no matter how unpleasant the message."

Liz conceded that many experts were asking, "How dare a member of the public speak out with such convictions?" But, she said, "It doesn't take a genius to discern the truth from spin. Why is thimerosal even in these vaccines? Why hasn't it been recalled? And why aren't parents being told about the truth by the CDC?"

The tourists in the back of the room looked dumbstruck.

Following the break, Burton introduced the government experts. They included Dr. William Egan, Dr. Marie Bristol-Power, and Dr. Roger Bernier, of the CDC's National Immunization Program. Burton wasted no time ripping into the bureaucrats.

"If this, *thim . . . thim . . .* How do you pronounce it?" he had to ask Beth Clay, working at his side. Clearly, this was still a new issue. "This thimerosal," he growled. "If it's not really a problem, then why are you phasing it out of vaccines?"

Lyn's heart began beating a little faster. She looked down the row. Liz and Sallie had the same reaction. They were smiling. The congressman had gathered his ammo. The former sergeant was poised for attack.

"Well . . ." Egan sputtered, "um, although we, um . . . although . . . I, or we, are not aware of any evidence . . . of any *convincing* data on—"

"We are talking about mercury!" Burton interrupted.

"Well, yes," Egan said, sounding defensive. "But we are nonetheless committed to removing all sources of mercury from children. And we are also concerned about the potential risk . . ." He was straying from the prepared script. "*Some* people are worried about data of exposure at low levels."

"Hmmm, low levels. That's interesting," Burton grinned. "My grandson got 62 times, *62 times,* the acceptable level. In one day!" He reminded Egan that an FDA panel had concluded in 1982 that thimerosal was "toxic, causes cell damage and allergic reactions, and isn't effective in killing bacteria. That was 18 years ago. And you keep saying there's no conclusive evidence?" He paused to chew on his glasses. "Why *is* that?"

"That report, Congressman, was referring to thimerosal in topical material, and in high concentrations," Egan said.

Burton couldn't help but interrupt again. "Oh! It's bad for them on the outside," he seethed, "so you give it to them on the *inside?*" Nervous laughter tittered across the room. Burton pressed on. "You know, Doctor, one of the things that concerns me, you say that mercury in vaccines hasn't been proven to cause this problem. Then how do you account for these dramatic rises? Do you think it's all genetic?"

"I . . . I don't know," pleaded Egan, looking almost hurt that Burton would ask the question. "I don't know the causes of the rise of autism."

"Well you've got to admit that it's a dramatic rise."

"It is dramatic. And I would agree with your assessment of it as 'epidemic.'"

"And mercury is a poison . . . *right*?"

"It's a neurotoxin. Yes."

"And the FDA and CDC are committed to phasing it out. Well, why not get rid of it immediately? Why not today? If you have a supply of non-thimerosal vaccines on hand to protect children, why are we continuing to put mercury into their bodies?"

Egan had no ready answer. The parents looked at each other in awe. Never did they imagine such a public chewing out of an FDA official, in the halls of Congress, no less. The day was turning out to be better than they hoped.

Another exchange, between Burton and the CDC's Roger Bernier, also let Burton showcase his defiance. Bernier had insisted that much of the mercury in vaccines had already been removed, and more was on the way out. "Last year at this time, a child could receive 187.5 micrograms of ethyl mercury from vaccines," Bernier said. "Today that maximum is down to 75 micrograms. We have now reached a point where six of the seven vaccines are free of thimerosal as a preservative, and we believe the seventh one [diphtheria-tetanus-acellular-pertussis] will be as soon as six to nine months now, which is in early 2001."

Burton was unimpressed. "Seventy-five micrograms," he repeated with unmasked scorn. And then he told the doctor: "1.5 micrograms is considered safe."

"I am not sure where you get that value, Mr. Chairman," Bernier fired back.

"For a thirty-three-pound child," Burton explained. "According to what we have found through our research, 1.5 micrograms is what is acceptable."

Bernier had no answer for this, except to repeat the now-familiar government mantra: "There is no data . . . ." He paused. "There is no *compelling* evidence at this time . . . of any harm that has come to any child from vaccines that contain thimerosal as a preservative." The parents thought Bernier was waffling, too. This was the same language Egan had used. Yes, there was data. It just wasn't "compelling" enough to warrant the removal of mercury.

"What a crock," Sallie whispered to Lyn.

Rep. Helen Chenoweth-Hage, a far-right Republican from Idaho who also has an autistic grandchild, agreed with Sallie, though she didn't quite phrase it that way. With her dark wavy hair, grandmotherly deportment, midwestern twang, and ah-shucks speech, she seemed like a schoolteacher scolding errant students.

"You guys . . . you *witnesses*. You know, you absolutely amaze me," she lectured the experts. "I wonder what the disconnect is, for Pete's sake! Did you listen to the same testimony I did?" Chenoweth-Hage began raising her voice to more than a grandmotherly decibel level. The room fell still. The tourists halted their shifting. Chenoweth-Hage pounded her finger on the desk. "And you're willing to tell us, with a straight face, that you are *eventually* going to phase this out?" She threw up her arms in exasperation. "Eventually? After we know that a small, tiny baby's body is slammed with 62 times the mercury it's supposed to have?" Now her arms were flailing.

"It doesn't make sense! No wonder people are losing faith in their government. And to have one of you tell us it's because mothers eat too much *fish*? C'mon! We expect you to get real." Her anger level rose even more. "We heard devastating testimony at this hearing. And this is the kind of response we get from our government *agencies*?" A thunderclap of applause echoed through the room.

In a prophetic pronouncement, Chenoweth-Hage warned the officials: "Just you wait 'til this gets in the courts. This case could dwarf the tobacco case, for Pete's sake. You know, if a jury were to look at this, the circumstantial evidence would be overwhelming. And we'd expect you to do something now, before that circus starts taking place." Scattered applause broke out again. "Denial is simply not *proper* right now!"

Lyn, Liz, and Sallie sat up in their chairs, elated. "Hooray for Helen," Liz whispered.

"Yeah," said Lyn, tears welling in her eyes. "You go girl. Give 'em hell!"

Caught up in the drama of the moment, Chenoweth-Hage pulled out the parents' mercury report and waved it above her head. "I have read this very excellent report by Sallie Bernard," she told the bureaucrats. "And I recommend that you get out of your paralysis of analysis and start by reading this. Folks! This passes the duck test, folks. It walks like a duck. It talks like a duck. It's a duck!"

The room erupted with clapping and hooting. Lyn noticed that the men in dark suits in the back of the room were now sprinting out into the hall, scowling as they dialed headquarters on their cell phones.

LYN REDWOOD went back to Georgia feeling victorious. Finally, some progress was being made. But pride quickly turned to paranoia.

Lyn noticed peculiar noises on her phone line. Whenever she would talk to other parents, or lawyers, or researchers, when she would say the word *autism* or *thimerosal,* her phone would rumble and click, as if a tape recorder were switching on. People on the other end of the line always assumed it was call-waiting making the noise. For a while, Lyn thought nothing of it. Barbara Loe Fisher—hearing the sound while on the phone with Lyn—told her about similar noises reported by parents in Texas after they had publicly taken on that state's mandatory birth dose of hepatitis-B vaccine.

"This is serious business," Lyn told Tommy soon after the clicks appeared. "And it really pisses me off that someone would listen in." But she added, somewhat hopefully, "I guess we really hit a nerve. Someone must be very upset at us."

Though she was starting to feel a little bit like Karen Silkwood, Lyn was not genuinely worried for her safety. But the phone clicks were creepy, and she wanted to find out if the line was tapped. She called the FBI.

"Well," the woman at the Atlanta Bureau inquired, "have you been threatened?" Lyn said she had not. "Then there's nothing we can do," the FBI woman replied. "Let me know if you get threatened and we'll look into it." By this point, Lyn felt as if every federal agency had let her down. Why should the FBI be any different?[100]

The Redwoods called a private debugging firm, which came to the house and checked out the lines. Nothing was amiss. "If you are being tapped," the inspector told her, "they probably did it down at the switching station." The phone company refused to allow the private inspectors into the station.[101]

Lyn had a friend in Washington with high-level access to government databases. He checked her home number against every list available, but it did not appear anywhere. If someone was monitoring her calls, it wasn't the government. Lyn suspected private industry. From that point on, she did all her autism-related business on a cell phone.

IF THERE WAS some peril to being a thimerosal activist, there was also comfort in numbers, however small the band of parents may have been. It was time for the Mercury Moms (and some dads, too) to formalize their relationship.

Liz drew up the papers of incorporation and filed with the IRS for tax-exempt status. There would be a board of directors, with Lyn as president, Sallie as executive director, Albert as secretary, Liz as legal counsel, and Heidi as treasurer. David Baskin would serve as scientific director, and Jim Moody would be the "Washington advocate." The group would be called the Coalition for Sensible Action for Ending Mercury Induced Neurological Disorders, or Safe Minds. It would be based out of Sallie's Cranford, New Jersey, office.[102]

A major order of business was how the new group could get its hands on the raw data in the Vaccine Safety Datalink analysis. Liz would begin drafting Freedom of Information Act requests to be filed with the CDC concerning all data and other information the agency had generated in its review. Safe Minds wanted access to all documents, including interagency e-mails among federal workers. And now that they knew about the secret Simpsonwood Retreat conference, the parents wanted the minutes from that meeting as well.

Lyn volunteered for another project. She had contacted a biochemist from the University of Kentucky, Boyd Haley, who had spent ten years researching the toxic effects of mercury in dental fillings and their possible link to Alzheimer's disease. Haley, who was chairman of the university's Chemistry Department, had incurred the ire of the American Dental Association for his theories, though they were backed up by published studies, including the one cited by the National Academy of Sciences.[103]

Haley had demonstrated how vapor from mercury in fillings could be released, through constant chewing, into the bloodstream and eventually the brain. Haley also showed that amalgams released enough mercury vapor to contaminate a large beaker with toxic levels of mercury in just twenty-four hours.

Haley hypothesized that mercury vapor from dental amalgams was slowly destroying brain tubulin and creatine kinase, two brain proteins vital to normal functioning that he said are dramatically sensitive to mercury inhibition. These proteins were found to be highly deficient in Alzheimer's patients, but not in healthy seniors.[104] And, based on his military experience, Haley had proposed that Gulf War syndrome might have thimerosal as a causal factor, given all the vaccinations that soldiers received prior to overseas assignment.

An obvious question presented itself: Why would some older people be susceptible to amalgam mercury, but not others? Haley thought it had to do with genetic susceptibility, as supported by a recently discovered gene that had been found to be a risk factor in Alzheimer's disease. Lyn found the idea fascinating. She wondered if the genetic susceptibility to mercury toxicity identified by Haley in Alzheimer's might hold a clue to the link they were looking for in autism.

Lyn contacted Haley, and he seemed eager to help. Lyn proposed, and the other parents concurred, that she would acquire several thimerosal-containing vaccines (using prescriptions written by Tommy) and ship them off to Haley, who would test them for toxicity. She would also urge Haley to apply for one of the vaccine-autism research grants that were under consideration by the MIND Institute.

Another pressing matter was that Safe Minds had been asked to send an envoy to an invitation-only brainstorming session on vaccines and autism being organized by Bernie Rimland, of Defeat Autism Now! and the Autism Research Institute. It was to take place in a few days' time at the Arizona Biltmore, a high-end resort in Phoenix. Lyn, though she wasn't thrilled about the prospect of Arizona in July, volunteered to go.

She was glad she did. Lyn got to know some of the leading lights of the movement—the renegade parents and doctor activists who would be key allies in the coming battle.

In addition to Bernie Rimland, Lyn spent time with Jeffrey Bradstreet, a doctor from Florida who ran a large autism treatment center; Stephanie Cave, the physician from Louisiana she had met at the Burton hearing; Amy Holmes, also from Louisiana and a parent of an autistic child, who worked with Dr. Cave on chelation studies; and Dr. Jeff Segal, a neurosurgeon who had quit his successful practice in order to conduct research that might one day help his autistic son, back home in Greensboro, North Carolina. Jane El-Dahr, the expert on autism and immunity from Tulane who had been in Atlanta for the May 15 CDC teleconference, was also there.

The think tank kicked off with everyone going around the table identifying themselves and their particular area of interest. Lyn was dismayed, but not terribly surprised, that most people wanted to discuss MMR, dietary interventions, and other issues. The Joint Statement of the FDA, the Public Health Service, and the AAP had been out for over a year, and no was talking about mercury. No one, that is, until Lyn's turn came.

Lyn delivered a forceful presentation on Will's case, on the mercury he received in vaccines, and on the acute neurotoxicity of mercury. She also told the group about the Verstraeten VSD data, which linked thimerosal to neurological developmental disorders.

When she finished, Lyn expected the conversation to turn back to MMR. She was pleasantly surprised. Sitting next to her was the tag-team of doctors Cave, Holmes, and El-Dahr, three supporters of the autism-mercury hypothesis. Cave and Holmes gave detailed accounts of children they had treated who excreted almost unimaginable amounts of mercury. The doctors said that every child had benefited in some way from chelation. Some had made miraculous recoveries. Their motor skills, memory, attention, immune function, and general well-being returned, sometimes fully, especially among younger kids who also received therapies such as Applied Behavior Analysis.

Amy Holmes said her own son Mike was doing "just great" following chelation. One year before, the boy could not talk. Now he wouldn't shut up. "He's become bossy," Amy said. "And I'll take bossy over mute anytime." In fact, Mike had officially shed his DMS-IV diagnosis of full-blown autism. It was simply gone.

Jane El-Dahr, the immunologist, spoke next. Vaccine mercury was most likely causing autism through two separate mechanisms, she said. The first was through direct neurotoxicity. Mercury was known to destroy certain brain and nerve cells that control motor and communication skills. This was likely to be what was happening in autistic kids.

The second mechanism was more complicated and indirect. Mercury is known to cause immune problems that set up an intricate chain of events that can damage the body in many ways. Various studies had identified immune abnormalities in 30 to 70 percent of patients with autism. There were three types of immune problems involved, and many autistic kids exhibited signs of all three:

1. *Immune dysfunction*—marked by chronic infections, not unlike patients with AIDS. Many kids she examined had presented with very high levels of cytomegalovirus, a virus known to cause damage in people with advanced HIV infection.
2. *Hypersensitivity*—a potentially dangerous allergic reaction to mercury mounted within the immune system.
3. *Autoimmunity*—in which autoantibodies produced by mercury exposure attack the brain and other parts of the body, much as in lupus.

Sensitivity to mercury ranged widely among individuals. In fetuses and developing infants, there was a ten thousand–fold increase in sensitivity as compared to adults. What's more, boys were four times more likely to be mercury sensitive than girls—the same ratio found in cases of autism. It was also roughly the same ratio for ADD, tics, speech delay, and most of the other neurological developmental disorders associated with increased thimerosal exposure by the CDC itself.[105]

The ability to eliminate mercury also varied widely among individuals. Dr. El-Dahr cited one study, which Lyn found especially intriguing, where newborn mice were virtually unable to excrete methylmercury. Again, it was the younger male mice who were the poorest eliminators of mercury, compared with older male mice or younger females.[106] The group listened intently. Lyn could sense that this was a turning point for the mercury theory. She looked over at Bernie. He seemed captivated.

And it wasn't over yet. The next day, one of the participants calmly announced he might have found a cause of autism.

His name was William J. Walsh, a biochemist and chief scientist at the Pfeiffer Treatment Center, a nonprofit research and treatment facility in Warrenville, Illinois, specializing in biochemical imbalances. Since 1989 the center had treated some sixteen thousand patients with behavior dysfunctions, depression, schizophrenia, learning disorders, and autism. Walsh and his staff had collected biochemical information from more than fourteen thousand patients. Most of them had striking abnormalities in specific biochemical building blocks needed for neurotransmitter production, transmission, and reception.

One particular building block was found to be especially dysfunctional, or possibly depleted, in autistic children, Walsh said.[107] It was a sulfur-based protein called metallothionein (MT), which performs a number of key functions within the body. A lack of MT could yield symptoms that are "strikingly consistent with autism."

Poor MT function would contribute to accumulation of heavy metals in the body, Walsh said. Metallothionein and its chemical cousin, glutathione, belong to a group of sulfur-hydrogen compounds known as "thiols." One of their main functions is to bind with mercury and other heavy metals before they can cross the blood-brain barrier, and eliminate them from the body. Thiols are, in a way, part of a natural, inborn chelation system that allows most people to endure increased exposure to heavy metals without noticeable harm. It is interesting to note that a synonym for *thiol* is *mercaptan,* from the Latin *mercurium captans,* or "mercury capturer."

Improper MT functioning, Walsh added, would impair healthy maturation of young brain cells. In the same way, the infant immune system and GI tract depend on the protein for proper development.

Walsh and his team examined blood, urine, and hair samples from 503 patients with ASD. They found an unusually high incidence and severity of "metal metabolism" imbalances in the children, suggesting an MT disorder.

One function of MT is to regulate the balance between copper and zinc in the blood. Out of the 503 patients Walsh examined, 85 percent (428) showed severely elevated copper-to-zinc ratios that were "far greater than that of any other population we have studied over the past twenty-five years." The average copper-to-zinc ratio in the ASD kids was 1.78. In the normal children, it was 1.15. "Careful analysis of the medical histories and chemistry data indicated that 499 of the 503 autistics (99 percent) exhibited evidence of a metal metabolism disorder," he announced.

And Walsh made one other very intriguing observation. "You've got 80 percent boys with ASD and 20 percent girls," he said. "What could that possibly have to do with autism? We found that testosterone suppresses MT, while estrogen enhances it."

Walsh was "certain" that metallothionein dysfunction was due to genetic error, he said. "Autism results from an inborn error of metal metabolism followed by victimization by an environmental insult such as toxic metal in the first two to three years." But a chicken-or-egg question remained. Did mercury exposure lead to MT dysfunction? Or did MT dysfunction make mercury more toxic? Further study was clearly needed.

"I'm a little dismayed by the public debate about whether autism is genetic or environmental in origin," Walsh concluded. "My data suggest that both sides are correct, since the metal-metabolism genetic error results in striking sensitivity to toxic metals."

. . .

MORE THAN A YEAR had passed since the FDA had asked drug companies to consider removing thimerosal from childhood vaccines. Given what they now knew about the preservative, Safe Minds decided to issue a formal written demand to ban mercury from vaccines and biologics and recall anything with thimerosal that still remained in clinics across the country. This would include a recall of the flu shot, which contained 25 micrograms of mercury and was "encouraged" by the CDC for pregnant women and children six months and older.

Safe Minds' first official letter was posted on July 31, 2000, to FDA chief Dr. Jane Henney. The letter, drafted by Liz and signed by Lyn, cited a litany of federal public health regulations that would prohibit the use of thimerosal in medical products.

"FDA should never have licensed vaccine containing thimerosal in the first place," they wrote. "The FDA has known at least since 1982 that thimerosal poses a serious health risk. Indeed, you have eliminated its use in many products."[108]

Given the known toxicity of mercury, "FDA could not have reasonably concluded that such vaccines were safe," the letter said. At any rate, public health laws prohibit the use of preservatives that are toxic to recipients. "The members of Safe Minds are shocked and alarmed by your inaction in the face of this clear threat to public health," they said. "Any inability or refusal on your part to immediately end the use of thimerosal is a clear and present danger to public health because of the long-term damage to the trust placed in you by the public and Congress." All doctors should be told that children exposed to thimerosal who develop autism, ADD, and speech delay "should receive prompt evaluation and treatment."

The letter achieved nothing. The FDA never had any intention of recalling thimerosal, which agency officials made abundantly clear. On August 3, Albert called Norman Baylor, a high-level vaccine regulator at the FDA. He wanted to know if the Safe Minds recall letter had been received, and how the agency intended to respond. He was given a bureaucratic brush-off, he told Sallie, Liz, Lyn, and Jim Moody in an e-mail. The letter was distributed throughout Baylor's department, Albert said. But Baylor saw "no reason" for another meeting, and had recommended against it.

"He said there is absolutely no need to recall vaccines containing thimerosal, since in the very near future there will be none left," Albert told the other parents. "Even if we go to court they will fight us on two grounds: by the time we get to court, there will be no vaccines with thimerosal; and no judge will allow a recall since it creates panic among parents for no reason. It would put the National Immunization Program at risk."

Two weeks later, the FDA's official rejection letter arrived at the Safe Minds office. Signed by Kathryn C. Zoon, Ph.D., a director at CBER, the letter was a dense four-page message of rebuke, refusal, and denial. Zoon began by insisting that there was no data to "provide convincing evidence of significant safety problems with the long-term use of vaccines containing thimerosal," and therefore "recall of vaccines or other drugs containing thimerosal is not warranted."[109]

"How about that," Lyn laughed sarcastically to Sallie. "There's no *convincing* evidence of *significant* harm from *long-term* exposure. What about *compelling* evidence of *moderate* harm from *short-term* acute exposure?"

Zoon had belittled Safe Minds for associating the apparent increase in autism with the rise in thimerosal exposure. "This is known as an ecological association," she said. "Ecological associations are generally not accepted as strong evidence of causality, because they do not link individual exposure to individual outcome." There were "many possible explanations" for the apparent rise in autism, she added, reciting the now-familiar reasons of better diagnosis and wider public awareness, though she did note that "dietary and environmental factors" might be at play.

Safe Minds did not accept the FDA's rejection. On August 22, a second letter was dispatched to Commissioner Henney. "We have provided your agency with documentation that more than satisfies the statutory standard for an immediate Class I recall," Safe Minds said, before launching an attack directly at the powerful agency. The autism epidemic was careening toward a "financial disaster for the health, social services, and educational systems in our country. Your agency will be held accountable. Do not magnify the thimerosal tragedy. Recall these toxic products immediately."[110]

OVER THE SUMMER, Safe Minds had taken on a new member who would prove to be an invaluable asset in critiquing the findings of the VSD analysis. His name was Mark Blaxill, the young father who attended the autism conference in Orlando back in 1998 and posted his musings on the FEAT list shortly thereafter. Mark lives in a three-story colonial home in Cambridge, Massachusetts, with his wife, Elise, and two daughters, Sydney and Michaela. Michaela was diagnosed in 1994 with PDD/autistic disorder.

Mark was senior vice president at the Boston Consulting Group, a world leader in devising corporate strategies for Fortune 100 companies. He brought to the table years of experience in the intricate complexities of statistical analysis. Like many people when they first hear about the mercury-autism theory,

Mark had been extremely skeptical. But over the summer, he started to take a much closer look at the analysis by Thomas Verstraeten, the Belgian epidemiologist who worked with the VSD team in Atlanta. Mark grew increasingly convinced that something was amiss. Like the other parents, he wondered why thimerosal was linked with some disorders, but not autism.

Mark worked closely with Sallie and Lyn to try to decipher what the VSD team had done with the numbers. Together they composed a list of questions that Safe Minds wanted to ask the Datalink team. Specifically, Lyn had been trying since the June 2000 ACIP meeting to meet with Verstraeten. They had a lot of questions:

- The researchers had included young children, from birth to three years of age, even though the average age of an autism diagnosis was 4.4 years. A diagnosis in the first years of life was very rare. Wouldn't this tend to water down the relative risk found among all children?

- Compared with the population at large, the VSD study found relatively few children with autism. In California, the full-blown autism rate was estimated at around 30 to 40 per 10,000 children. Using the CDC's own figures, Mark Blaxill calculated the autism rate at the two West Coast HMOs to be just 11.5 per 10,000. Had they missed or somehow eliminated all those other cases? What else could explain this dramatic underascertainment?

- Verstraeten and the VSD team only looked at exposures up to three months of age. By not extending the study out to six months of age, they missed an additional exposure of 62.5 micrograms of mercury. Why wasn't this additional exposure considered?

- Nearly 17 percent of the children had been excluded from the study because of "perinatal" or "congenital disorders." What was the rationale for this, and how might it affect the total outcomes?

- The researchers did not look for outcomes like PDD-NOS and Asperger's syndrome, even though they are autism spectrum disorders. This meant that children like Will Redwood would not have been counted. Why not?

- Prenatal use of Rho(D) immune globulin was not taken into account, even though fetal exposure to mercury was known to be more harmful than postnatal exposure. Why was this additional mercury exposure not considered important?

• The study's design called for a Phase II segment to confirm the findings, in which neuropsychological tests of selected children were to be conducted. Why was this not done?

• Instead, in Phase II, the researchers went outside the VSD to purchase a small database from the Harvard Pilgrim HMO to compare outcomes there with their original findings. But the study population at Harvard Pilgrim was significantly smaller (fifteen thousand children), which would lower its "statistical power" and thus weaken the signal for outcomes. Why did they choose to go this route, and why did they select Harvard Pilgrim, which had been placed under state receivership after teetering on the verge of bankruptcy just a few months earlier, partly because of problems with information systems and record keeping?.[111]

IN EARLY NOVEMBER, Thomas Verstraeten finally agreed to meet with Lyn. He set the date for the tenth, three days after the hotly disputed election between Al Gore and George Bush. Soon the country would be plunged into a desperate electoral stalemate as lawyers for both sides fought over Florida's all-important votes.

As the nation went to the polls on November 7, 2000, Liz Birt filed Safe Minds' first Freedom of Information Act request. The group was seeking a flood of documents from the federal health bureaucracy, namely "all material, including drafts, in whatever form utilized or developed by the consultants engaged by CDC and by its employees." They also requested all correspondence leading up to the Simpsonwood review, and all materials "in whatever form, utilized or developed by CDC and FDA personnel regarding the use of thimerosal as a preservative in vaccinations."

It would be months before Safe Minds was issued the first batch of documents. Without the paperwork, they were flying blind when it came to forming an intelligent critique. They suspected statistical manipulation, yet had no proof. But they did have plenty of questions. Lyn prepared her list very carefully prior to meeting Verstraeten.

On November 10, as the Florida fiasco unfolded before a riveted nation, Lyn drove to a featureless office park on the edge of Atlanta, where National Immunization Program staff worked in an unmarked cinderblock building set among young pine trees.

The Belgian researcher received Lyn warmly in his tiny cube of an office, which lacked both windows and fresh air. It was beginning to seem as if everyone who worked in public health was condemned to labor in dark, cramped quarters. On his crowded bookcase, Lyn noticed pictures of Verstraeten with his kids. She smiled and, almost reflexively, took out her wallet and showed him photos of Will. She also showed him a picture of a boy with pink disease, taken from a book published in the 1950s. Verstraeten was impressed by how alike they seemed.

The two were going to hit it off, Lyn thought. They sat down for an intensive two-hour conversation. Verstraeten patiently went over the VSD study with the young mother from Tyrone. He spoke softly and deliberately, without rushing or looking at his watch. There was no attempt to condescend, and his sympathy for Lyn seemed genuine.

"Please bear in mind that these are preliminary analyses," he began. "They should not be treated as our final findings." Verstraeten also confessed that he had been "confused" by the study and its ambiguities. "Some days I look at the data and I'm convinced that there is a problem," he said, "and on other days I think there is nothing."[112]

This is a good guy, Lyn thought to herself. He's not just spitting out the company line. This is no CDC villain.

Lyn's biggest question was why there was such a preponderance of younger kids in the study, who were far less likely to be given an autism diagnosis. Verstraeten told her that the latest cycle of data had just come in, with an update of diagnoses on the same children one year later. He said the number of cases with autism had gone up. "Can I get a copy of that update?" Lyn asked eagerly. Verstraeten was conflicted. He wanted to share it with Lyn, he said, but needed to wait until the new data was fully analyzed and approved for release.

Another problem Lyn saw with the original data was that, if a child were referred outside the HMO for an evaluation, the diagnosis might not appear on his or her HMO chart. "How many pediatricians actually diagnose autism?" she asked. Verstraeten said he did not know. "Most kids I know were diagnosed by specialists, not by their pediatricians," Lyn said. "I can't think of many children who were diagnosed inside an HMO."

Lyn was also concerned about kids who dropped out of the HMO but remained in the database. "For example, a child can drop out of the HMO at two years of age if his parents move or change jobs," she said, "which is too young to have been diagnosed with autism. But even if he drops out, he's still included in the overall data, which will skew the results." She asked Verstraeten if he could look only at kids who were continuously enrolled throughout the entire study period, 1992–1998, because they would be at least six years old by now. He agreed to do so.

Lyn also asked why the investigators had purchased outside data from Harvard Pilgrim to do their follow-up confirmation study, instead of conducting neuropsychological evaluations on selected children, as called for in the original study design. To her amazement, Verstraeten agreed that going to Harvard Pilgrim was a mistake. The sample size was too small to achieve enough statistical "power" to detect subtle differences in outcomes. "We should have just examined the children as originally planned," he said. "It would have been more decisive."[113]

Verstraeten walked Lyn down to the lobby. She was feeling quite good about the encounter, even a measure of affection for the earnest European. Searching for her keys, Lyn found a bag of homemade cookies her mother had baked and sent off with her. She pulled them out and handed them to Verstraeten.

"Here, my mom made these. They're chocolate chip. Please take them as a gift for all your time and trouble. And don't worry," she said, grinning, "I didn't poison them."

ON DECEMBER 23, 2000, shortly after the electoral dust settled and the Supreme Court confirmed George W. Bush as president of the United States, Bush named his new director of the Office of Management and Budget. It was Mitchell E. Daniels, Jr., the senior vice president for corporate and marketing strategy of Eli Lilly, one of the Republican Party's most generous corporate contributors.

Daniels, once an aide to Ronald Reagan and a former leading staffer at the conservative Heritage Foundation, had little hands-on experience in budgetary or financial matters, and no background in accounting.

Apparently this was a purely political appointment. Even the *Wall Street Journal* raised an eyebrow. "The President-elect's cabinet picks have been so corporate-friendly that some Republicans refer to the incoming administration as Bush-Cheney Inc.," a December 26, 2000, article in the pro-business paper said. "At a time when issues of enormous concern to the drug industry are ripe for action, George W. Bush has ensured that the industry will have one of its own in an influential position in his administration." With Daniels, Bush picked someone from an industry that was "sure to be in the hot seat in Congress as it moves to consider adding prescription drug benefits to Medicare."[114]

The parents did not pay much attention to the appointment. The grueling year was finally limping to a close. There had been so much to do, they had somewhat lost track of Washington. That inattention would soon change.

7. Mounting Evidence

PRESIDENT GEORGE W. BUSH took office on a dark, rain-swept afternoon in January 2001. It was enough to ward off some, but not all of the protestors who gathered in Washington to denounce the election's shaky outcome. The next day, Bush installed his cabinet, including Mitchell Daniels, who was also to be appointed to the president's Homeland Security Council and the National Security Council.

The year was off to an uncertain beginning for the nation. For the parents, it would be an epic year, in ways they could not yet conceive. It would herald the first thimerosal lawsuits against Eli Lilly and the vaccine makers; it was the year that thimerosal took a seat in the deliberations of the mainstream medical establishment.

The Institute of Medicine, a respected branch of the National Academies, had been contracted with by the Department of Health and Human Services and the CDC, at the request of Congress,[115] to convene two new hearings on vaccines and autism. The first would be in the spring, on MMR, and the second in July, on thimerosal.

One issue that still needed settling was the debate over whether the autism "epidemic" was real or not. Despite dramatic numbers coming out of California, many researchers insisted that most, if not all of the increase could be explained away by expanded diagnostic codes for autism-related disorders, greater public awareness, and even migration patterns. Families with autistic kids might have moved to places like California to avail themselves of the range of services available there to the disabled.

Before they could argue that autism was triggered by environmental factors, the parents would have to show that actual case rates were indeed on the rise. Mark Blaxill was the natural point person for the mission. He spent his entire 2000 holiday season and much of January poring over epidemiological data collected from a number of autism population studies—not only in California, but in other industrialized nations like Japan, the UK, Denmark, and Sweden.

Because of his training and expertise, Mark knew that looking at total case numbers alone revealed very little about the actual *incidence* of autism in any given area. What mattered was not the number of new cases reported every year, but the number of children diagnosed with autism for each year of birth.

For example, in California (which only tracks "classic" cases), Mark wanted to know if more kids born in a certain year, say 1995, had been diagnosed as autistic by age five than kids born in 1994 or 1993. It was the only way to show an increase in the actual incidence rate, and not just a rise in the total cumulative numbers. Once he broke down the figures by birth "cohorts," Mark found significant increases in the number of diagnoses with each successive birth year.

To Mark it seemed risible for anyone to refute the obvious: autism rates were going through the roof. He labeled the phenomenon "Epidemic Denial," and set out to deconstruct the mentality of the antiepidemic theorists, who insisted that the true incidence of disease had remained static.

What could account for such denial? "The vaccination movement is sacred, untouchable," Mark told the other parents. Government researchers inside the CDC or FDA "are in it for the satisfaction, the sense of mission. They want to go after disease, and vaccines are the way to go." The notion that vaccines might cause harm, even to a minority of kids, "threatens the very core of what these bureaucrats believe in," he said. "This whole apparatus is there to do good, to defend children. The scientists, the bureaucrats, the public health people, the pediatricians, all of them are dedicated to the proposition that they will serve the health of young children with these interventions. The notion that the interventions are harmful is unthinkable."

This canon of beliefs dovetailed perfectly with modern science's near-religious faith in all things genetic, especially in the age of the human genome project. "The gene theory becomes obsessive, but without proof it becomes part of the mantra," Mark said. "Everyone wants it to be genetic. They want it to be a problem that the genome can solve. They all think, 'It's a nice disease with clearly genetic clues. And we'll crack it. Give us money and we'll find the answer. We'll be the heroes that solve this genetic disorder.' "

The possibility that environmental factors might be at work, even with an underlying genetic component, presented "very inconvenient facts for these folks," Mark continued. "Theirs is a clean, neat model. It explains everything. It justifies their lives. It justifies their careers. It produces no guilt, no liability. It's the march of progress, the practice of good medicine, the future of technology. And it's all threatened by this one little fact. So they attack it. It must be wrong. It *must* be."

In early February, as if to prove Mark's point, an editorial appeared in the journal *Pediatrics,* published by the American Academy of Pediatrics, titled "Is There an Epidemic of Autism?"[116] The author, Dr. Eric Fombonne, a renowned child psychiatrist from the Institute of Psychiatry in London, had little doubt that the answer was no. This by inference, of course, indicated that there was no environmental root of the disease.

"The so-called epidemic of autism has prompted investigators to search for a cause," he wrote. "While some studies have suggested that a vaccine routinely given to infants may be responsible, others have found no association." As for the rising numbers in California, Fombonne dismissed them as mishandled, misinterpreted data: the report did not account for wider diagnostic criteria, nor did it consider California's population growth, much of it due to immigration.

Fombonne suggested that the number of Californians with autism, even after they were broken down by year of birth, remained more or less the same for each birth cohort. Autism was a serious problem, he admitted, more serious than previously believed. But it wasn't on the rise. "There is no need to raise false alarms of putative epidemics, nor to practice poor science to draw the attention to the unmet needs of large numbers of seriously impaired children and adults," he wrote. "The magnitude of the problem had clearly been underestimated in the past."

"Underestimated?" Mark grumbled when he read the editorial. Did Fombonne really mean to suggest that tens of thousands of older kids and adults who should have been diagnosed with autism years ago were now walking around literally undetected? Where *were* all these people? And why did there seem to be so many more kids with autism today than anyone, including seasoned schoolteachers, could ever recall before?

Mark composed his own letter, posted on the FEAT site, in which he accused Fombonne and others of inventing what he called the "Hidden Horde Hypothesis." Fombonne's contention that autism rates were higher than previously thought but that no one had realized it until now "requires that there are large numbers of children that were undiagnosed with autism that are now unrecognized as autistic today," Mark wrote. That would mean that there were anywhere from 150,000 to 650,000 undiagnosed children with autism (not including adults, which would triple the number) at large in America. But the official count of the total childhood autistic population (enrolled in the IDEA program nationwide) was 53,000. "This raises the commonsense question: where could one possibly locate all these undiagnosed people with autism? For Fombonne to reject a generation of epidemiological research, he must be able to prove that these undiagnosed cases exist. There is no credible evidence to support this claim."[117]

WAS AUTISM really treatable? Lyn Redwood was beginning to think it was. If the disease and its related disorders were, as she believed, the result of infantile mercury poisoning, then maybe something could be done not only to extract the metal but also to reverse the damage she thought it had caused.

She wasn't the only one asking this question. Bernie Rimland, the "Father of Autism" from DAN! and the Autism Research Institute, who had convened the think tank in Phoenix the summer before, had also become convinced that thimerosal was a factor in the disease. Rimland now believed it was vital to standardize a protocol for safe and effective chelation therapy, dietary interventions, and related treatments that could help reverse some of the damage the metal had caused. He invited twenty-five people for yet another brainstorming session to run from February 9 to 11 in Dallas, to build consensus on the safest, most effective steps toward mercury detoxification and repair. Lyn was asked to represent Safe Minds.

Lyn was also charged with surveying parents on the autism-mercury list— which she and Sallie had set up online—about chelation and their experiences with the unproven therapy. She asked what type of chelating agent they used, at what schedule and dose levels. She asked for a description of each child's physical and mental response to the therapy. She also asked for urine, hair, or stool test results to document the types and amounts of metal each child excreted.

The Dallas meeting had its share of prickly disagreements, but a consensus did emerge. The doctors at the meeting had collectively treated well over three thousand patients for heavy metal poisoning. Some fifteen hundred of them were autistic children, and the doctors said that no other treatment had brought about the degree of improvement found with chelation. When the meeting ended, Rimland issued a statement saying that a consensus paper on mercury detoxification would be ready by May 2001.[118]

A NEWCOMER had sat in on the Dallas meeting, a petite, soft-spoken woman in her mid thirties with short brown hair. Her name was Melissa Miles, and she was an attorney for the Dallas-based law firm of Waters & Kraus. The firm was known for successful litigation of asbestos cases. Now Andy Waters, a partner, wanted to pursue legal action against Eli Lilly and the vaccine makers. He had asked if Miles could sit in on the meeting. The young female attorney got to know Lyn at the session, and the two hit it off.

Lyn had already been approached by a number of attorneys, some of whom had flown into Atlanta to review the merits of her case. She was the mother with the most information and they wanted to pump her for it in order to help their clients. Some seemed sincere, some seemed like ambulance chasers, but Lyn helped them all. She had not, however, thought about filing a suit of her own. She had been so busy these past months, there had been no time to contemplate court action, nor had she talked it over with Tommy. Besides, she thought, the evidence against thimerosal was still new and unproven. It was probably too circumstantial, at this point, to hold up in trial.

But Lyn was impressed with Melissa. The young lawyer thought the Redwoods had a good case. Her boss Andy Waters concurred. He told Melissa he wanted to "expose the lack of concern for our most vulnerable citizens, our infants," and Lyn liked the way that sounded.

After Lyn got home from Texas, Melissa contacted her by e-mail. She was interested in Lyn's prenatal exposure from immune globulins, but wanted to know about the full range of vaccines that Will received. Melissa also noted that there were three coal-fired power plants not far from Tyrone. She wondered if Georgia Power, the local utility, might also be listed as a defendant in the case.

A few days later, Liz Birt met with Andy Waters. Andy was tall and slender, with light brown hair. Clever and charming, Andy was known for his ability to whip a jury into torments of compassion for the aggrieved. His firm had won some impressive cash awards in asbestos cases. Liz liked Andy. He was the kind of aggressive lawyer she could relate to. Andy told her he wanted to cobble together a coalition of firms around the country to take on the thimerosal cases under the umbrella of Waters & Kraus.

Liz thought it was a great idea, but she was beginning to grow weary of the fight. The idea of spending years more trudging through courtrooms, taking depositions, and cross-examining drug executives and FDA officials was exhausting just to think about.

"I'm pooped," she said to Lyn one day. "Sometimes all of this is too much for me to handle emotionally. But I feel responsible for seeing this through, seeing how it plays out for the children and their families. I would do anything for a normal life."

It was an emotion that most parents of an autistic child feel at some point. But if there were a silver lining, Liz said it was Safe Minds. "I think that God has brought all of us together on this road," she told Lyn. "I love you."

Lyn was moved to tears. "I love you, too!" she said. "Will's disability has brought sorrow into my life, but meeting people like you, Sallie, Albert, Heidi, Rick, Bernie, and so many others—I never would've made it through this without your support!"

Maybe, Lyn speculated, "one day our lives will return to normal and we can lie around on the couch all day and eat bonbons."

"You think?" Liz laughed, in spite of herself.

The next week, Lyn called Melissa Miles. The Redwoods had decided to litigate. They would file suit in Georgia state court, and wanted to be represented by the Atlanta firm of Evert & Weathersby, which had signed on to the Waters & Kraus consortium. It wasn't an easy decision. Tommy did not want to include Will's physicians in the suit. He only wanted to go after the corporations. He convinced Lyn that the doctors themselves were innocent. They didn't know about the danger of thimerosal. But the companies did.

Technically speaking, the Redwoods were not eligible to sue in state court. As parents of a vaccine-injured child, they were required by law to first file a claim through the federal government's Vaccine Injury Compensation Program (VICP), though this provision was disputed by some lawyers and legal experts. Also known as the Vaccine Court, as discussed earlier, the program was established by Congress in 1986 to pay damages to people who could prove they were harmed by immunization. Congress intended it to be a no-fault, nonadversarial payment scheme that was swift, flexible, and less costly than civil tort.

FOR THOSE FAMILIES that are eligible, Vaccine Court claims are managed by a Special Master. Department of Justice lawyers represent the Secretary of Health and Human Services, who becomes a codefendant in each case. Medical costs of illness are covered, while compensation for death or injury is capped at $250,000. Pharmaceutical companies pay none of this. The funds come from a 75-cent-per-vaccine surtax.

All plaintiffs in vaccine injury cases are supposed to file in Vaccine Court before taking any other legal action. If their petitions for relief are denied, or if they are unhappy with the results, they may then file a lawsuit in civil court.[119]

The prospects for success in Vaccine Court are bleaker than Congress intended. Of the 8,074 petitions filed between 1988 and 2003, only 1,790 won compensation (3,842 cases were dismissed, and the rest were still pending by 2004). And while payments for medical costs and other damages are fairly generous (in 2002, they averaged $772,675), they are nowhere near the millions of dollars that civil trial juries are known to award in medical cases, especially when children are involved.[120]

The Redwoods would gladly have filed in Vaccine Court, but there was one very big hitch. The program had a statute of limitation of just three years, and the clock started running on the date of injury (onset of diagnosis). Will had been diagnosed in 1995, six years earlier. There was no way they could file a claim. Civil court was the only option left open. But in order to go directly to civil court, the plaintiffs and their attorneys would have to find a loophole.

Andy Waters believed he had found the loophole. Vaccine Court had jurisdiction only over companies that manufactured the vaccines themselves, as well as the doctors who administered them. But thimerosal, Waters put forth, was an *additive* to vaccines, not an integral ingredient of the shots themselves. By this logic, thimerosal suits were not bound by Vaccine Court rules. It was a novel but potentially risky approach.

Over the next few weeks, Lyn continued funneling information to the Dallas attorneys. Waters was especially interested in Thomas Verstraeten's VSD analysis. He and Melissa wanted to file a Freedom of Information Act petition to obtain the raw data. Lyn told them that Safe Minds had already put in that request. But she offered to stay in close contact with Verstraeten himself, if possible.

"Let me try to contact him first. He thinks I'm 'just an upset parent,'" she said. "An attorney would only increase their resistance to releasing information."

Lyn also put Andy Waters in contact with Boyd Haley, the University of Kentucky Chemistry Department chairman. "I love this guy!" she told Melissa. "As difficult as this has been, it's people like Boyd who truly search for the truth, no matter how unpopular the position. He's given me faith that we will prevail."

Then she wrote to Boyd. "After much frustration trying to get CDC, FDA, AAP and NIP to take our concerns seriously about thimerosal, we have decided to move forward with a products liability case here in Georgia," she said, adding that Waters was the lead attorney. "I know we are up against tremendous force, but I feel this firm has the knowledge and experience we need to be successful."

Lyn asked Haley if he would fly to Dallas to brief the attorneys. "Boyd, you said one day that you would help give me the mallet to beat FDA over the head with," she said. "Well I'm ready to start swinging! I hate that this has gotten to this point, but they will never admit any harm unless the issue is placed in the courts. They are ruthless."

Time was not on the families' side. There was talk in Washington of closing the legal loophole Andy had learned. Lyn wanted to file as soon as possible. "The attorneys are trying to move quickly on this because they are afraid that the vaccine manufacturers are going to ask Congress for immunity," she told Boyd. He was happy to help, and he flew to Dallas to meet with Andy, Melissa, and the other attorneys.

In March 2001, Waters & Kraus filed the first ever thimerosal civil suit in the United States, on behalf of a Texas family by the name of Counter, in the District Court of Travis County, Texas.[121] It got local and national press attention.

"The symptoms of mercury poisoning are, in many cases, identical to the symptoms of autism," Waters & Kraus said in a statement, adding that "a significant number of individual cases against the vaccine industry will be filed in the near future."[122]

THE FEDERAL VACCINE COURT needed fixing, many parents believed. Critics said that government lawyers fought each case tenaciously, as if their own money were at stake. Cases dragged through the program for months and sometimes years. The burden of proof was excessively high. Lawyers for the families were not compensated until a case was settled. Without these interim fees, they were put at a terrible disadvantage against the full-time government attorneys and their staffs. Even when petitioners did manage to win a settlement, some still had to battle the court-appointed administrators who doled out the award money. In some cases, stricken families were nickel-and-dimed over things like new leg braces for a growing child with polio.[123]

The court was so unlikely to award damages that a sizable surplus had collected in the fund, which had swollen to more than $1.6 billion. In 2000 some $144 million in revenues came in from the 75-cent vaccine tax, and another $75 million were generated in interest. But total payouts for the year were just $45.3 million, plus another $9.5 million for administrative costs.[124]

The excess was an outrage to antitax crusaders in Congress. In early 2001 they introduced a measure to slash the vaccine surcharge to 25 cents. Their bill was supported by the drug industry and by local governments, which purchase vaccines in bulk.

"The surplus is dwarfing the claims paid from the fund," wrote sponsors Rep. Ron Lewis (R-KY) and Rep. Karen Thurman (D-FL) in a "Dear Colleague" letter. "HHS officials are unaware of anything that would result in an increased number of claims."[125]

But Health and Human Services officials were well aware that new thimerosal claims were entering the vaccine compensation system each month. Thousands, potentially tens of thousands more cases that still met the statute of limitations could follow. With vaccine injury payouts averaging eight hundred thousand dollars, it might only take two thousand successful cases to wipe out the entire fund.

Even as some lawmakers tried to gut the Vaccine Injury Compensation Program, others were trying to make it more user-friendly. On February 14, 2001, Rep. Dave Weldon, the Republican doctor from Florida, introduced the Vaccine Injured Children's Compensation Act of 2001 (VICCA), which was cosponsored by Rep. Jerrold R. Nadler, from the Upper West Side of Manhattan, one of the most liberal Democrats in the House. The measure would extend the statute of limitations to six years and ease the burden of proof. It would also cover interim attorney fees and earmark money for training and counseling of parents and their severely ill children.[126]

"This program must recognize that strict scientific proof is not always available," Weldon and Nadler wrote in their own "Dear Colleague" letter. "Sometimes it is difficult to prove a direct causal relationship. We believe it is important to err on the side of the injured child."[127]

Parents and their advocates saw the Weldon bill as a step forward. Barbara Loe Fisher and the National Vaccine Information Center got behind the bill, and so did most attorneys with clients inside the VICP. But for people like the Redwoods, the bill would be meaningless. Yes, it would open up the vaccine program to thousands more families, but not to theirs. Again, Will had been "injured" for just over six years. He would still be ineligible to file.

This conflict would later become a bone of contention among some parents. When Bill Frist proposed a similar measure, Lyn reluctantly wrote an e-mail to Barbara Loe Fisher explaining why she could not support the bill. "I understand it is a tremendous improvement over what we had," she said. "But is it fair to all those that have been injured over the years? No, it isn't. And that's what I have struggled with. I just can't tell a parent with a child born in 1997 that they do not have the same rights as parents of a child born just one day later. I feel trapped in this 'Greater Good' scenario. It is just something that I personally cannot compromise."

THE INSTITUTE OF MEDICINE meeting on thimerosal had been set for July 16, in Cambridge, Massachusetts. The parents would need to convince IOM officials that their side of the mercury-autism hypothesis merited a full hearing. They knew it would be a landmark meeting, and they were determined to testify. This left them with just a few months to sift through and catalog all the evidence they had gathered to date. They needed to present their findings in a rational, scientific manner.

A good deal of their argument would center on alleged flaws in the Vaccine

Safety Datalink analysis. Safe Minds was becoming increasingly suspicious that CDC officials had somehow manipulated the data to achieve an outcome they desired: one that played down, or eliminated entirely any "signal" of an association between thimerosal and autism.

Lyn remained in contact with Thomas Verstraeten. Meanwhile, Mark had slogged through the study's complicated methodology, as presented by the researcher at the June 2000 meeting of the Advisory Committee on Immunization Practices. He was beginning to piece together what he believed the CDC officials had done with the study, and when.

But the parents still had very little to go on. None of the FOIA requests that Liz had filed with the CDC and FDA had yet come through. They were still flying semiblind. More documentation was needed if they were to prove their allegations of government malfeasance.

Liz fired off a flurry of correspondence about her prior requests. Each letter became more specific in its demands. One missive to the CDC, dated May 21, 2001, requested the following documents: (1) minutes taken during the meeting held at the Simpsonwood Retreat, (2) the raw database of the Vaccine Safety DataLink and the most currently available updates to the medical records of children studied, (3) all internal memoranda, including e-mails, between CDC employees and independent contractors, employees of the National Immunization Program, members of ACIP, employees of the FDA, HHS, NIH, and its related agencies, and representatives of vaccine manufacturers "regarding the use of thimerosal containing vaccines and neurodevelopmental delays."[128]

Over the spring of 2001, more data to implicate thimerosal kept filtering in. It was all duly cataloged into the swelling evidence of harm that the parents had gathered for their presentation at the Institute of Medicine.

Thimerosal Warning in Russia. Searching for thimerosal toxicity studies on PubMed, an online search engine of medical journals, Sallie came across an abstract for a study done in 1983 in the Soviet Union, of all places. Apparently the Russians had harbored serious concerns about thimerosal. In fact, the USSR banned its use in childhood vaccines during that decade. Sallie managed to track down a hard copy of the article, which was printed in Russian. She sent it to Liz, who knew someone who could have it translated. Nearly twenty years earlier, Soviet scientists had warned about "the toxic action of ethylmercury-based preparations, which kills and damages cells at the site of injection, thus inducing the formation of autoantigens whose effect on the body cannot be predicted." It said that thimerosal was not only highly toxic to cells, but capable of actually changing cell properties. "The use of thimerosal for the preservation of medical biological preparations," the study said, "especially those intended for children, is inadmissible."[129]

"I can't believe it," Liz told Lyn when she read the paper. "The Communists figured this out years ago, and here we are with our wonderful free enterprise system, banging down the doors to be heard."

Crossing the Blood-Brain Barrier. Conventional wisdom held that ethylmercury, because of its extra carbon group, was too large a molecule to pass through the blood-brain barrier, which protects the brain and nervous system from exposure to environmental toxins. But a study in the journal *Neurotoxicology* by W. Slikker, Jr., from the FDA's National Center for Toxicological Research, said flatly that "thimerosal crossed the blood-brain and placental barriers and results in appreciable mercury content in tissues including brain." Even though the FDA had approved this "therapeutic" product, Slikker wrote, it was an example of the "need for further study of important ingredients of therapeutic agents that have both benefits and potential associated risks."[130]

Brain Damage in Canada. Another study, this time from a team at the University of Calgary's Faculty of Medicine, found that mercury exposure—even in amounts as tiny as one micromolar, or one-thousandth of a microgram—leads to direct degeneration of brain neurons. The findings were presented in a cover story in the April edition of the British journal *NeuroReport*.[131] The researchers had also produced a breathtaking time-lapse video, recorded with a microscopic camera and posted on the journal's Web site. It clearly showed that when micromolars of mercury came into contact with neuronal axons (the branchlike structures that pass electronic impulses on to the next nerve cell) the axons shriveled like hair being singed by fire.

The report illustrated how "mercury ions alter the cell membrane structure of developing neurons," wrote Fritz Lorscheider, professor of physiology and biophysics at the University of Calgary. The discovery provided "visual evidence of our previous findings that mercury produces a molecular lesion in the brain." Mercury damage was induced in "microtubules" of snail brain neurons. These tiny spindles within cells are similar in all animals, including humans. The team found that mercury ions attach to a neuron and cause its microtubules to disassemble or break down, stripping the neuron of its protective membrane. These unprotected neurons then shrivel and tangle together into a formless mass, no longer able to function normally, no longer capable of transmitting electronic impulses.

It was only an "in vitro" (test-tube) study. But given what Slikker had written about ethylmercury crossing the blood-brain barrier, it seemed plausible that some brain cells would have been exposed and presumably shriveled by the same mechanism seen on the video. Watching the video made Lyn sick. All she could think about was that horrible spindle disintegration process going on millions of times, whenever Will was exposed to mercury. For the parents, the video was tough to watch.

But the parents were also heartened by the study. "It's unbelievable!" Liz said. She had unearthed another report showing that mercury was a strong inhibitor of brain microtubular assembly in cows. "These substances are the same across species, whether snail, cow, or man," she told the group. "This is more proof that thimerosal is the culprit in the failure of neurons to properly develop in autistic children."

Gulf War Syndrome and Mercury? Through her growing national contacts, Lyn had met a former Air Force captain, a pilot in the 1990 Gulf War, named Frank Schmuck. Like most Gulf War veterans, Schmuck had received a series of vaccines before deployment. At one point, he got several shots in one day. Many contained thimerosal. When the war ended, Schmuck returned home to become a commercial airline pilot. But over time he started feeling sick. He had unexplained, severe weight loss, GI inflammation, neurological damage, short-term memory loss, and a tumor on his liver. The symptoms grew so debilitating that he removed himself from flying status.[132]

Eventually Schmuck was diagnosed with Gulf War syndrome, a vague cluster of complaints mysteriously afflicting thousands of returnees from the war, as well as post-traumatic stress disorder. He was evaluated by an environmental medicine specialist who found a level of mercury in his hair of 14 parts per million (5 ppm is considered to be a diagnosis of mercury toxicity). Schmuck underwent intensive chelation therapy, and copious amounts of mercury poured from his system. His symptoms began to improve almost immediately. The Department of Veterans Affairs, after reviewing Schmuck's medical records, reclassified his illness as mercury toxicity. When Schmuck reviewed his own records, he was shocked to find that he had been injected with some 800 micrograms of mercury in his military vaccines. He had also been given thimerosal-containing immunoglobulin, to boost his immune response to the shots.

After nearly a year of chelation, Schmuck's cognitive (reaction ability, awareness), memory (retention ability), and intellectual (reason, deductive ability) capacity had increased from 66 to 95 percent. By March of 2001 he was taken off disability. Not long after that, the FAA restored his commercial pilot's license. Schmuck also retained a law firm in Andy Waters's coalition and filed suit against the vaccine makers and Eli Lilly, charging them with fraudulent misrepresentation, fraud and deceit, negligence, product liability, illegal and deceptive business practices, and loss of consortium.

Thimerosal as Environmental Hazard. In early 2001, the National Institute for Environmental Health Sciences updated its statement on thimerosal toxicity. The information was part of a safety guide for lab researchers. It warned that thimerosal was "toxic by ingestion and inhalation," and also an eye irritant. When heated to decomposition "it emits very toxic fumes of mercury, sodium oxide, and sulfur oxides." In case of a spill, lab workers were told to seal contaminated clothing in a vapor-tight plastic bag and evacuate the room. Symptoms of thimerosal exposure were nausea, liquid stools, pain, heart and liver disorder, deafness, and severe uncoordination. Acute poisoning could cause gastrointestinal irritation, renal failure, and death. Other early signs included loss of speech, writing, and gait, inability to stand or carry out voluntary movements, occasional muscle atrophy, difficulty understanding ordinary speech, irritability and bad temper progressing to mania, stupor, coma, mental retardation in children, anxiety, mental depression, insomnia, hallucinations, and central nervous system effects.[133] Again, Lyn thought this could have been taken from a text on autism.

Mercury-Induced Autism in Japan. In 1977 a team from Fukushima Medical College began an autism prevalence study in the province of Fukushima-ken. It was the largest study of its kind, and it remains the largest population screening for autism outside the United States. Researchers found an autism prevalence rate of 2.33 per 10,000, not a particularly high number by current standards. But the authors took the extra step of segregating the diagnoses by birth year (an unusual practice at the time) from 1960 to 1977. The number of autistic children born between 1960 and 1965 was very low, between zero and three per year. But among children born in 1966 (the year of a large mercury spill in the area), the number began to rise rapidly into the teens, reaching a maximum of 21 per 10,000 in 1972—among children who were five years old at the time of the screening. Mark Blaxill examined the data and calculated that the prevalence rate rose from 1 per 10,000 before the mercury spill to almost 7 per 10,000 afterward.[134] It was the first time anyone had identified a documented increase in autism rates following a major environmental mishap. If mercury in fish had been implicated in autism (and not just milder neurological disorders), why couldn't mercury in vaccines be to blame as well?

Boyd Haley's Lab Work. Also in early 2001, Safe Minds' new academic ally, Boyd Haley of the University of Kentucky, had begun to conduct a number of lab experiments on the toxicity of thimerosal, using the vaccine samples that Lyn had furnished. Haley told the parents that thimerosal broke down when exposed to light, releasing its ethylmercury at a rapid rate. This finding reminded Lyn that in very busy clinics, vaccine vials were often placed on the counter in the morning, where they remained exposed to light for most of the day. Boyd had used brain tissue to monitor the viability of tubulin (the protein component of microtubules), to test both the light-degraded and the intact forms of thimerosal. The thimerosal without exposure to light caused over 80-percent inhibition of tubulin, but the solution exposed to light caused a nearly 100-percent loss of the protein. Boyd was not surprised to find higher toxicity in the "photolyzed" vaccine. And he also found that methylmercury was not as toxic to tubulin as the ethylmercury released from thimerosal after exposure to light. This contradicted conventional wisdom on the two forms of organic mercury.

Next Boyd compared identical vaccines with and without thimerosal to see if there was a difference in neurotoxicity. He discovered that the mercury-laced shots were tenfold to a hundredfold more toxic than those without thimerosal. There was one outstanding exception: the preservative-free MMR vaccine. It was as toxic as the thimerosal-containing vaccines. There was something in MMR that inhibited enzymes and brain proteins, but Boyd could not determine what it was, lacking enough MMR vaccine in his lab. Finally, Boyd told Safe Minds he was working with a doctor friend from New Zealand named Mike Godfrey. Dr. Godfrey shared Haley's interest in the APO-E4 gene, and agreed that it was a risk factor in Alzheimer's disease. He had looked for the gene in autistic children and found a huge preponderance of them with APO-E4, indicating that a genetic risk factor leading to the inability to eliminate toxins might at least partly explain the neurological aspect of autism.[135]

THE FULL STORY about what the Vaccine Safety Datalink team did to conduct the analysis—and why—may never be known. Were their motives purely scientific, or was something more sinister at play? Did they purposely set out to manipulate the data and bring down the relative risk of autism and other disorders, as the parents were beginning to believe? Or were they simply trying to achieve the greatest clarity and least statistical "noise" that they could, as the researchers and their defenders insisted?

Lyn, Liz, Sallie, Mark, Teresa, Jane El-Dahr, and others had spent months going through the Verstraeten study. But without access to the documents they had requested, the parents could only speculate on how investigators reached the conclusion that there was no statistically significant association between thimerosal and autism, and inconclusive associations with other developmental disorders.

In advance of July's Institute of Medicine meeting, Safe Minds sent their concerns in letter form to the IOM immunization committee. It was an attempted preemptive strike against what they knew the government side would be presenting.

The parents wanted to know why the disease rates were so much lower in the HMOs than in California as a whole. Had the researchers inadvertently missed these cases? Or, as the parents suspected, had they "cherry picked" data to lower the overall rate of autism and other adverse outcomes?[136]

The underascertainment of case rates was not insignificant. Though the CDC reported that the "capture rate" of all cases was 90 percent, Safe Minds said it was far lower. In the two HMOs, the CDC found a combined autism rate of about 12 per 10,000 children. But California statistics at the time showed a statewide rate of 30 to 40 per 10,000. Attention deficit rates were also much lower in the HMOs—34 per 10,000—while the CDC itself reported that the nationwide rate in the same age group was around 300 to 600 per 10,000.

The Safe Minds letter, signed by Lyn, plainly accused the CDC of lowering the total number of diagnosed cases of NDDs. In the original Davis report of 2000, the number of children identified with autism was 153, she said. But one month later, at the CDC's June vaccine advisory committee meeting, Verstraeten had reported that the number of cases—in the same study—was just 67. Developmental neurological disorders, meanwhile, dropped from 3,702 in the Davis abstract to 1,743 in the ACIP presentation. ADD fell from 346 cases to just 158.

"I must ask what manipulation occurred to the data which resulted in over half of the population of children with autism, developmental neurological disorders, and attention deficit to fall out of the database," Lyn wrote to the IOM.

Then there was the troubling question of using so many young children in an autism surveillance study. The researchers noted that most children were under three years of age at the end of the follow-up period. They must have known there would be very few autism outcomes among the one- to three-year-olds, but included them anyway.

This would be akin to conducting a study of marriage trends among young people. If one looked at twenty- to thirty-years-olds, one would find many wedded couples, and the marriage "rate" would be relatively high. But what if ten- to twenty-year-olds were added to the mix? There would be roughly a doubling of the study population, but very few additional married couples. The rate would drop precipitously. Then imagine including one- to ten-year-olds (a preposterous idea), and the rate tumbles further.

Jane El-Dahr observed that it was likely that parents of children with disabilities might not have selected these particular HMOs in the first place. "I don't know about the level of services provided by Kaiser, but most families with disabled children pick health plans based on the level of payment of services for their child's needs," she told the group. "If kids with disabilities are not enrolled in these HMOs at the same rate as the diagnoses appear in the population, this is a worthless database."[137]

There were many other flaws, the group contended. When a child was diagnosed with any of the outcomes, this would be considered a statistical "end point" and the child would no longer be followed to see if any other problems were diagnosed.

"Does this mean that once a diagnosis such as speech delay was made, the child was removed from the database?" Lyn asked in her letter to the Institute of Medicine. "If so, subsequent diagnoses would not be counted. Using these criteria would definitely result in an under-reporting of diagnoses such as autism, which may first present as a speech or language delay or neurodevelopmental delay. Could this be the reason for the decreased incidence of these findings in the population studied?" Indeed, if Will had been enrolled in the VSD study, or Matthew Birt, or Bill Bernard, they would never have shown up on the charts as autistic.

Will's initial diagnosis had been language delay.

Then there was the complex issue of the study's statistical "power." In the science of statistics, larger pools of data always produce more accurate results by reducing the margin of error (which, in the parlance of number crunchers, is referred to as the 95 percent confidence interval, or 95 percent CI—meaning that analysts are 95 percent certain that the true number lies somewhere between the low and high ends of the margin of error). In a political poll, a larger sample size will typically have a slimmer margin of error. A survey of 1,000 voters will have more statistical "power" than a poll of 100 voters. Indeed, if you were to sample only 100 voters, the difference between support for candidate A and candidate B could well be due to chance. It would have very low statistical power. If the difference in votes fell within the wide margin of error, the results would not be considered "statistically significant."

The number of kids studied at one HMO, Northern California Kaiser, was fairly high at about 70,000. But in the second HMO, Group Health Collective of Puget Sound, there were only 16,000 children. The same was true for the third HMO, Harvard Pilgrim, in Massachusetts, whose data the CDC bought to compare with the results from the West Coast children. For this reason, the Kaiser numbers had much more power than those of Group Health or Harvard Pilgrim. Given this unevenness, the relative risks for an adverse outcome found at Kaiser were statistically significant. In the smaller HMOs, similar risks for outcomes were sometimes found, but the data failed to meet the criteria for significance. The margin of error (95% CI) was wider—the low end of the range fell below a relative risk of 1.0.

Speaking of Harvard Pilgrim, why would the CDC go outside its own massive database and purchase data from another source, to verify what was found in the first two sites? And why buy such a small database?

Moreover, the only outcomes that were investigated at Harvard Pilgrim were the ones found to be significant in the initial assessment: ADHD, speech delay, language delay, and tics. Autism was not even looked at because the first phase of the study had not found statistically significant outcomes for the disorder. Harvard Pilgrim had also come under financial constraints related to internal problems with its data. In January 2000, the HMO was placed under state receivership.[138] "We question if the problems with their information systems could possibly impact the VSD database analysis collected at this HMO," Lyn told the IOM in the letter.

"If the CDC were principled," Mark said to the group, "if they cared about the truth, if they were saying, 'This is a plausible hypothesis and we need to give it the best shot to figure out what's going on,' they would have done this very differently. It all leads me to believe this is deliberate. They are doing this to make the signal go away."

ON JUNE 15, 2001, Liz Birt finally received a reply from the CDC to her FOIA requests. The internal agency documents were ready to be picked up from headquarters in Atlanta. The agency refused Liz's request to waive the processing fees of $1,563.90. Even worse, the CDC denied Safe Minds' request for access to the raw VSD data for independent review, citing patient confidentiality. "We are unable, at this time, to protect the rights and privacy of the persons in organizations participating in the VSD, while at the same time sharing this information with outside groups such as Safe Minds."[139]

But there was a considerable concession. "Wishing to share information to the extent feasible," the letter said, "CDC invites Safe Minds and their science consultants to meet with CDC scientists to develop an analyses plan for the VSD data set, which could be mutually agreed upon and carried out to answer the questions of greatest interest to Safe Minds." The agency offered to conduct the analyses at no cost. "CDC hopes that Safe Minds will accept this offer," it said, "as CDC continues to explore more permanent mechanisms for sharing scientific data with outside parties."

"Mechanisms!" Liz scoffed as she read the letter. "We're supposed to ask them what to look for, and they will run the numbers and get back to us? I don't think so. They're hiding something. We need the raw data."

A few days later, Lyn drove into Atlanta, with a check furnished by Sallie, to retrieve the materials from CDC headquarters. She was handed a cardboard box filled with reams of documents, including hundred of e-mails between officials of the CDC, the FDA, the Academy of Pediatrics, and other organizations. The group would not have time to review everything before the Institute of Medicine meeting.

One document was worth an early look, however. It was the unpublished minutes from the closed-door review conducted on June 7–8, 2000, at Simpsonwood.

The Simpsonwood meeting had been convened by the CDC's National Immunization Program, which brought in eleven consultants and forty-nine other "resource specialists and observers" from state and federal health agencies, universities, medical academies, and the vaccine-producing drug companies. The intent was to review the VSD analysis to determine if there were a "signal" between thimerosal and developmental disorders and if so, how strong. The group was also asked to recommend next steps for the investigation.[140]

Simpsonwood is set amid a Georgia pine forest along the Chattahoochee River, which flows lazily through the western outskirts of Atlanta. The medium-frills compound (it's spartan, but with pool and tennis courts) is run by the North Georgia Conference of the United Methodist Church. The retreat's Web site calls it a "Christian ministry of hospitality offering a serene setting for renewal, reflection, relaxation, and enrichment of the mind, body, and spirit through Jesus Christ." Secular groups are welcome, except those "inconsistent with the Christian ideals inherent in this purpose."[141]

Lyn flipped through the 260-page transcript, dense with the jargon of epidemiologists and statisticians. She knew it was important, but it also looked deadly dull. The Redwoods were about to head out for a week's vacation in Florida, and Lyn rather reluctantly tossed the heavy report into her luggage, sarcastically thinking what terrific beach reading it would make.

When she got to Florida, Lyn read the first five pages of Simpsonwood and she was hooked by the gripping accounts. The document kept her up at night, crying, as she read how "consultants" to the CDC said that alarming indications of thimerosal's dangers could—at least in theory—be whittled down to next to nothing. The minutes confirmed the worst of what Lyn and the parents had suspected, she thought.

As soon as she got home, Lyn made copies of the report and sent it to Liz, Sallie, Mark, and Jane El-Dahr.

The CDC officials had said nothing to the parents about it, but they had in fact been making preliminary—and confidential—findings of an association between thimerosal and adverse outcomes. They knew it when they held their teleconference with Safe Minds back in June 2000, but kept mum about it. In fact, the officials had convened the high-level, unpublicized conference on the disturbing findings. Many critics would later allege that the Simpsonwood meeting was held to rubber-stamp a white-washed and watered-down report.

A summary of the Simpsonwood proceedings, somewhat contradictory in nature, was written by Dr. Paul Stehr-Green, an associate professor of epidemiology at the University of Washington. Dr. Stehr-Green failed to mention the fact that some participants had expressed reservations about the VSD team's methodology. He left the impression that any prior concerns about thimerosal were overblown, and that no evidence of harm had been found. And yet, even after the data underwent several "reanalyses," there remained a "slight tendency for groups with higher exposure to thimerosal-containing vaccines to have higher rates of the same neurobehavioral outcomes."[142]

On the other hand, the level and consistency of statistical significance of these findings was "unimpressive" and most consultants thought them weak at best.

At the same time, "the implications of this issue were profound and, therefore, further investigations should be pursued with a degree of urgency," he said, and ended his confusing summary by adding there was "nearly universal agreement" that the results "do not offer adequate evidence to support (or refute) the existence of causal relationship."

The minutes were far more revealing about the actual debate that took place. CDC officials were concerned there might be a problem associated with thimerosal. "What if the lawyers get hold of this?" one participant had asked at Simpsonwood. "There's not a scientist in the world who can refute these findings." Moreover, it appeared that the CDC was highly reluctant to offend the drug industry. One doctor at Simpsonwood wrote to colleagues afterward that CDC was "not in favor of expressing a preference for a particular vaccine (i.e. thimerosal free) for fear of alienating the other manufacturers and disrupting a free market economy."

Lyn said she was "stunned" by it. Liz said the minutes showed "just what a mess we are in."

Sallie was furious. She had had it with the CDC. "What is disgusting about this meeting," she wrote the group, "is that we met with the whole CDC contingent one week after Simpsonwood. We had given them our paper 2 1/2 months earlier, in April 2000. Yet, they never breathed a word of Simpsonwood at our meeting. Instead, they handed us VSD findings which said there was NO correlation with developmental disorders, and, even though we were known community advocates with an interest in the issue, we were not invited to Simpsonwood. Yet the whole gang from the vaccine manufacturers was there. These people play by different rules than everyone else, I guess because they've gotten away with it for so many years."

For Mark, the minutes were like "reading a novel I couldn't put down," he said. "They are hiding something." The purpose of the meeting was for the CDC to cover its tracks through a weekend of rubber-stamping, he guessed. "The investigators are legitimately worried. This isn't just Tom V, but also Bob Davis and even guys like Chen and DeStefano. They seem to have invited an easy crowd, the vast majority of whom are absolutely aching to find ways to dismiss this 'signal' if they can."

The dynamics of the meeting "discouraged any and all criticisms of the analysis," Mark said. It "suppressed important supporting comments, reached conclusions that were inconsistent with the data presented, and pointed to some seriously flawed next steps." Within days, Mark had written a harsh critique of Simpsonwood, suggesting that there was more doubt and dissent than Stehr-Green indicated in his summary. His six-page review, called "The Governance Problem," charged the following:[143]

1. There was an active interest in suppressing the signal in any way possible.
2. There was widespread interest in concealing the information in the study.
3. There had been clear, previous pressure to suppress the inquiry.
4. The constant praise for Verstraeten was careful and for the record, but supportive comments by consultants were clearly unwelcome.
5. There were clear moments at which conflicts of interest were apparent.
6. Numerous errors and omissions surrounded the science.

At the meeting, the CDC arranged for two researchers "to find ways to argue that data showing a signal was invalid," Mark wrote. "Dr. Robert Davis examined the accuracy of the data, and Dr. Philip Rhodes [a CDC statistician] devised a number of ways to manipulate the sample to achieve a less significant result."

Rhodes had suggested that one way to suppress the signal was to restore the thousands of children with congenital disorders who were excluded from the study. He argued to restore these cases, "which would serve to add 'noise' that could obscure the signal," Mark wrote. Rhodes himself had said, "All those kids that Tom has excluded, I have thrown them in. I think there is a clear argument that is going too far, but that further brings things down. So you can push, I can pull. But there has been substantial movement from this very highly significant result, down to a fairly marginal result."

Throughout the meeting, doubts were raised from a number of quarters about the study's merits. One of the biggest skeptics was Verstraeten himself. When he first came to the CDC, only one year before, he said, "one of the things I knew I didn't want to do was studies on toxicology or environmental health. I thought it was too confounding. It's very hard to prove anything in those studies. Now it turns out that other people also thought that this study was not the right thing to do."

Then he announced, "I will present the study nobody thought we should do."

Apparently the Simpsonwood group never thought their comments would be made public, and Verstraeten's candor grew with each passing hour. At one point he admitted that the preponderance of younger children had corrupted the results, dragging down the rate of outcomes.

"One thing that is for sure, there is certainly an under-ascertainment of all of these cases," he said. "Some children are just not old enough to be diagnosed. So the crude incidence rates are probably much lower than what you would expect, because the cohort is still very young."

And yet, Verstraeten said, there were clear warning signs in the data that implicated thimerosal. This was especially true with speech delay, the most common disorder found, and for which the trend had been "highly statistically significant."

Verstraeten had also separated out premature babies and looked at their outcomes. Among these smaller infants, who received many more micrograms per kilogram than normal babies, outcomes were not only statistically significant, but the risk was high. Verstraeten had looked at two groups of preemies whose total mercury exposure in the first year differed by just 25 micrograms. Children in the higher exposure group were two or three times more likely to have an adverse outcome than those in the lower exposure group. "The ones that got more thimerosal are at a higher risk," Verstraeten said, though he did note that the sample was quite small.

There seemed to be one consistent theme in what Verstraeten was saying. It did not matter to what extent the data was "pushed" or "pulled," the associations for neurological disorders and thimerosal exposure simply would not disappear. "You can look at this data and turn it around," he said, "and look at this, and add this stratum, and I can come up with very high risks. And I can come up with very low risks, depending on how you turn everything around. You can make it go away for some and then it comes back for others."

And then he dropped something of a bomb. "So the bottom line is, okay, our signal will *simply not just go away*" (italics added).

Verstraeten offered three possible explanations. "My first hypotheses is [that] it is parental bias. The children that are more likely to be vaccinated are more likely to be picked up and diagnosed. Second hypothesis, I don't know. There's a bias I haven't recognized, and nobody has yet told me about it," he said. "Third hypothesis: It's true. It's thimerosal."

Verstraeten was then asked if the thimerosal hypothesis was biologically plausible. "When I saw this, and I went back through the literature, I was actually stunned by what I saw," he replied. "Because I thought it is plausible. So basically to me that leaves all the options open, and that means I can not exclude such a possible effect."

His warnings seemed to fall largely on deaf ears. Most consultants concluded that the signal was weak and not significant. There was one conspicuous exception. His name was Dr. William Weil, "an old pediatrician," he told the group, from East Lansing, Michigan. Dr. Weil was also representing the Committee on Environmental Health of the AAP. Unlike his colleagues, Weil saw a clear connection between exposure and outcomes.

"The number of dose related relationships are linear and statistically significant," he lectured his colleagues. "You can play with this all you want. They are linear. They are statistically significant. The increased incidence of neurobehavioral problems in children in the past few decades is probably real."

Dr. Weil was particularly concerned about high-dose versus chronic exposure. "Like many repeated acute exposures, if you consider a dose of 25 micrograms on one day, then you are above threshold," he said. "And then you do that over and over to the same neurons. It is conceivable that the more mercury you get, the more effect you are going to get."

Weil also cautioned his colleagues that the brain and central nervous system are not fully developed at birth. They continue developing for months postpartum. These first months of life provided a critical window for damage. "The earlier you work with the central nervous system, the more likely you are to run into a sensitive period for one of these effects," he said. "It changes enormously the potential for toxicity. There's a host of neurodevelopmental data that would suggest that we've got a serious problem. To think there isn't some possible problem here is unreal."

Finally, the renegade said, he worked in special education in the public schools. "The number of kids getting help in special education is growing nationally and state by state at a rate we have not seen before," he said. Then, in a challenge to the genetics crowd: "The rise in the frequency of neurobehavioral disorders is much too graphic. We don't see that kind of genetic change in thirty years."

Weil wasn't the only one troubled. Dr. Richard Johnston, a pediatrician and immunologist, said the study "leads me to favor a recommendation that infants up to two years old not be immunized with thimerosal containing vaccines." Then he made a startling admission: "My gut feeling? It worries me enough. Forgive this personal comment, but I got called out at eight o'clock, and my daughter-in-law delivered a son. Our first male in the next generation, and I do not want that grandson to get a thimerosal-containing vaccine until we know better what is going on."

Some participants seemed concerned about their reputations. Dr. John Clements of the World Health Organization warned that research results would have to be "handled." He correctly predicted that "through the freedom of information," the data would be taken by others "and used in ways beyond the control of this group. I'm very concerned about that as I suspect it's already too late to do anything regardless of any professional body and what they say."

Others worried about lawsuits. Dr. Robert Brent, a pediatrics professor at Thomas Jefferson University in Delaware, said that "because of the nonsense of our litigious society, it will be a resource to our very busy plaintiff attorneys when this becomes available. They don't want valid data. They want business, and this could potentially be a lot of business." At another point he added: "The medical legal findings in this study, causal or not, are horrendous."

And, Brent warned, "You could readily find a junk scientist who would support the claim with 'a reasonable degree of certainty.' But you will not find a scientist with any integrity who would say the reverse with the data that is available. So we are in a bad position from the standpoint of defending any lawsuits. I am concerned."

Toward the meeting's end, all twelve consultants voted on whether more research was needed. Nearly all of them voted affirmatively. Then they were asked to rate the probability that there was a relationship between thimerosal and neurological problems, on a scale of 1 to 6. Eleven of them rated the probability as low, at 1 or 2. But the twelfth consultant rated it as a 4. It was Dr. Weil. His dissent was rebuked by Dr. David Johnson, of ACIP, who told him, "You are across the line! You are across the line toward the strong."

SIMPSONWOOD was powerful stuff. The parents were itching to share the record with anyone who would listen. Sallie knew the minutes had the potential to be explosive. "We need to strategize about how to use these Simpsonwood minutes to our best advantage," she wrote to the group days before the

IOM meeting. "I know we're all really pissed off. But let's think rationally about the best approach." She suggested sending the IOM committee the minutes, along with a critique.

"They can see that we see the data was manipulated, and we're not going to let it go," she said. "And we can ask the committee to be sure to ask Verstraeten about some of these issues, so he can't hide. We can make sure the IOM knows we will eventually get hold of the raw data, so the truth will come out anyway. They might as well dig it out themselves so they don't look like fools and hurt their long-term credibility."

There was a lot of work left before the IOM meeting. Boyd Haley, the Kentucky chemistry chair, and Jeff Bradstreet, the Florida pediatrician who treated kids with chelation, had been invited to present. Safe Minds members wanted their own voices heard, too. They pressed the committee to allow Lyn, Sallie, Mark, and Jane to testify.

"Lyn and I are concerned that the list of presenters selected to date is heavily weighted to those who will espouse the official government position of 'no evidence of harm,' " Sallie complained in another letter to the committee.[144] "This view is wrong and is not supported by the available evidence." She urged the committee to include Safe Minds; "otherwise the IOM will send a signal to the public that it is not interested in producing an unbiased report."

Sallie then upbraided the CDC and FDA. "Research on this issue will be carried out by the very agencies implicated in allowing thimerosal to continue in vaccine," she said. "This is a blatant conflict of interest, of the same vein as tobacco companies investigating smoking and lung cancer. We respectfully request that the recommendation be made that the above agencies and those who regularly conduct research for them not be allowed to be involved in future studies."

The committee agreed to have Mark and Jane testify. Sallie and Lyn could speak during the public comment session. The group braced for a grueling day in Cambridge.

ONE DAY before Lyn left for Massachusetts, attorney Roger Wilson drove out to Fayetteville, Georgia, to file the Redwoods' liability and negligence lawsuit in the Superior Court of Fayette County. Defendants included Wyeth Lederle, GlaxoSmithKline, and Aventis Pharmaceuticals, which made Will's shots, and Southern Company and Georgia Power Company, which operated coal-fired power plants in the area around Tyrone.

"The defendants have facilitated delivery of poisonous mercury into Will Redwood's body," the complaint said. This was done "by virtue of the drug companies having used a preservative which is more than 49% mercury by weight in their vaccines, and by virtue of Southern Company and Georgia Power having released mercury and other heavy metals into the air in particulate form for inhalation and other ingestion following deposition in the fields and streams around the Redwood residence.

"The mercury contamination combines with and compounds other exposures to cause permanent and disabling injury to Will Redwood. Each exposure was unnecessary and preventable," it said. "Will Redwood's parents were not informed that their son's vaccines contained [mercury]. Had they been given the option of paying more for a mercury-free vaccine, they would have taken this option. The cost of a mercury-free vaccine was only cents more."

The drug companies were "well aware that mercury is a neurotoxin and is highly toxic to the human system," the suit said. "By the time Will Redwood first received a thimerosal-containing vaccine, the defendants had actual knowledge that thimerosal was hazardous when introduced to humans." Will required special education and training as well as intense medical monitoring. His injury would "in all likelihood impair both the quality and the duration of his life." Meanwhile, Lyn and Tommy "suffered great personal emotional injury and grief as a result of his regression from a normally developing child into a severely impaired individual."

The Redwoods were suing for unspecified damages to cover past and future costs of medical expenses, emotional distress, and loss of consortium, which the lawsuit said included, "the care, comfort, and society of their child." They sought retaliatory damages, too. "Plaintiffs request proper and adequate punitive damages," the complaint said, "to punish and to deter defendants from a similar course of conduct in the future."[145]

ON A BRILLIANT SPRING MORNING in Cambridge, several dozen people gathered in a small auditorium at the Charles Hotel in downtown Cambridge, not far from Harvard Square. The Safe Minds parents buttressed themselves for a tough day of debate with some of the nation's leading experts on mercury poisoning, childhood disorders, and epidemiology.

It was IOM day.

The committee chair, Dr. Marie McCormick, who was also head of Maternal and Children's Health at the Harvard School of Public Health, was a middle-aged woman who came across—to the parents at least—as stern. The parents had taken to calling her "Church Lady" after the priggish Dana Carvey character on *Saturday Night Live*. "She is definitely hostile to our side," Mark had told his wife, Elise. "But we are determined to get our points across no matter what."

Lyn settled in to listen, alongside Sallie, Liz, Mark, and so many others with whom she had formed a comfortable bond.

The morning session went quietly enough, Lyn thought. Leslie Ball, the FDA pediatrician, reviewed her work in determining mercury exposure levels in children, and the safety guidelines established by different federal agencies. She was followed by two doctors from the University of Michigan, Gary Freed and Marjorie Andreade, who spoke on public perceptions of vaccine safety, government policy on thimerosal, and different ways to reduce vaccine mercury.

So far, so good, Lyn thought. Little was presented to dispute the mercury-autism theory. Then came a round of speakers who fell securely inside the Safe Minds camp. Jane El-Dahr reviewed the points raised in the Safe Minds paper on mercury poisoning and autism. She discussed how mercury can impair immune function and talked about the autoantibodies that can attack the brain.

"When I first started to review the immunology literature in this field, I was struck by the fact that every researcher who has looked for an anti-brain antibody of any kind of children with autism has been able to find it," she said. "I could not understand how this could occur. It was not until I heard about the idea of mercury and went to that literature and looked, that I found the explanation."[146]

Mercury causes diffuse damage to the nervous system by altering a number of key proteins. These altered proteins produce autoantibodies. The same antibodies found in people and animals exposed to mercury were also found in autistic children, she said.

And the antibodies perpetuate themselves, even if exposure stops. "Once mercury has bound to protein so the immune system recognizes it as foreign it is not necessary for the metal damage to continue for the autoimmune response to be perpetuated," she said.

Jeffrey Bradstreet, from the International Autism Research Center, presented his data on 221 children with ASD (183 boys and 38 girls) treated at the center. He found that 87.3 percent of them excreted mercury in their urine following chelation. Compared with control subjects, the autistic children were excreting on average 500 percent more mercury. Both groups had received the same thimerosal-containing vaccines.

When it came time for Thomas Verstraeten to present his VSD finding, the Belgian investigator opened with a surprising announcement. "As of eight A.M., European time, I have been employed by a vaccine manufacturer," he said. He had been hired by GlaxoSmithKlineBeecham to work at their offices back in Belgium.

It had been a year since Verstraeten presented his findings to the Advisory

Committee on Immunization Practices meeting in Atlanta. Since then, the VSD study had undergone yet another "reanalysis," as more children and more diagnoses were logged in the HMOs. But in this reanalysis, the team examined the two West Coast HMOs separately.

A year before, when the two were combined, the team had found a statistically significant risk of 1.64 for neurodevelopmental disorders. But now, with them separated because one HMO was small and lacked power to show statistical significance, Verstraeten said the results were no longer consistent. The same was true for speech and language delays. (The team had stopped looking at autism outcomes altogether.)

Verstraeten said there were arguments for and against an association between thimerosal and adverse outcomes. "What is an argument for the true effects? For some of the estimates, we found high statistical significance. Some of these associations are biologically plausible, and for some, we saw a dose response."

The argument against the theory, again, was that the findings were not consistent between HMOs. The larger HMO provided higher statistical power than the smaller one, but Verstraeten failed to name this discrepancy as a possible explanation for the inconsistent findings. "In phase one of our analysis, we found several significant associations between thimerosal and neurodevelopmental disorders," he said. "However, in an analysis in a smaller and independent data set, we could not confirm those associations for speech or language delay and ADHD."

Albert Enayati, who had driven up from New Jersey with his autistic son, Payam, lashed out at Verstraeten during question time. "You are having great difficulty putting everything together," he said. "To me this is a national emergency. Why should the whole nation be held hostage by a number of individuals at CDC?" He said that Safe Minds wanted the data itself, not other people's interpretations. "We have asked you repeatedly, not once, not twice, not three times, that we want to look at the raw data," he said. "We want an independent epidemiologist to look at the data, and you continue refusing us. If you have full confidence in what you are doing, what is wrong that an independent researcher could look at the data and come up with a fair assessment of what you are doing? You are just bringing the value of CDC lower and lower. As it is, the parents have zero confidence in the Centers for Disease Control immunization program. This type of behavior makes it one hundred percent worse."

Dr. Robert Chen, head of the VSD team, rose to challenge Albert. He said the HMO records were private. Release of the information would hurt business interests. "These are proprietary health care information systems, and we have to respect that," Chen said. "These HMOs are doing this for the public good, in terms of being able to collaborate and work with us, and they cannot basically allow their competitors to have that general release. We are trying to figure out a compromise mechanism."

The question of methylmercury versus ethylmercury also arose. Dr. George Lucier, former director of the Environmental Toxicology Program at the National Institutes of Environmental Health Sciences, said the methyl form remains in the blood longer than ethyl and was thought to cross the blood-brain barrier more efficiently. Ethylmercury was thought to be more toxic to kidneys.

But according to a study submitted to the IOM by the independent expert Laszlo Magos (who did not testify in person), ethylmercury is converted to inorganic mercury in the blood of animals at twice the speed of methylmercury.[147] There was evidence to suggest that inorganic mercury, once it crosses the blood-brain barrier, remains in the brain indefinitely. Since ethylmercury is converted to the inorganic form more quickly, this could suggest that it causes more long-term damage.

Official government policy was to treat ethyl and methyl mercury as equally toxic. Dr. Lucier said that ethylmercury was "slightly less toxic." But, he added, "the database for ethylmercury is weak, which creates considerable uncertainty in risk assessment. Ethylmercury should be considered equally potent." Lucier believed that both forms could accumulate in children, both during and after pregnancy. "Ethylmercury exposure from vaccines added to dietary exposures to methylmercury probably cause neurotoxic responses which are likely subtle in some children," he said.

As evidence, he discussed a study from the Faroe Islands, a cluster of windswept outcroppings belonging to Denmark, halfway between Iceland and Norway. During whaling season, the islanders eat huge amounts of whale meat, which contains high levels of methylmercury. Children born to mothers whose hair concentrations reached 10 to 20 parts per million were found with neurological deficits, especially in memory, attention, and language.[148]

He said that by adding ethylmercury exposure, even after averaging it out for several months, safety limits could have been reached to the point where "I don't think you can conclude anything but that there is a probability. And when I say it is probable, I mean it is somewhat greater than fifty percent for some individuals who have already elevated mercury levels; who may be genetically at risk."

Enough children were born at the "cusp" for toxic effects, he said, "that any additional exposure beyond that seems to me very likely to cause a neurodevelopmental effect. I'm not saying this is going to be a huge effect or happen in all the individuals. It is likely to be subtle, but it is likely to happen in some individuals."

Mark Blaxill's turn came next. "Something is happening here," he began. "I don't think any of us would claim to know exactly what, but your mission is the advancement of science. The history of science is often advanced by the anomaly, the trend that no one can explain using conventional theories." The committee was listening intently. "Infants have been exposed in an interesting contour to sharply higher amounts of mercury, thimerosal-containing vaccines, starting around 1990," Mark said. The timing of the increase in autism rates and rising mercury exposure from vaccines coincided.

The California data really got attention. Mark put up a slide to show rising levels of mercury in vaccines from 1990 to 1998 and the corresponding increase in autism cases. Because there is a lag time between vaccination and diagnosis, Mark overlaid the case rates in two-year lapsed time. They closely followed increased thimerosal exposures.

"We are seeing an anomaly, and no one has a good explanation for it," Mark said. "The reason it has not been addressed is because it is uncomfortable. One of the reasons it is uncomfortable is that the hypothesis we are discussing today is not an issue of infectious disease or even genetic disorders, but iatrogenic [physician-induced] disease."

Neal Halsey, who came last, seemed, to Lyn, to border on remorseful. When he realized the levels that children were being exposed to, his initial reaction had been surprise and disbelief, he said. "There still are a number of people involved in vaccines who have the disbelief that this could possibly be a true safety issue. But the calculations are correct."

So why had vaccine experts not taken note of the total mercury burden? Because vaccines were labeled as having a thimerosal concentration of .01 percent, "which in my mind and many other peoples' mind, this is a trace, trivial, insignificant amount," he said. But mercury exposure guidelines were in micrograms. "I did not, and others did not, go through the calculations," he continued. "I do believe that if the labeling had included the dose in micrograms, someone would have picked this up earlier than it was picked up. There is no doubt in my mind about that. I feel badly that I didn't pick it up."

Halsey pointed to a glaring inconsistency in U.S. mercury policy. In March 2001 the FDA advised women of childbearing age not to eat shark, mackerel, swordfish, and tilefish. Swordfish contains about 28.5 micrograms of mercury per ounce. He asked why a mother could not eat "a three or four ounce meal of swordfish, but yet her baby, which weighs about one twentieth of what she weighs, can have 62.5 micrograms on a given day?" he asked. "We would have lost credibility enormously in the eyes of the public if change hadn't been made."

Halsey went on to challenge the VSD study, in particular the purchase

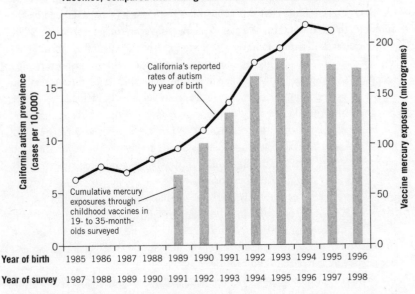

FIGURE 4. Rising levels of cumulative mercury exposure from childhood vaccines, compared with rising incidence of autism in California.

California's reported rates of autism by year of birth

Cumulative mercury exposures through childhood vaccines in 19- to 35-month-olds surveyed

Left axis: California autism prevalence (cases per 10,000)
Right axis: Vaccine mercury exposure (micrograms)

Year of birth: 1985 1986 1987 1988 1989 1990 1991 1992 1993 1994 1995 1996
Year of survey: 1987 1988 1989 1990 1991 1992 1993 1994 1995 1996 1997 1998

Source: Presentation by Mark Blaxill, Safe Minds, to meeting of Immunization Safety Review Committee, Institute of Medicine, Cambridge, Massachusetts, July 16, 2000.

and use of the Massachusetts data. He claimed that some people had seen no effect at the Harvard Pilgrim HMO thereby refuting the hypothesis: "Well, that is really not true. I don't know what the real power is of that study to say that there really isn't an effect there." His own interpretation, Halsey said, was that the data were inconclusive, but still "suggestive of an effect from thimerosal."

During public comment, Sallie rose to speak. "We heard today there is a very good chance that these kids have been damaged," Sallie said. "Where is the research? This finding on thimerosal came out in July of 1999. In the two years since, there has been nothing done to look at treating these children." Parents had initiated their own studies on chelation, she said, "but we don't even know if chelation is going to work. Where is the research going to start? When is science going to focus on this, take it seriously and do something about our kids?"

When the day was over, many parents left with a cautious smile on their face. "We got our message across," Mark said. "I was surprised the other side didn't bring out their top guns, only mid-level people. It seemed they weren't putting up a very big fight." Mark then invited the group to the Blax-ill home for beer, pizza, and a little good cheer.

Lyn was pleased. "IOM was incredible!" she wrote later to Rick Rollens. "The government looked very bad, all the science was on our side. Even folks who were presenters who we did not think shared our views, did."

8. Damn Lies and Statistics

TWO YEARS HAD PASSED since the Joint Statement on Thimerosal had been issued, and for the first time, Liz, Lyn, and Sallie felt as if they could take a small breather from their thimerosal crusade during the summer of 2001. The years had taken a toll, on the women, their families, even their marriages. There had been too many papers, too many medical meetings, rallies, congressional hearings, and late-night conference calls to allow for anything close to a normal life. Not that life with an autistic kid could ever be normal.

The stress was hitting Liz Birt and her family the hardest. Matthew was sick almost all the time again. She had tried chelation therapy, but it only seemed to make him sicker. Once, just a few days after a treatment, Matthew had a grand mal seizure at school and was rushed to the hospital. It could have been an episode of epilepsy, which ran in Liz's family. But after that, she didn't try chelation again.

Liz's marriage was disintegrating. The year before, her husband had told her she needed to curb her autism activism for the sake of everyone else in the household. She was spending too much time on the road, at meetings, in the law libraries. He was concerned. She needed to be home with the kids.

One afternoon at home, out of earshot of the children, he complained to Liz that she was "obsessed." He worried that she was spending too much time trying to nail "those" people. Maybe, he added, one needed to be a little "obsessed" to reach one's goals, but not to the point of being a bad mother. Liz knew he had a point. But fighting this fight, she felt, was the same thing as taking care of Matthew, who was still sick, still not talking. Recently he had taken to climbing atop high bookshelves and curling up like a cat.

Lyn Redwood desperately needed to spend more time with her family as well. Tommy would grimace wearily at her nonstop activism, and the children missed her.

But some of Lyn's work was starting to show dividends. Will seemed to be getting better. Lyn wasn't sure if it was the ABA-style therapy, the chelation, the dietary interventions she was trying, like high-dose vitamin B-12 therapy, or a combination of these things.

"Will is making steady progress," his teacher wrote in his first grade end-of-year report. "He smiles daily, he is well mannered and anxious to please." His reading comprehension was quite good, though his math concept skills were poor, and he still showed patterns of disability. Most of his learning was still rote in nature, recalling information rather than actually processing concepts. But he was improving, and Lyn and Tommy were delighted.

In July, Will and Lyn flew to Tampa to visit her mother. Lyn had arranged an appointment with Dr. Jeff Bradstreet, at his clinic in Palm Bay, a two-hour drive away. Bradstreet gave the boy an exhaustive workup, including repeated blood tests and a screening of Will's organic urinary acids. Bradstreet was finding many commonalities in the urinary acids of autistic children, and Will was no exception.

Bradstreet found the presence of highly unusual bacteria, for which he prescribed antibiotics. Will also had low levels of coenzyme Q, glycerin, and glutathione, a sulfur-based protein and one of the body's natural chelators. Bradstreet prescribed a course of IV glutathione, to be repeated every six months and supplemented with oral glutathione.

The vitamin B-12 levels in Will's blood were almost off the charts. Lyn had been giving Will high-dose oral B-12 every day for over a year, so it stood to reason. But many children have ultrahigh B-12 serum levels, not because of dosing, but because their tissue for some reason was not absorbing the nutrient. One way to test for this was to measure the level of methylmalonic acid. High levels of this acid meant the B-12 was not being absorbed, and Will's levels were very high.

Bradstreet also found the presence of autoantibodies to myelin basic protein (which helps insulate nerve cells), another common trait in autistic kids. What's more, Will had a very low ratio of sulfur to creatine in his urine, which indicated a sulfur depletion, also common in autism. Meanwhile, his copper levels were highly elevated, which was consistent with

what Bill Walsh was finding in his research on metal metabolism and depletion of metallothienein, another sulfur-based protein that binds with mercury to eliminate it from the body. Finally, Bradstreet prescribed oral
selenium tablets daily. "It is the best ongoing defense against residual brain
mercury," he told Lyn.

As the summer settled into its quiet rhythms, the work of Safe Minds did
not stop entirely. The quest for access to the VSD data continued. Dan Burton backed the parents in their mission. On July 28, 2001, he wrote to Dr.
Walter Orenstein, director of the CDC's National Immunization Program, requesting all the raw data from VSD and Harvard Pilgrim, plus updates on
medical records and patient chart reviews. "We understand that names of
these children need to be redacted," Burton wrote, adding that children's
birth dates could also be changed to reflect only month and year of birth.[149]

But the CDC refused to release the data to anyone. On August 6, Liz ap-
pealed the decision. "Because of the harm done to the process of scientific inquiry by your unreasonable delays and withholding," she wrote, "we seek an
expedited appeal with respect to the wrongfully withheld VSD data." The
CDC's refusal to release the information was "contrary to the traditional
practice in the scientific community of making raw data publicly available so
that other researchers can confirm—or refute—the conclusions reached in
your studies," Liz said.[150]

The CDC's decision to block access was "based on the entirely improper
use of hiding the truth about the connection between thimerosal in vaccines
and developmental delays, including autism, from the general public, parents
of afflicted children who could seek immediate treatment, the press and Congress," she said.

Liz said the CDC had "skewed and sanitized the data" to make the study
conform to a "predetermined bias that there is 'no proof' that thimerosal is
harmful."

It took almost a year for the CDC to issue a formal rejection of Liz's appeal. Agency officials concluded that release of the data, even with names removed, would "constitute a clearly unwarranted invasion of personal
privacy."[151] There were still ways to determine the identity of the patients,
which would be a serious breach of legal and ethical codes.

And the CDC cited another reason. It was opposed to releasing data until
the VSD study was published in a medical journal. The analysis contained
"preliminary findings" that were "pre-decisional." Release of the data would
interfere with the agency's "deliberative and decision-making process." Critics said this argument was bogus. Data is data, they countered. Data cannot
be altered through the "deliberative process."

The CDC had not closed the door entirely, however. A few weeks later, officials from the CDC and IOM invited Safe Minds to send three of its members to Washington for a small planning meeting in which the CDC would instruct the IOM to oversee a reanalysis of the VSD data. Safe Minds was invited to discuss a "statement of task" for the project, and to air its concerns over any new studies.[152] No industry representatives would be invited. It was a serious, generous offer. Safe Minds accepted. Lyn, Liz, and Sallie would fly to Washington for the meeting, which was scheduled for Thursday, September 13, 2001.

Two days before the meeting was to take place, the unimaginable happened. The World Trade Center lay in a toxic, smoldering heap and the Pentagon had a ghastly slice cut from it, like some giant stone pie. The country reeled in grief. The nation's business came to a virtual standstill for several on-edge days, as Americans kept their bloodshot eyes glued to the news.

On September 13, no one was flying anywhere. The IOM briefing was canceled.

The terrorist attacks of September 11 altered everything in America. The atrocity even influenced the thimerosal controversy. The sudden threat of terrorism, and especially bioterrorism, would transform the national discourse on vaccine injuries, and the civil liability of drug companies that supply the nation's immunization arsenal. In the post 9-11 world, pharmaceutical companies would likely be called upon to produce vaccines against horrors like smallpox and anthrax. In return, they would clamor for protection against vaccine injury lawsuits, especially in cases involving thimerosal.

THREE WEEKS after the attacks, with the national media still fixated on global terrorism, the IOM committee released its findings. The report was shared with reporters on October 1 through a conference call, rather than in person, due to post-attack travel considerations. The committee staff extended a rare offer to Lyn, Sallie, and Barbara Loe Fisher to listen in on the call. They were also sent advance copies of the report.

The committee report was hardly a solid win for Safe Minds. But it did not rule out the possibility that thimerosal in vaccines could cause neurological damage. "Although the hypothesis that exposure to thimerosal-containing vaccines could be associated with neurodevelopmental disorders is not established and rests on indirect and incomplete information," the report said, "the hypothesis is biologically plausible."[153]

Lyn and Sallie were pleased with this. They knew that establishing plausibility was the first step toward proving causation. And the IOM echoed many of the points Safe Minds had been making. Plausibility evidence, while "indirect," included:

1. High-dose thimerosal exposures are associated with neurological damage.
2. Toxicological and epidemiological literature establishes methylmercury, a close relative, as a toxicant to the developing nervous system.
3. Children who received the maximum number of thimerosal-containing vaccines were exposed to ethylmercury in amounts that exceeded some federal guidelines for methylmercury.
4. Some children could be particularly vulnerable to mercury due to genetic or other differences.

On the other hand, much of the available evidence discounted plausibility:

1. Low-dose thimerosal exposure in humans has not been demonstrated to be associated with effects on the nervous system.
2. Neurodevelopmental effects have been demonstrated for prenatal but not postnatal exposures to low doses of methylmercury.
3. Toxicological information on ethylmercury, particularly at low doses, is limited.
4. Thimerosal exposure from vaccines has not been proven to result in mercury levels associated with toxic responses.
5. Symptoms of mercury poisoning are not identical to those of autism and other NDDs.
6. Autism is thought to originate primarily from prenatal injury.

The IOM was either unable or unwilling to determine whether causation—as opposed to plausibility—had been shown. "The evidence is inadequate to accept or reject a causal relationship between exposure to thimerosal from vaccines and the neurodevelopmental disorders of autism, ADHD, and speech or language delay," the report said. Critics on both sides derided what they perceived to be scientific waffling.

The panel acknowledged that concerns over thimerosal would not simply evaporate. The preservative was still found in vaccines given to children, including the tetanus and flu shots. It was also in an "unknown quantity" of Hib and DTaP vaccines still on shelves and being used by doctors. And many foreign countries, especially in the developing world, depended on thimerosal as a preservative for multidose vaccines.

The continued presence of mercury in vaccines could "raise doubts about the entire system of ensuring vaccine safety," the report warned. "Late recognition of the potential risk" could contribute to a "perception among some that careful attention to vaccine components has been lacking." The committee found "significant reasons for continued public health attention to concerns about thimerosal."

The panel's list of recommendations was impressive. Much of it echoed what Safe Minds had been demanding for some time. The committee called for the use of thimerosal-free DTaP, Hib, and hep-B vaccines, "despite the fact that there might be remaining supplies of thimerosal-containing vaccine available." To Lyn and Sallie, this was tantamount to a recall. Score one for Safe Minds, they thought.

The panel also called on "professional societies and governmental agencies" to review policies about thimerosal use in products other than vaccines given to infants, children, and pregnant women. Other sources of thimerosal exposure, such as Rho(D), should be identified, and fetal exposure to mercury through maternal fish consumption should also be considered.

As for actual research, the IOM called for case-control studies to "examine the potential link," and population studies to "compare the incidence and prevalence of neurodevelopmental disorders before and after the removal of thimerosal from vaccines."

The panel called for research into how children metabolize and excrete metals, "particularly mercury." It called for theoretical modeling of ethylmercury exposures, "including the incremental burden of thimerosal with background mercury exposure from other sources." And, to the parents' surprise, the IOM supported "careful, rigorous and scientific investigations of chelation when used in children with neurodevelopmental disorders, especially autism."

The press release that accompanied the report likewise seemed balanced and straightforward, Lyn and Sallie thought. "Link Between Neurodevelopmental Disorders and Thimerosal Remains Unclear," the headline said.[154] "Current scientific evidence neither proves nor disproves a link" between thimerosal and neurodevelopmental disorders, the release said. But, it noted: "Mercury can build up in the body with each additional exposure, whether from vaccinations or other sources, such as fish consumption. It is medically plausible that some children's risk of a neurodevelopmental disorder could rise in part through increased mercury exposure from thimerosal-containing vaccines."

Because safety guidelines were established specifically for methylmercury, the report added, it wasn't clear if "additional exposure from ethylmercury could result in an unsafe cumulative level."

Lyn and Sallie thought the tone of caution was impressive. But committee chair Marie McCormick didn't seem to think so. In the press release, she opined that the IOM report "should be reassuring news for parents."

Clearly, there was a difference in philosophy. The committee saw the thimerosal glass as half full, Lyn and Sallie thought, while Dr. McCormick seemed to think of it as half empty, if not completely dry. Lyn grew more agitated as McCormick read her remarks and answered questions from reporters. The data "did not show a consistent dose-response relationship, that is, the more you got the more the risk was increased," she said. A reporter from *USA Today* asked if that was an argument against plausibility. McCormick said yes.[155]

But VSD data had indeed shown a statistically significant relationship between rising exposure levels and increased risk at the largest HMO. Yes, there was a dose-response relationship, but it was not "consistent." The two smaller HMOs, while reporting a dose-response relationship, did not meet the criteria for statistical significance.

McCormick also told the reporters that thimerosal exposures in children were "very low," that thimerosal in vaccines had not been "proven to be dangerous," and that the hypothesis that it was, was "not supported by clinical or experimental evidence." But she failed to note that the hypothesis was not disproved by the evidence, either.

Word of McCormick's press conference quickly spread. "I understand from Sallie that Church Lady was somewhat less than honest during the press conference (big surprise there . . . !)," Jane El-Dahr e-mailed Lyn later that day. "I got Liz a voodoo doll for her birthday. I think I know who the inaugural person stuck full of pins will be."

Lyn concurred. "I am still so pissed," she wrote back. "As soon as it ended I called Beth Clay, and then Church Lady herself! I ranted at them for about 15 minutes and said that since this direct misrepresentation of the report has happened, now it warrants investigation! I am out for blood here! It takes a lot to get me really pissed off, and she has done it."

SAFE MINDS would have to challenge Dr. McCormick on her assertions, in addition to offering a reply to the report itself. Sallie thought they should praise the IOM committee "overall, in tone," because its recommendations were "what we've been saying for over a year." But she also wanted to "blast the fact that they couldn't find the evidence conclusive one way or the other," she said. "The evidence is all over the place. Essentially, they discounted everything that wasn't published, though they said they looked at it. The findings are schizophrenic. How can their recommendations be so good, yet they find the evidence inconclusive?"

The IOM was "very worried," she surmised, "and they're sending their own signal to the medical community that thimerosal is a real problem. They are telling them that further research will make the evidence conclusive, and to be prepared."

Mark had a slightly different take. "We need to celebrate victory here," he said. "The text of the document reads favorably. Their recommendations are quite comprehensive and very good. We should say that they effectively support our entire research agenda.

"What we got," Mark added, "is the best we could have hoped for."

Media accounts of the IOM report tended to take the thimerosal peril seriously, while also echoing the document's muddled, glass-half-full conclusions. "Vaccines May Pose Mercury Hazard for Kids," warned one headline in *USA Today*.[156]

" 'Infants and children should not get vaccines with thimerosal,' says an Institute of Medicine report," the article began. But then again, it continued, no "proof" of harm had been found, and it quoted Dr. McCormick's opinion that this was "reassuring news." On the other hand, the IOM panel "couldn't dismiss possible problems related to thimerosal."

Harmful or not, thimerosal was "still on the shelves in some clinics," the article warned. "Parents should ask that their child receive thimerosal-free vaccines. But if unavailable, they should still get the vaccinations for their child."

Within days, Safe Minds had completed its official response and distributed it on a publicity news wire service. The group was "pleased that the IOM report acknowledges the biological plausibility," they said, before questioning the report for not going far enough. "We believe that no child should get any mercury-containing vaccines," they added. "We are renewing our call for the immediate removal of remaining stocks of childhood thimerosal-containing vaccines still on shelves. In addition, we ask that research be conducted into how to identify and repair mercury damage in children."[157]

Lyn also complained directly to the Institute of Medicine about the "pervasive pattern of misrepresentation" by Dr. McCormick in her press conference remarks. Her words "seemed more to reflect the position of a public relations director for the National Immunization Program than the chair of an impartial review committee," Lyn said. "Quite frankly, we are deeply concerned by her conduct."[158]

"Thimerosal has not been proven safe," Lyn added. "We are getting quite tired of repeating the mantra that 'absence of evidence is not evidence of absence.' But given Dr. McCormick's determined spin in the other direction, we have little choice. The kind of ideological bias Dr. McCormick has displayed is the essence of conflict of interest. Indeed, it is because she evinces the zeal of the true believer that we consider her unfit to continue in the role of chair."

Meanwhile, the American Academy of Pediatrics echoed Dr. Mc-Cormick's sunny outlook on the findings. The academy issued a press release on October 1, to coincide with the report. "IOM Report on Vaccines Should Reassure Parents—Children Should Be Vaccinated," the headline said.[159] "No evidence currently exists that proves a link between thimerosal-containing vaccines" and autism or other neurological developmental disorders, the release continued. Like Dr. McCormick, AAP president-elect Dr. Louis Z. Cooper was quoted as saying that parents "should be reassured about the safety of vaccines," while children "should be immunized according to the recommended age-appropriate schedule."

Lyn fired off another letter, this time to Dr. Cooper. The academy's statement "left me wondering if we had read the same report," Lyn said. "Pediatricians pay sizeable dues to be members of the American Academy of Pediatrics and rely on your organization to keep them up to date on research and policy that impact their practice. In my opinion, the 55,000 members of AAP deserve a refund."

Lyn complained that four "highlights" of the IOM report were virtually ignored by the AAP: "1) There is insufficient evidence to support or refute the safety of thimerosal in vaccines; 2) The association between thimerosal and neurodevelopmental disorders is biologically plausible; 3) Thimerosal should be removed from medical products; 4) Further research is necessary."

"Instead of relaying these balanced set of facts, your press release focused on misleading statements," Lyn charged. "The American public, partially due to advances on the Internet, is now able to access documents like the IOM report and read the findings themselves. They will no longer tolerate cherry picking of reports to portray a false sense of security. Shame on you AAP!"[160]

WITHIN DAYS of the IOM announcement, a second round of FOIA documents arrived from the CDC. This time a box was mailed to Liz's home (the family had since moved to the leafy North Shore suburb of Wilmette).

No one will ever know what would have transpired if Safe Minds had obtained these documents before the IOM held its meeting, for the information they contained was explosive. When the box arrived, Liz was getting ready for a DAN! conference. She stuffed some of the papers into her carry-on, thinking they would make for good plane reading. Liz had no idea how good they would be.

About an hour into the flight, Liz took out the documents. There were scores of e-mails between officials who had been privy to the VSD study in its early days. But one document stood out from the rest. It was a thirty-page

FIGURE 5. Relative risk + 95% CI of *autism* after different exposure levels of thimerosal at 3 months of age, NCK and GHC.

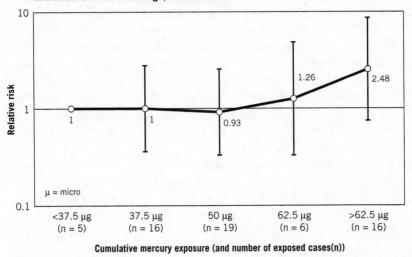

Relative risk

10

1

0.1

1   1   0.93   1.26   2.48

μ = micro

| <37.5 μg | 37.5 μg | 50 μg | 62.5 μg | >62.5 μg |
| (n = 5) | (n = 16) | (n = 19) | (n = 6) | (n = 16) |

Cumulative mercury exposure (and number of exposed cases(n))

Source: Thomas Verstraeten, et al., Graph 3 from "Thimerosal VSD study, Phase I—Update 2/29/00," internal report of the National Immunization Program, CDC, February 29, 2000.

report, stapled together and titled "Thimerosal VSD Study, Phase I—Update 2/29/00." At the top of each page were the words "CONFIDENTIAL—DO NOT COPY OR RELEASE."[161]

Liz had never seen this one before. In fact, few people outside the CDC even knew it existed. Liz was infuriated that the government would have kept something like this confidential. She thumbed through the report until she arrived at the results section. When she read the part about autism, she almost gagged on her peanuts. Children in the two HMOs who received the most mercury, more than 62.5 micrograms, at three months of age were almost *two and a half times* more likely to develop autism, with a relative risk of 2.48, than those in the lowest exposure group.

"Holy shit!" Liz shrieked audibly, without realizing it. Startled passengers turned to stare. The woman next to her looked petrified. "They knew!" Liz said. "Those bastards knew, and . . . and . . . they covered it up!" Just as the woman was about to change seats, Liz regained her composure and offered an apology.

Then she settled in to read. No wonder this was never released. In February of 2000, the CDC knew it had a grave problem, she thought. They were sitting on a relative risk of 2.48, and must have realized that if they went public with it, all hell would break loose. So what did they do? It simply looks like they started playing with the numbers until they got that risk down to 1.69, which is what they presented at that ACIP meeting back in June 2000.

On closer inspection, Liz saw that the 2.48 relative risk was just shy of being statistically significant: the low end of the margin of error (95% CI) fell slightly below the risk of 1.0. No matter. This was big. It was the closest thing to a smoking gun anyone had found.

There was more. Authors Verstraeten, Davis, and DeStefano explained that they had considered exposures at one and three months because "at this age, the central nervous system is still immature and more susceptible to mercury."

Among the children studied, they found "increasing risks of neurological developmental disorders with increasing cumulative exposure to thimerosal." They also found "similar increases" for the risk of developmental speech disorder, autism, stuttering, and attention deficit disorder, though these increases were not statistically significant.

"We can state," it said, "that this analysis does not rule out that receipt of thimerosal-containing vaccine in children under three months of age may be related to an increased risk of neurological developmental disorders."

When Liz returned home, she sent copies of the documents to her Safe Minds colleagues. She also sent a copy to Andy Waters, the lawyer in Dallas.

Nothing in the papers could be construed as incontrovertible proof of any deliberate manipulation or cover-up. But there were some revealing e-mails showing that at least some officials were worried about the early results emerging from the data.

Some messages appear without context, rendering them a bit vague and even cryptic to the outside reader. Take, for instance, the e-mail that Verstraeten sent on December 17, 1999—midway through his initial analysis—to Davis and DeStefano.[162]

"It just won't go away," the subject line read. Verstraeten did not specify what "it" was, but one could reasonably assume he meant the "signal" between thimerosal exposure and certain outcomes.

In the memo, he said, "all the harm is done in the first month," without defining what the "harm" was. And he ended with this plea: "Some of the relative risks increase over the categories, and I haven't yet found an alternative explanation. Please let me know if you can think of one."

On March 9, 2000, Verstraeten sent another e-mail to Davis and DeStefano, again showing concern that thimerosal had damaged at least some of the kids. Looking at the diagnosis "neurologic developmental delay," he had found a "relationship with increasing numbers of Hib or DTP" vaccines, both of which typically had contained thimerosal. "This does not make sense," wrote Verstraeten.[163] "A cumulative effect seems more reasonable for a toxic substance like mercury than for a biological agent like a vaccine, I would think." This indicated that thimerosal was the problem, not the vaccine.

Verstraeten also noticed that the risk of developmental delay began to drop among children who, for whatever reason, failed to get their first Hib and DTP shots before three months of age. He said it confirmed his "hypothesis" that it didn't really matter "whether a kid gets thimerosal in the second or third month of life. What matters is not getting it before the third month, after which the implications gradually diminish."

Ten days later, Verstraeten raised yet another red flag. He had selected a number of patient charts for use in an internal audit of data from Northern California Kaiser. They included charts for ten premature infants. Some preemies had received a series of four DTP-Hib combination shots, with a total of 100 micrograms of mercury. The others received the vaccines separately—four DTPs and four Hibs—with a total of 200 micrograms of mercury. He found a stunning relative risk of 5.0 among the high-exposure group, compared with kids who received the combination vaccines. The finding was "very extreme," he said. "It warrants closer examination of these diagnoses."[164]

Verstraeten was not the only one with concerns. On April 26, 2000, Coleen Boyle, an official in the CDC's Division of Birth Defects, sent her own comments on the study to Frank DeStefano. She echoed the study's critics by pointing to the preponderance of younger children in the pool, as this would dilute the relative risks for many outcomes. "Since most of the diagnoses are generally not picked up until the second or third year of life, had you considered eligibility criteria of at least 18 months or two years?" she asked. "What happens if you do this?"[165] They were good questions.

Boyle was also worried about the low rate of adverse outcomes found in the study, compared with the general population. "For me, the big issue is the missed cases and how this relates to exposure," she said. "Clearly there is a gross underreporting." The VSD figures showed that 1.4 percent of the kids had a speech or language problem, she said. But national surveys had revealed rates of 4 to 5 percent. Meanwhile, attention deficit/hyperactivity disorder (ADHD) was found in less than 1 percent of the VSD children, even though other reports said that the rate in the general population was more like 3 to 10 percent.

The acquisition of the Harvard Pilgrim data was another cause for concern. To begin with, the HMO relied on diagnostic codes that were entirely different from those used at the original two HMOs. It would be difficult to make direct comparisons between the Massachusetts outcomes and those diagnosed on the West Coast. Just as worrisome, there was very little variation in the thimerosal exposure levels of the children in the database, which was "bad because you also have no internal heterogeneity that would allow us to differentiate the thimerosal effect from other effects," as Verstraeten wrote to a Harvard Pilgrim executive.[166]

Finally, there was a lot of buzz about Simpsonwood. A detailed account of the weekend was issued by one of the participants, Dr. Thomas Saari, to dozens of colleagues around the country. His reviews were mixed.

The general consensus at Simpsonwood had been that there was little evidence, if any, of harm. Even with high bolus doses, total mercury levels "still appeared to be far too low to cause problems," Saari wrote. On the other hand, there was "sufficient data to suggest a signal (nay an association) that further study is warranted," he said, adding that roughly half the consultants "felt ambivalent" about the results. "If a signal exists at all," he said, "the likelihood that thimerosal is the culprit is weak."[167]

But then he contradicted this by observing that "the effects on neurodevelopment don't appear until total mercury doses from vaccines exceed 50mcg per visit."

Saari discussed how the data was "recalculated to look for raw relative risk rates and trends." But despite these efforts to remove the "confounding" factors, risk rates were "unchanged or actually somewhat higher."

"The associations," he said, "simply would not go away."

In the end, the consultants proposed a number of follow-up studies. But there was little enthusiasm at Simpsonwood for this idea. Many believed that "little more could be gained in manipulating the current CDC study further," Saari said. He added that some attendees felt "this study should never have been done, because it was bound to create this controversy."

Verstraeten was not pleased with Simpsonwood either. He was discomfited that some participants had wanted to compare data from injected doses of ethylmercury to data on ingested methylmercury from the Faroe Islands studies. Such comparisons, he said, were irrelevant and probably invalid.

On July 14, 2000, Verstraeten wrote to Philippe Grandjean, the lead investigator in the Faroe Islands study, about his misgivings.[168] "I apologize for dragging you into this nitty-gritty discussion, which in Flemish we would call 'muggeziften,' " he said. "I know much of this is very hypothetical. Personally, I would rather not drag the Faroes into this thimerosal debate, as I think they are as comparable to our issue as apples and pears, at the best."

Verstraeten fretted that many experts did not "seem bothered by comparing apples to pears." Their attitude seemed to be that "if nothing is happening in these studies, then nothing should be feared of thimerosal."

"I do not wish to be the advocate of the anti-vaccine lobby and sound like being convinced that thimerosal is or was harmful," he said. "But at least I feel we should use sound scientific argumentation and not let our standards be dictated by our desire to disprove an unpleasant theory."

And there was another very interesting e-mail that Liz came across. It was sent by the CDC's Walter Orenstein to Roger Bernier, asking if maybe Sallie Bernard and the folks from New Jersey should be invited to the [Simpsonwood] review."[169] Liz never found the response, but she knew what the answer had been.

MARK BLAXILL was the first to take aim at the secret VSD documents. "Liz just faxed me the initial Phase I analyses from CDC," he told Lyn. "I spent some time going through the data (love those plane flights). I believe it demonstrates a major error in the CDC's use of the data that led them to understate the autism risk."

More than 34,000 new patients had been added to the sample between this initial analysis and the one that was shared publicly at ACIP in June 2000. "The vast majority came from two relaxations in the exclusion provisions," Mark wrote.[170] The initial sample excluded 19,300 children who appeared not to be continuously enrolled, but were considered to be continuously enrolled in the later sample. "This represented a 9.3 percent increase in the inclusion rate for the later sample. This may be a problematic inclusion."

The researchers had also excluded from the initial report 13,300 other children with congenital/perinatal disorders, only to add them back in the later sample. This led to an additional 15.2-percent increase in the inclusion rate, according to Mark. "The incorporation of these previously excluded children *sharply* changed the profile of both the autistic and the NDD samples," he said, and went on to suggest that "this offers the possibility for fraudulent manipulation."

Since so many younger children were included, the relative risk of autism was guaranteed to go down. "In essence the CDC made the same mistake many do when they count cases of autism: they failed to account for the length of time it takes for a typical case of autism to get diagnosed and find its way into the system," Mark wrote. "They simply assumed that a case of autism will show up as frequently in a cohort of one-year-olds as in a five-year-old cohort. The literature clearly shows the opposite. This flawed assumption leads them to some major errors."

Mark was right about the statistics. Among the youngest 40 percent of kids, there was not a single report of autism. "It may therefore be possible that the relative risk for the 3–5 year old group may exceed 4.0 times," Mark surmised. "But I can't say this for sure without knowing more about how they calculated relative risk."

Lyn identified another problem. Older children often "disenrolled" from the HMOs, leaving the database younger still. "This may be OK if you are looking at allergic reactions to a vaccine, but not for long term outcomes like delayed neurotoxicity," she said. "We have to get to the bottom of this VSD data and have Burton hold a hearing, and then a Department of Justice investigation—they knew what they were doing!"

ANDY WATERS, the attorney from Dallas, decided to go public with the secret VSD documents he had received from Liz.

"We are now in possession of a previously unreleased confidential report authored by CDC scientists," he announced to the media on October 16, 2001.[171] The report "clearly demonstrated that an exposure to more than 62.5 micrograms of mercury within the first three months of life significantly increased a child's risk of developing autism. Specifically, the study found a 2.48 times increased risk of autism. U.S. courts of law have generally held that a relative increased risk of 2.0 or higher is sufficient to substantiate that a given exposure causes disease."

· Waters noted in the press release that lead author Thomas Verstraeten had "since left the CDC and is now employed by GlaxoSmithKline, a manufacturer of thimerosal-containing vaccines for many years that is a defendant in numerous suits pending nationwide." He called on Glaxo to permit the deposition of Verstraeten, "in order to understand if conflict of interest issues may have played a role in the CDC's decision to keep this report confidential, and specifically, their failure to reveal it to the IOM."

The report, and the fact that it was kept from the public, was "shocking, but unfortunately not surprising," Waters said, given the "political influence of pharmaceutical companies and the tremendous liability they face if they are forced to compensate thousands of families for the costs of care that these children require."

THE DAY after Waters made his announcement, the CDC's Advisory Committee on Immunization Practices convened a regularly scheduled two-day meeting in Atlanta. Thimerosal and the IOM report were featured topics on the agenda. On October 17, 2001, Sallie flew in to attend, alongside Lyn.

At the meeting, the CDC announced that it had conducted a random survey of the remaining supply of thimerosal-containing DTaP, Hib, and hep-B vaccines within its own massive distribution system. Among the sixty-six thousand doses examined, only 5.5 percent contained thimerosal.[172]

But when it came time for public comment and Lyn got up to speak (by now ACIP members were used to the stubborn mother), she lectured the panel about the secret VSD report. "As early as December 1999, senior CDC personnel knew of a signal, a relative risk of autism and thimerosal exposures greater than 62.5 micrograms at three months of age equal to 2.48," Lyn said. Safe Minds, she announced, would call for a "Congressional and United States Attorney's office investigation into the generation and alteration of these reports, including but not limited to subsequent oral testimony by Roger Bernier of CDC reporting an 'inconclusive relationship' between the administration of thimerosal-containing vaccines and neurodevelopmental disorders."

The committee members stared blankly at Lyn, or shuffled papers nervously. "Parents will no longer blindly trust the health of their children into the hands of individuals who are indifferent to their fate and make calculations based upon an undefined 'greater good' hypothesis," Lyn continued.

"It may be too late for those children who have already suffered irreversible harm from thimerosal-containing vaccines, but the individuals here today can take steps to perhaps save even one child, and that child's family, from the nightmare diagnosis of a developmental disability," she said. "This will be judged as one of the greatest public health tragedies of our nation."

9. War on Four Fronts

FOR THOSE PUSHING the mercury-autism agenda forward, the diverse threads of the fight would come together in 2002. Four major battlefronts had emerged, all inextricably linked.

There was the scientific battle, still simmering in university labs and private clinics, at major conferences, and in the pages of peer-reviewed journals as each side collected and used its own data to advance its argument and attack opponents.

There was the legal battle being waged in civil courts around the country, where judges deliberated over hearing the thimerosal cases or remanding them to Vaccine Court. Regardless, Andy Waters had begun discovery in his first civil suit. The documents he possessed would help forward his argument of liability, fraud, and malfeasance on behalf of Eli Lilly and a handful of other companies.

Next, a political battle had emerged in Congress over how to reform the Vaccine Injury Compensation Program, who should be allowed into the VICP, and what the burden of proof and financial awards should be.

Finally, in the bureaucratic battle, parents would take on the two most powerful health agencies in the country. They would pursue the Centers for Disease Control for the Datalink numbers and probe more deeply into what the Food and Drug Administration knew about thimerosal's toxicity, and when. They would also help Dan Burton's staff investigate the FDA's sluggishness in removing a known neurotoxin from vaccines.

For Safe Minds, the scientific front could not have been more crucial. Without hard data to support their arguments on science, prospects for victory on the legal and political lines would evaporate. The year was to bring some extraordinary scientific findings. Although none of them on their own could be construed as "proof," taken together, the body of evidence began to yield a clearer picture of how thimerosal might affect normal childhood development.

The University of Kentucky's Boyd Haley, a scholar of mercury for over a decade, had begun to test the toxicity of thimerosal-containing vaccines in his lab. In early 2002, Haley wrote to Lyn, who had procured the vaccines for his study, about his early results. He and his team had taken mouse neuronal cells in culture and exposed them to a variety of substances, including thimerosal (in the same 0.01 percent solution found in vaccines); aluminum, another vaccine component; and neomycin, a common antibiotic widely used in pediatrics and found in the MMR vaccine.

Haley measured the percentage of neurons that were still alive after exposure to each substance over a twenty-four-hour period. There was also a control group of unexposed neurons. Nearly all control cells were still alive after twenty-four hours. In the aluminum-exposed group, about 90 percent of the cells had survived, and in the antibiotic group, survival was 80 percent. But among neurons exposed to thimerosal, only 30 percent were still alive after twenty-four hours.[173]

What really struck Haley was the *synergistic effect* found after combining thimerosal with the other chemicals. When thimerosal was mixed with aluminum and neomycin, survival rates after twenty-four hours plummeted to less than 10 percent. When the cells were exposed to all three substances, none survived after twenty-four hours.

Haley and his colleagues wanted to test another idea: given the 4 or 5 to 1 male-to-female ratio of autism, ADD, and other developmental disorders, what effect might testosterone and estrogen have on mercury toxicity? Estrogen, Haley found, actually had a protective effect on cells. Among neurons exposed to thimerosal and estrogen, most were still alive after twelve hours. But with the testosterone-thimerosal combination, the opposite was true. Cells died *a hundred times faster* than those exposed to thimerosal alone.

Haley's research on testosterone was consistent with a study by Dr. Simon Baron-Cohen, a renowned autism expert and professor of developmental psychopathology at the Autism Research Centre of Cambridge University. Baron-Cohen measured testosterone levels in the amniotic fluid (which surrounds the fetus within the uterus) of women. The children were then followed up after

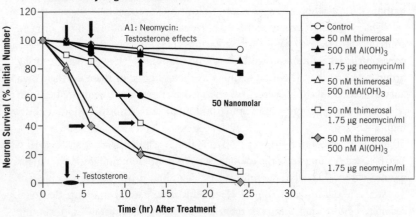

FIGURE 6. Synergistic Toxicities

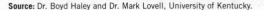

Source: Dr. Boyd Haley and Dr. Mark Lovell, University of Kentucky.

birth. All were typically developing, but those children with higher concentrations of testosterone in their amniotic fluid made less eye contact with their mothers at one year old and were slower to develop speech at eighteen months old. They also found it harder to socialize when they started school at four years old and tended to have narrower interests, compared to children with less fetal testosterone. Fetal testosterone is produced by the fetus itself and is produced in greater quantities by the male fetus. But even within males or within females, there are considerable individual differences in how much fetal testosterone is produced, and this seems to be associated not just with differences in social behavior but also with masculinization of the brain itself.[174]

Haley thought this was a clear sign of a hormone-based gender risk factor for mercury toxicity, but he worried that the scientific community would not see it that way. "Just watch," he told Lyn, "now the drug companies will state that testosterone causes autism."[175]

Meanwhile, Dr. Amy Holmes, the pediatrician who chelated autistic patients with her partner, Dr. Stephanie Cave, was investigating mercury levels in baby hair. Most people in the mercury-autism camp, including Dr. Holmes herself, assumed that the findings would show that autistic children had higher levels of mercury in their hair than typical kids. After all, Will Redwood's hair had been loaded with the metal.

Dr. Holmes had been collecting hair samples from baby haircuts (taken at fifteen to twenty-four months) of children with autism spectrum disorder at the clinic. She also persuaded the parents of two dozen healthy children to donate hair samples. For good measure, she sent a sample from her own baby haircut, and one from her autistic son, to a lab for analysis.

What the lab found made little sense. Even though the ASD kids and the controls were exposed to the same levels of thimerosal in their vaccines, the controls had far *greater* amounts of mercury in their hair than the ASD group. Among the ASD kids, higher functioning children had more hair mercury than low-functioning kids.

As for her own baby hair, it came back showing mercury levels at a fairly high 4.9 parts per million, even though Holmes had only received a total of 50 micrograms of ethylmercury from her childhood vaccines, decades earlier. But baby hair from her son, who had been exposed to nearly 250 micrograms of mercury, had only a tiny amount of the metal—just 0.35 ppm.[176]

When Holmes and Stephanie Cave first saw the results, they thought the technicians must have switched the samples accidentally. They had expected to find the opposite results. Then Dr. Holmes talked things over with Boyd Haley.

"Now all of this makes perfect sense," she told the Safe Minds group. "Boyd said that if you give two people an equal amount of mercury and then measure their blood and hair levels several months later, the person with the higher hair level is the one who actively excretes mercury and has less risk of toxicity."

Boyd Haley and Mark Blaxill agreed to team up with Holmes to write a paper on the findings, which were accepted for publication by the peer-reviewed *International Journal of Toxicology*.[177]

And the team made another remarkable finding: In the normal children, elevated mercury levels in hair corresponded to the number of dental amalgams in the mother. In contrast, the autistic children had exceptionally low mercury levels, even if the mother had a mouthful of fillings. "This clearly shows that autistic children do not handle mercury like normal children," Haley told the parents. "The most straightforward explanation is that autistic children are a subset of the population that can't excrete mercury very well."

Dr. Holmes had found another intriguing result. Her own baby hair had a copper-to-zinc ratio of 0.8, right in the middle of the normal range. But her son's hair had a ratio that was 300 percent higher, or 2.5. This finding was consistent with the metallothionein theories of Bill Walsh, the researcher who had reported similar copper-to-zinc imbalances in autistic children at the Phoenix DAN! conference. Walsh had attributed the imbalance to a genetically induced dysfunction of metallothionein. He surmised that MT dysfunction, which was more common in boys, blocked the excretion of heavy metals.

The Holmes study also dovetailed quite well with the work of Dr. Jeffrey Bradstreet, the Florida M.D. who reported that ASD kids excreted five times more mercury in their urine after chelation than controls. Taken together, the Holmes and Bradstreet studies strongly suggested, but did not prove, that normal kids continually shed mercury through urine, hair, and feces, while autistic children naturally retain it in organs and tissue. Only when "challenged" with chelation, the argument went, was the built-up mercury in autistic kids finally expelled.

Amy Holmes conducted a second study, in which she compiled data on children with autism who had chelation therapy for at least four months. She documented their progress as measured in memory, cognitive function, social interaction, and other markers. Among the youngest kids (one to five years), 35 percent showed "marked improvement" (little or no autistic symptoms) and 39 percent showed moderate improvement, while 11 percent had only "slight" improvement, and 9 percent showed no progress. Among six- to twelve-year-olds, one-third had marked or moderate improvement, though after age twelve, the improvement fell dramatically:[178]

The implications of these findings were twofold. If removal of mercury led to improvement in autism-related symptoms, didn't it stand to reason that mercury played some role in the creation of those symptoms? And if chelation therapy was more effective in children under six, wouldn't it behoove the government to investigate it as a treatment for autism as quickly as possible?

NOW THAT the "confidential" VSD report had finally seen daylight, the parents and their attorneys worried that the drug companies and their political beneficiaries, most of them Republican, would move decisively against the rising tide of litigation.

They were right. In early February 2002, Safe Minds learned that lobbyists from Lilly, the vaccine makers, and the Pharmaceutical Research and Manufacturers of America (PhRMA) were making the rounds on Capitol Hill, with a list of demands couched in a barely veiled threat. The lobbyists warned that vaccine makers were being driven out of the business, largely due to the high cost of litigating injury cases (even though most were settled within VICP, where taxpayers foot the bill).[179] This dwindling total of suppliers had created a number of vaccine shortages, including a dearth of DTaP shots.

In a world of terrorism, the lobbyists cautioned, the stakes were higher than ever. Drug companies might be asked to assemble millions of doses of vaccines against smallpox, anthrax, or bubonic plague. But a clear and

FIGURE 7. Comparison of chelation treatment results—improvement in symptoms of children with ASD, based on age.

	Improvement (%)			
Age	Marked	Moderate	Slight	None
1–5	35	39	15	11
6–12	4	28	52	16
13–17	0	6	68	26
18+	0	0	25	75

Source: Dr. Amy Holmes.

growing danger hovered on the bioterror horizon. The threat wasn't Osama bin Ladin or Saddam Hussein. It was those outrageous thimerosal lawsuits. The companies wanted total litigation protection. They wanted all civil cases to be dismissed and funneled into VICP, but only *if* they were within the statute of limitations; they wanted to bar families from "opting out" of VICP once they entered; and they wanted to maintain the statute of limitations and limit awards for death or injury. This would leave most families with no further recourse whatsoever.

By late winter, two competing congressional bills to "reform" the Vaccine Court were introduced.

The first bill, in the House, was introduced by Dan Burton, with Henry Waxman signing on as the unlikely lead cosponsor. The National Vaccine Injury Compensation Program Improvement Act of 2002, better known as the Burton-Waxman bill, grew from similar legislation introduced a year before by Dave Weldon and Jerrold Nadler.[180]

Its most important provision would change the statute of limitations from three to six years, and offer a "look-back" window for families to enter the VICP if they had previously been excluded by the statute of limitations. This was critical to plaintiffs like the Redwoods, whose son had been vaccinated more than six years earlier. Even if the statute were extended, he still would not automatically be eligible, but a look-back window would offer them the same chance at compensation as other families.

The Burton-Waxman bill would also raise compensation for "future lost earnings" of injured children and increase compensation for vaccine-related deaths from $250,000 to $300,000. It would compensate families for counseling costs, create a guardianship to administer awards, and cover interim attorney fees and legal costs.

The second bill, backed with considerable political muscle, would be introduced in April by Sen. Bill Frist of Tennessee, and ignite a controversy of its own.

IN EARLY 2002, CDC vaccine officials announced their willingness to open the Datalink to outside research. But there were conditions. Anyone wishing to look at the guarded database would first have to jump through a series of bureaucratic hoops. And even then, gaining complete and unfettered access to the raw data (purchased and maintained at taxpayer expense) was not going to happen.

Under the rules proposed by the CDC, access to the database would be granted only to bona fide scientists with institutional affiliations working on approved and funded studies.[181] In other words, parents and lawyers need not apply.

Researchers who qualified would have to submit a detailed proposal to the CDC, a summary of the study, and a list of the exact data files they wished to examine, including data sets previously studied by VSD staff. The CDC was clearly unwilling to let researchers comb willy-nilly through the data, trawling for trends that others might have missed.

Next, interested researchers would have to divulge the "specific hypothesis of vaccine safety to be examined," and provide a full explanation of methods to be used, including any "proposed analytic strategies" for tabulating the results. Such requests gave the CDC great leeway for accepting or rejecting proposals.

That was not all. When and if CDC approval was granted, researchers would then have to ask the Institutional Review Board (IRB) of each participating HMO for access to their data. This hurdle was not only time-consuming, it provided for the rejection of access outside of government.

Once approval was obtained from each IRB, documented proof would need to be furnished to the CDC. After paying a fifteen-hundred-dollar access fee, researchers could then, and only then, apply to view the data, but only that data that had been specifically prerequested.

Next, researchers would have to travel at their own expense to the CDC's Research Data Center in Hyattsville, Maryland, where the Datalink was maintained. They would have access only when the facility was "available," and only when CDC staff were on hand to "monitor" their work.

Once the researchers arrived, they would be sent to a computer workstation, which staff would preload with the requested files. Only three outside researchers would be allowed access at a time, and they needed to sign an agreement to "maintain the confidentiality of the data they will analyze."

The researchers would not be permitted to take notes on anything they saw during the session. Pencils and paper would be forbidden, as well as cell phones, pagers, "or other devices that would allow them to communicate with persons on the outside." After government programmers ran the requested numbers, the outside researchers would be provided with a computer printout of the results, but nothing else. Even then, all "output" would be subject to close review before its removal from the computer room.

Safe Minds had no intention of letting the proposed rules take effect without a fight. Nor had the group abandoned its efforts to get the data through the Freedom of Information Act, even though this avenue had so far yielded nothing. Jim Moody, their Washington legal counsel, sent a blistering letter to the FOIA office of the Public Health Service, which oversees the CDC. The integrity of the scientific process "demands that raw data be freely available to ensure proper replication," Moody said, adding that he would seek "appropriate sanctions for your wrongful withholding of the VSD data."[182]

Moody informed the government that Safe Minds had obtained documents that showed an "appalling cover-up of an epidemic of vaccine-related disorders." He said that CDC staff, in testimony before Congress, "deliberately distorted data to conceal the possible link between mercury-containing vaccines and disease."

The libertarian lawyer then betrayed his distaste for big government in a flourish of rhetorical drama. "Perhaps hundreds of thousands of children have been poisoned by toxic vaccines mandated by government agencies so desperate to obtain the supposed benefits of universal vaccination that they failed to perform their basic statutory responsibility," Moody wrote. "Public confidence in vaccines may be another casualty, as much from the cover-up as the unsupportable decisions to mandate unnecessarily toxic vaccines in the first place."

WHEN DAN BURTON began looking into the vaccine-autism controversy in 1998, he and his staff knew they would eventually need to publish a report on what they had found. To that end, Beth Clay was pulling the divergent strands of the inquiry together. A key piece of the investigation was to look into the FDA's initial thimerosal review.

Liz was desperate to assist, and she offered her time and legal skills to the effort. Burton agreed to let her volunteer. Liz began by going back over the testimony of FDA officials at previous committee meetings. She was especially interested in what Dr. William Egan had said at the July 2000 hearing, when Burton asked him when the FDA first became concerned about mercury in vaccines. Egan had said that the "major concern" began somewhere around May of 1999.

Was that really likely? Liz had discovered an article, published back in 1986 in the journal *Adverse Drug Reactions and Acute Poisoning Review,* which said that thimerosal "may present problems occasionally in practice. It is therefore now accepted that multidose injection preparations are undesirable and that preservatives should not be present in preparations."[183] The article was written by A. K. Winship, who at the time was senior medical officer in the UK's Department of Health and Social Security.

"It is my understanding that [Winship] would be in a similar position as a top administrative officer of our FDA," Liz wrote to Burton on March 7, 2002.[184] "I cannot believe, based upon articles such as this, that the FDA did not know that thimerosal was a problem in vaccines before May of 1999. If a senior official in the UK stated as a matter of fact in 1986 that multi-dose preparations were undesirable because of thimerosal, what were our FDA officials doing? Here we are 15 years later and the FDA has not mandated that thimerosal be removed from all vaccines, nor has it acted to recall pediatric vaccines containing thimerosal. I find the conduct of FDA officials reprehensible."

As further evidence of Egan's purported malfeasance, Liz recalled that he had been asked by Rep. Helen Chenoweth-Hage about FDA studies to prove thimerosal's safety. Egan had no good answer, mostly because no such study existed.

"There was a long history of the use . . . the safe use of thimerosal . . ." he had said. "You know . . . in vaccines, since they were . . . since it was first introduced. And at that time [1990] there was no data to suggest that the added mercury from the introduction of those new vaccines would be harmful."

Liz found Egan's statement "patently false," she wrote. "By 1990 there was a mountain of evidence that thimerosal was unsafe." In 1987, for instance, the Commission of the European Communities initiated a research project of known or suspected "spindle poisons," including thimerosal. And in 1993 an article in *Mutation Research* said thimerosal was a "strong inhibitor of microtubular assembly," an essential process for proper neuronal development.

"Again, I find it incomprehensible that officials at our FDA could have overlooked this research," Liz wrote. "If they did so, they are grossly incompetent. As you can see, much was known about thimerosal prior to 1999. I am sure that through the process of subpoenas we will discover much more. I am extremely distrustful of individuals at CDC and FDA. They have a history of outright lying. When possible, they engage in the distortion of facts to suit their purposes."

. . .

ANDY WATERS'S coalition of law firms continued to swell, as attorneys for families outside the VICP's statute of limitations brought their cases forward in civil court.

It was a rocky road. Many cases, including the Redwoods' suit in Georgia, had been shunted back and forth between state courts (the preferred venue of plaintiffs, because of higher damage awards and more sympathetic juries) and federal courts (preferred by drug companies, for the opposite reasons). Many judges ruled that plaintiffs had to apply for compensation in Vaccine Court first, before taking their cases to civil court. The fact that many of these families were ineligible to enter the VICP didn't matter.

Some judges, however, agreed to hear the cases before them, including some within the Waters & Kraus coalition. Discovery in these cases could get under way.

As part of the discovery process in the Counter case (the first private lawsuit alleging a thimerosal-autism connection) Waters & Kraus received forty-six boxes of internal Lilly documents. Inside, Waters found a seventy-year-old paper trail of evidence that Lilly knew about thimerosal's dangers and had relied on bogus clinical data to maintain approval for the preservative.

Waters decided to go public with the information. The documents "clearly demonstrate that Lilly's thimerosal product was known as early as April 1930 to be dangerous," he said in a March 17 news release.[185] But Lilly, "in its apparent eagerness to promote and market the product," secretly sponsored a 1930 toxicity study on patients already known to be dying of meningococcal meningitis. Doctors injected 22 patients with high levels of thimerosal and then monitored them for toxic effects. Most died within days, from meningitis. Thus, no adverse thimerosal effects were observed.

"Lilly cited this study repeatedly for decades as proof that thimerosal was of low toxicity and harmless to humans," Waters said. "They never revealed to the scientific community or the public the highly questionable nature of the original research." Instead the company "made every effort to corrupt the medical and scientific literature [by] arranging to publish the results of its questionable secret study."

Remarkably, this 1930 study of 22 dying patients was the only data on the safety of thimerosal ever submitted by any drugmaker to the FDA.

Despite Lilly's repeated claims that thimerosal was safe, many researchers had sent the company documents dating back to the 1930s, each raising a red flag about thimerosal. Lilly was advised repeatedly that their conclusions of low toxicity were wrong, Waters said.

For example, a 1935 letter from the director of biological services of the

Pittman-Moore Company to Dr. Jamieson of Eli Lilly, alerted the company that "we have obtained marked local reaction in about 50 percent of the dogs injected with serum containing dilutions of Merthiolate [thimerosal] varying from 1 in 40,000 to 1 in 5,000 . . . no connection between the lot of serum and the reaction. In other words, Merthiolate is *unsatisfactory as a preservative for serum intended for use on dogs* [italics added]."[186]

As further evidence, Waters offered the following timeline:

1947 Article received by Lilly: "No eruptions or reactions have been observed or reported to Merthiolate [thimerosal] internally, but it may be dangerous to inject a serum containing it into a patient sensitive to Merthiolate."

1948 Article received by Lilly: "Merthiolate is such a commonly used preservative for biologicals, plasma, cartilage, etc., that it would seem important to determine whether harm would result following its subcutaneous or intravenous injection in skin sensitive individuals."

1950 New York Academy of Science article, "Mercurials as Antiseptics"—"[are] toxic when injected parenterally and cannot be used in chemotherapy."

1963 Article received by Lilly: "There is another point of practical significance: does the parenteral injection of Merthiolate-containing fluids cause disturbances in Merthiolate-sensitive patients? It is known that persons that are contact-sensitive to a drug may tolerate the same medications internally, but it seems advisable to use a preservative other than Merthiolate for injections in Merthiolate-sensitive people."

1967 Lilly's Medical/Science Department requests that the claim "nontoxic" on thimerosal labels be deleted in the next printing run.

1972 The *British Medical Journal* reports cases of skin burns resulting from the chemical interaction of thimerosal and aluminum. "Mercury is known to act as a catalyst and to cause aluminum to oxidize rapidly, with the production of heat," it said.

1972 Article received by Lilly: Merthiolate in vaccines caused six deaths—"The symptoms and clinical course of the six patients suggest subacute mercury poisoning."

1976 Lilly responds to Rexall Drug Company's efforts to place the following warning: "Frequent or prolonged use or application to large areas may cause mercury poisoning." Lilly objects to the "connection of our trademark with the unjustified alarm and concern on the part of the user which the statement is likely to cause.

We are not aware of any instance of 'mercury poisoning' after decades of marketing this product. This is because the mercury in the product is organically bound ethylmercury as a completely non-toxic nature, not methylmercury."

1983 Additional language is added to some labels: "If you are pregnant or nursing a baby, seek the advice of a health professional before using this product."

1991 Lilly ceases manufacture and sale of thimerosal. Licensing agreements demonstrate continued profits from the product until at least 2010.

1999 Lilly prints a new Material Safety Data Sheet (or MSDS) for lab workers and emergency personnel on proper procedures for handling thimerosal. The preservative, it says, can cause: "Nervous System and Reproduction Effects; Effects of exposure include fetal changes; Mercury poisoning may occur; Exposure in children may cause mild to severe mental retardation; Hypersensitivity to mercury is a medical condition aggravated by exposure; Hazardous substance, toxic waste disposal."

THE LILLY DISCOVERY DOCUMENTS brought Andy Waters to a novel legal strategy. Instead of suing for strict product liability, he would go after the companies for fraud, negligence, and other damages. His strategy was tested when Lilly filed a motion to dismiss the Counter case in Texas. Lilly lawyers argued, among other things, that the company could not be liable because the company neither made nor distributed thimerosal.[187]

Waters conceded this point in his counterargument, but insisted that Lilly should still be held liable for "foreseeable' harm caused by its *own conduct*."[188] Its "manipulating of the medical literature and concealing the dangers of thimerosal" left the company liable for "negligence, misrepresentation, fraud, and conspiracy, among others," he asserted.

Eli Lilly "purposefully and maliciously altered scientific literature and hid the true dangers of thimerosal in vaccines with full knowledge that children would suffer mercury poisoning," he continued. The company "knowingly and recklessly made false material representations to the FDA, physicians, consumers, and the general public," with "every reason to expect its misrepresentations would be relied on by doctors, drug companies, and eventually parents and pediatricians."

The motive was money, Waters alleged. "Lilly continues to profit from its sordid history with a product it knew should never have entered the stream of commerce," he said. A 1999 company memo showed that Lilly would profit from thimerosal marketing and sales "in 40 nations throughout the third world for many years into the future. This profiteering was unconscionable," he concluded. "There is no social utility in permitting a company to callously disregard the well being of children [to] maximize profits through misinformation and deceit. Social values and policy considerations *require* that companies like Lilly be held financially responsible for the injuries they cause."

IN APRIL 2002, a Vaccination Injury Compensation Program reform bill that was decidedly different from the Burton-Waxman version was introduced on the Senate side by Bill Frist, the Republican from Tennessee. Frist, a heart-lung transplant surgeon elected in 2000 to his second term, was a rising star in the GOP. Close to the White House and a hunting buddy of Bush adviser Karl Rove, Frist reportedly was on Bush's list of possible running mates in the 2000 presidential campaign.

Frist was the ranking minority member of the Public Health subcommittee of the Senate Health, Education, Labor and Pensions Committee. The chairman, Ted Kennedy, worked closely with Frist on issues like AIDS in Africa. Still, the two butted heads on many other subjects. Frist gained national attention during the anthrax scare of 2001 by calmly explaining the disease to an anxious public. He had since become the White House point person on bioterror issues in the Senate. He was also chairman of the National Republican Senatorial Committee, where he helped construct the GOP takeover of the Senate, in November 2002.

When the Frist bill was introduced, it seemed to be a reasonable piece of legislation aimed at improving the user-friendliness of the VICP, while also guaranteeing the national vaccine supply. Frist called his bill the Improved Vaccine Affordability and Availability Act. Like Burton-Waxman, it extended the statute of limitation to six years, raised the death benefit to $300,000, and provided counseling for affected families.[189]

But on closer inspection, the parents found cause for alarm. Frist offered no look-back window. Anyone injured in 1996 or earlier would be ineligible for compensation. Nor did the Frist bill provide interim legal and attorney fees or guarantee increased compensation for "future lost earnings."

Perhaps most troublesome, Frist would shut the door to civil court for most cases. As the law stood now, plaintiffs had three options (some would call them "loopholes") for filing suit outside the VICP. They could file a claim on their own behalf, as opposed to their children, for "loss of consortium and society." Secondly, they could join a class-action suit seeking costs for "medical monitoring" of their kids.

Or they could sue the makers and distributors of thimerosal by claiming that it was an "adulterant or contaminant" to vaccines, not a component of the shots themselves. The distinction was crucial. Vaccine "adulterants" were not covered under the VICP. Thus, Andy Waters argued, thimerosal cases belonged in civil court. (Even so, most judges had stayed their thimerosal cases until the VICP issue was resolved.)

The Frist bill would sew up these loopholes. It would eliminate the right to parental claims in civil court until *after* the family went through the vaccine program (a program for which many would remain ineligible). It also barred class-action suits.

As for thimerosal itself, one section of the bill stated that an "adulterant or contaminant shall not include any component or ingredient listed in a vaccine's product label." Thimerosal was always on the vaccine label.

Frist went on the offensive to promote his legislation (encouraged, perhaps, by the ten-thousand-dollar campaign contribution that the drug lobby, PhRMA, gave his political action committee the day after he introduced the bill).[190]

Many parents expected Frist to couch his argument in the context of national vaccine shortages, and he did not disappoint.

"With five of the nine recommended childhood vaccines and some adult vaccines in short supply, it is essential that we take action to address the underlying causes of these shortages," Frist said in a statement.[191] "The threat of liability and the cost of unwarranted litigation once again pose challenges to the stability of our vaccine supply. Just one of the pending lawsuits in the United States seeks $30 billion in damages, while the total global value of the vaccine market is only $5 billion."

Frist said the number of companies licensed to sell vaccines in the United States had dwindled to just four (two of which were European-owned). His bill would "ensure that unwarranted litigation does not again destabilize the vaccine market causing the few manufacturers licensed to sell vaccines in the United States to leave the market."

Frist's answer was to force plaintiffs into the VICP "before initiating a lawsuit." But the senator failed to mention that thousands of families were ineligible for the program—precisely those families whose children had been vaccinated throughout the early 1990s, when the list of vaccines on the childhood schedule had been dramatically increased.

SCOTT AND LAURA BONO, the parents from Durham, North Carolina, whom Lyn had met at the April 2000 Burton hearings, were among the most vocal parents leading the fight against Bill Frist. Scott and Laura were not Safe

Minds members, but they were in utter agreement when it came to thimerosal and the mission of the Safe Minds parents.

The Bonos' twin daughters, Ashley and Dillan, were born in 1987, and their only son, Jackson, arrived in March 1989. His regression from normalcy into autistic symptoms, including acute gut problems, mirrored that of so many other affected kids. Jackson was also prone to escape, and the Bonos had to seal every window in their large house and install an alarm that sounds every time an outside door is opened.

Jackson had been diagnosed with PDD-NOS in 1990 at nineteen months, and in September 2000 he was additionally diagnosed (Laura would say "correctly" diagnosed) with mercury poisoning. The Bonos had spent over five hundred thousand dollars—about three hundred thousand of which was paid by insurance money and the rest from their retirement savings—for all the special medical care, testing, and education their son required. He had been to some one hundred doctors and countless clinics. Thousands of dollars more were spent repairing or replacing everything that their often out-of-control son had destroyed.[192]

In early 2002, the Bonos were preparing to file a civil lawsuit. Jackson's "date of injury" was 1990 and he was ineligible for the VICP. Even if the statute were extended to six years, Jackson would still not be eligible without the look-back window offered in the Burton-Waxman bill. He would not be eligible under the Frist version.

Laura would dedicate much of the coming three years to fighting Frist and his vaccine legislation. She began by organizing a letter-writing campaign among parents around the country. Laura sent her own communication to North Carolina's conservative senior senator, Jesse Helms.

"Senator Frist is proposing a bill that will significantly tie the hands of parents who believe their child was hurt by vaccines," she told Helms. "To not be able to sue the pharmaceutical manufacturers is NOT allowing United States citizens their day in court." Families were overwhelmed, she said, "struggling to find therapy and medical interventions. They often go bankrupt and are divorced due to the strain."

. The question of whether vaccines were to blame, or whether parents were mistaken, was not the argument, she said. "The point is, it is completely wrong for the Senate to decide to rob parents of their day in court! And what if vaccines did cause the explosion of autistic children that the CDC has now deemed at 'epidemic' proportions? Then I'd say you, as a Senator, should lead the way for North Carolina to also join suit to reclaim North Carolina funds that have been spent on these children through the schools, Medicaid, homes for the disabled, etc. These funds could possibly dwarf the tobacco lawsuits in all states. Let the courts decide. Not the Senate."[193]

. . .

FOR TWO YEARS, Dan Burton had been rattling his saber over access to the VSD data. He wrote to the CDC demanding the records and endorsed Safe Minds' repeated but unsuccessful FOIA requests. Exasperated, he and members of his staff hinted that they would use the power of subpoena, if needed, to get the information.

The staff, who normally maintained good relationships with the political appointees within Health and Human Services, strained those friendships when told that the HMOs were threatening to withdraw from the program if the VSD data was turned over to the committee. In one conversation, Beth Clay would ask the HHS congressional liaison staff if they were going to tolerate being "blackmailed"—the threats made by these companies were extortion. Beth reminded the HHS staff that the data had been "bought and paid for by the American taxpayer. This data belongs to the American public and should be available for independent evaluation. . . . One of the tenets of good science is replication and independent verification . . . [and] only by having outside researchers access the data, could these findings ever be confirmed."[194]

CDC officials stood fast. Protection of the HMO patients' privacy was paramount, they said. And even if the names, addresses, and Social Security numbers were redacted, identities could be revealed through careful cross-checking of birth dates and dates of medical care, such as hospitalization. The potential "outing" of patients would devastate people being treated for things like HIV or mental illness.

Making the records public, moreover, would damage the integrity of the entire VSD program. Participating HMOs, fearing lawsuits from members and opposed to the release of "proprietary" information, were adamantly against the idea. They had threatened to pull out of the program if patient records were released, the CDC said.

But those concerns were not enough to throw Burton off the trail. His staff had prepared a draft subpoena, ordering the CDC to produce all records collected under the Datalink project.

A copy of the draft subpoena was sent to Waxman. Despite his cosponsorship of the VICP bill, Waxman was angry with the chairman. In a letter to Burton, the Democrat from Los Angeles excoriated the Republican from Indianapolis, and Safe Minds as well.

"I urge you to reverse course," Waxman told Burton, warning that a subpoena "could lead to the collapse" of the VSD.[195] Ironically, this would end the ability to monitor vaccine safety. HMOs were ready to bolt from the program if patient records were revealed, Waxman cautioned. "Concern was heightened last summer after a group called Safe Minds filed a request under the FOIA act for raw VSD data," he said. That prompted the HMOs to demand "explicit assurance" of control "over any new uses and distribution of their data" which would constitute a "profound violation of medical privacy."

Patient identity, Waxman said, could be breached "with ease." One HMO employee tried out this scenario, using his own daughter as a test case. With her birth date and the knowledge that she had recently sprained an ankle, an HMO analyst was able to find her records among the millions of unidentified patients in the whole VSD system.

Parental efforts to obtain the data were unwelcome, too. "Representatives of Safe Minds claimed in the presence of my staff that a refusal by CDC would be met by a subpoena from you," he said. "Your subsequent subpoena threats led investigators at the participating HMOs to realize that even CDC's protection may not be able to guarantee the confidentiality of the records."

For good measure, Waxman echoed Senator Frist and the White House by reminding Burton that the VSD was "critical" for monitoring the safety of smallpox vaccinations, "and can also serve as a valuable tool for monitoring other bioterrorism threats." He urged Burton to accept the CDC's data-sharing plan and abandon the slippery slope to subpoena. And yet, despite "this reasonable solution which does not compromise patient confidentiality and would protect the future of the VSD," he chided Burton, "you have yet to abandon your subpoena threats."

LIZ BIRT'S LIFE was falling apart. In May of 2002, she filed for divorce. It was the last step in the steady decline of the marriage. They had tried counseling, but it was a miserable failure. The gap between them had grown too wide, and the rift would never heal. Her husband had slowly come to distance himself from Liz's autism crusade and hence from her. He was weary of her warring and wary of vaccines, government cover-ups, and evil drug companies out to poison hapless babies. He'd had enough.

Liz thought he was somehow threatened by her dedication to the cause. "It's because I'm doing something more important than he is doing," Liz told Lyn one day. "He used to be interested in what was going on, but that has stopped. He's not as connected to it, he's not as outraged as we are."

Liz's husband accused her of harboring more love and affection for Andy Wakefield and the Mercury Moms than for her own family. She had a psychological problem, he suggested, in which she was only able to bond with people in diverse geographic areas.

"What he doesn't understand is that when you go through hell with people and your kids are all horribly sick, you bond with those people," she told Lyn. "It's like being in a concentration camp: you rely on each other to get through it."

It was going to be a messy divorce. The once-happy couple entered into mediation but failed to agree on any kind of financial settlement. When talks broke down, Liz learned that he was going to sue for sole custody of all three kids. He said she was an unfit, mentally unstable mother. It almost destroyed her. Liz went into psychotherapy and was prescribed antidepressants.[196]

The divorce quarrel would drag on for years. In the meantime, Liz needed a paying job after all that volunteer time she had spent doing research for Dan Burton's staff. The chairman offered Liz a salaried position. She was hoping for some other type of work, but she also wanted to help. Burton had subpoenaed documents on the 1999 FDA literature review of thimerosal and the events leading up to the Joint Statement. Beth Clay sent thousands of the papers, copied onto CDs, to Liz for her review. It took Liz hundreds of hours, camped out in the basement of her home, to read all the internal FDA messages. They reminded her of what Safe Minds had found in the CDC e-mails during Simpsonwood and the early days of the Verstraeten study. Once again, she thought, a claque of health officials was confronting an ugly secret and grappling with what they should do about it.

While the CDC staff had been uneasy about a signal that wouldn't "go away," the FDA's anxiety apparently was over the unsettling recognition that no one had bothered to add up the total amount of mercury being injected into kids in the 1990s. Nobody had asked if levels were creeping toward something worrisome. No one had wondered why thimerosal still had full FDA approval when the only safety study had been done in 1930, using dying patients. And apparently, no one had asked why an FDA panel, in 1982, wrote that thimerosal was toxic to cells and unsafe for over-the-counter products, yet the FDA never removed it from vaccines. The agency had unquestionably failed in its most fundamental duty to ensure that every medical product it approves was shown to be safe and effective.

As at the CDC, there were people inside the FDA who were questioning whether they had dropped the ball when it came to thimerosal.

Liz summarized the subpoenaed FDA e-mails in a May 21 memo to Burton. The most incriminating, she said, were several messages sent to colleagues from Dr. Peter Patriarca, director of the Division of Viral Products at the FDA's Center for Biologics Evaluation (CBER), just before the Joint Statement's release in July 1999.

On June 29, 1999, Patriarca wrote about an "interim plan" to remove thimerosal from vaccines.[197] The plan had "been in place for many years," he said. "We just need to 'speed up' the existing plan, not create a new interim plan." Obviously, Liz thought, the FDA knew long ago that thimerosal would have to be removed. But after so much delay, the agency still had not acted decisively. What was this "interim plan," she wondered, and why was it never implemented?

As Dr. Patriarca pointed out, it would have been simple for someone to do the math. Adding up the mercury contained in vaccines was not exactly "rocket science," he scoffed, adding, "Conversion of the percentage of thimerosal to actual micrograms of mercury involves 9th grade algebra. What took the FDA so long to do the calculations? Why didn't the CDC and the advisory bodies do these calculations, while rapidly expanding the childhood immunization schedule?"

It was a terrific question, Liz thought. She hoped Burton would find an answer.

Dr. Patriarca had also mused to colleagues about the pros and cons of the Joint Statement. One advantage was that it would "force manufacturers to develop 'crash' programs" for thimerosal removal. To Liz, this was a sure sign of bureaucratic spinelessness. "It is abundantly clear that the manufacturers were dragging their feet and no one at the FDA was willing to force them to take thimerosal out," Liz said in her memo to Burton. She suggested that Burton call Patriarca to ask him for "a copy of the FDA's plan for thimerosal removal. He refers to it, so it must exist."

Patriarca had e-mailed another message on July 2, 1999, exactly one week before the Joint Statement was released, with a "heads-up" to coworkers that, he conceded, had not been cleared by superiors.[198] The FDA's "greatest point of vulnerability" was that the thimerosal review "could have been done years ago, and on an ongoing basis, as the childhood immunization schedule became more complex." And he reminded everyone that the calculations were uncomplicated. Then he offered this assessment of the bureaucratic pickle in which the FDA found itself: "I am not sure if there will be an easy way out of the potential perception that the FDA, CDC and immunization policy bodies may have been 'asleep at the switch' regarding thimerosal until now."

Liz described another e-mail from someone she said "sounds like a voice of reason." It was sent by Susan Ellenberg, director of the Office of Biostatistics and Epidemiology at CBER, on June 28, 1999.[199] Ellenberg weighed the risks and benefits of abruptly taking thimerosal out of the vaccine supply. On the one hand, swift action might lead to a "non-orderly" transition to mercury-free shots, where vaccines for some children would be delayed until replacements were ready. On the other hand, removing thimerosal could potentially prevent a lot of misery in children.

Ellenberg warned it would be unwise to be "dismissive of the scientific evidence available," in case it turned out that thimerosal "truly does cause neurotoxicity in the amounts currently being given." The FDA risked making one of two errors, she warned. It would be wrong to move quickly to remove thimerosal if it turned out to be harmless. And if there was a problem with thimerosal, it would be wrong to move too slowly.

"I don't think we know which error would produce worse outcomes," she said, noting that half of all infants were exposed to thimerosal "at unacceptable levels." If 10 percent of those children suffered "some level of neurological deficit as a result," it would cause more injuries than waiting six to nine months for mercury-free vaccines.

Liz Birt was keen to keep working on the investigation, and Burton agreed to keep her on as a professional staff member. For the rest of the year, Liz would spend many long days and nights each month in Washington. She toiled for hours on end in a small windowless room in the bowels of the Rayburn Building, combing through stacks of boxes crammed with documents from the FDA, Eli Lilly, and the vaccine makers.

DAN BURTON had already presided over six hearings on vaccines and childhood disorders, earning him the affection of many parents. But his badgering of federal vaccine officials had rankled some influential people, not only on Capitol Hill but within the drug lobby and certain circles at the White House, where the antiterrorism drumbeat was sustained at a breathless tempo.

Burton was implacable. In April his committee had hauled in officials from the NIH and CDC and grilled them on the paltry federal research dollars earmarked for autism. The CDC's budget provided just $11.3 million for autism, while $62 million went to diabetes and $932 million to AIDS. At the NIH, $56 million had been allotted for autism, while diabetes got $688 million and AIDS spending reached $2.2 billion.[200]

Burton had nothing against AIDS or diabetes research, but he demanded more money for the "growing autism epidemic." He joined with autism groups in calling for an additional $120 million in NIH autism research and another $20 million at the CDC.

In June of 2002, Burton was interviewed by a television reporter named Valeri Williams, from WFAA-TV in Dallas. Williams had conducted an unusually thorough investigation on thimerosal, covering the story perhaps more aggressively than any U.S. journalist. Burton, she said, told her he would bring criminal charges if "it's proven the government agencies were involved in a cover-up." On camera, Burton said it didn't matter "whether it's a private company or a government agency. If they know they're harming somebody and they continue to let it happen, they should be held accountable."[201]

"Government accountability," Williams reported, "is something that parents of autistic children have been asking for years." She said that health officials had "squirmed uncomfortably in their seats" during Burton's autism hearings, as "more evidence emerged suggesting that they misled the public. Burton repeatedly asked FDA and CDC officials what they knew and when they knew it."

Not everyone interviewed agreed with the mercury theory. Dr. Jane Siegel, a professor of pediatrics at University of Texas Southwestern in Dallas and a former member of the CDC's Advisory Committee on Immunization Practices, insisted there was "no data thus far that's been looked at to prove that there's a connection, that there's a causative relationship." But Williams pointed out that, just two years earlier, the CDC *did* conduct a study showing a 2.48 relative risk for autism. The study, Williams noted, was stamped "Do Not Copy or Release."

Siegel explained that the report wasn't released because it was merely a draft. "Until they're final and ready for publication, they're always considered a draft, not to be widely distributed," she said. "This preliminary information could be distributed, and that could do harm." So why was it marked "Confidential, Do Not Release," rather than simply "Draft"? Williams asked. "I think we're mincing words," Siegel said.

Williams then said that the CDC had eventually released a public report, but the findings were much different. "The new study was amended with different data, which lowered the autism rate," she said. Siegel had no reply, at least not on camera.

The next night, using the documents obtained by Andy Waters, Williams tore into Eli Lilly.[202] Lilly officials declined an interview, but they did send an e-mail asserting that the company's "primary concern is for patient safety." It noted that Lilly had discontinued its sale or use of thimerosal ten years ago, but didn't stop other pharmaceutical companies from taking over the production of the vaccine preservative.

The parents loved Williams's reporting, but her superiors apparently did not. A few months later, she told Lyn that the station had commanded her to end the investigation. Williams wondered if the top brass feared her reports would upset drug companies, who bought millions of dollars in ad time to promote their products. By the end of the year, Williams was gone from WFAA and her news reports were pulled from the station's Web site.

ELI LILLY'S considerable investment in the political fortunes of George W. Bush had yielded another dividend. On June 11, the White House announced the appointment of Lilly president and CEO Sidney Taurel to the Homeland

Security Advisory Council. The council would provide President Bush with post-9/11 advice on national antiterror matters "from experts representing state and local government, the private sector, public policy experts and the non-profit sector," a White House statement said.[203]

It was a prestigious, powerful, and secretive body. The fifteen slots were highly coveted. Joseph J. Grano, Jr., chairman and CEO of UBS Paine Webber, was named to head the council, indicating the degree to which the private sector would be called upon to shape the nation's new security profile. In addition to Taurel, other big business appointments included Kathleen Bader, a top executive at Dow Chemical Company, and James Schlesinger, chairman of the MITRE Corporation and senior adviser for Lehman Brothers, in addition to his prior stints as secretary of energy and defense, director of the CIA, and chairman of the Atomic Energy Commission. (Another member, Paul Bremer, would later become the administration's point man in Iraq.)

The panel meets behind closed doors and does not release minutes or other records. Christopher Logan, a writer for *Congressional Quarterly,* reported in 2002 that "this little known group has already held sway over important homeland security issues."[204] But the council had "flown so low under Washington's normally sensitive political radar" that government watchdogs "admitted ignorance of the group's activities," Logan wrote. "It's one of Washington's best-kept secrets."

The panel's first task was to review the administration's "critical infrastructure protection plan," Logan said, adding that 85 percent of all facilities under review were owned by the private sector. "Members of the advisory council are reviewing policies that could have beneficial and detrimental effects on their own companies," he said. "The council resembles Vice President Dick Cheney's Energy Task Force, a utilities-heavy group that met behind closed doors and excluded citizen input or media requests for agendas and minutes of its meetings."

There was another important but unreported appointment made the same day Taurel was named to the council. Lilly announced in a statement that Dr. Gail Cassell, vice president of scientific affairs, had been appointed to the Council on Public Health Preparedness, a panel that reported directly to HHS Secretary Tommy Thompson on bioterror, which presumably included discussions on vaccines. Also that day, Cassell assumed a new role with PhRMA, to provide the drug lobby with "scientific leadership for the development of the industry's bioterrorism strategy."[205]

The same Lilly statement also noted the company's generous support for the CDC. Lilly had given more than two million dollars to a CDC bioterror program to improve surveillance for emerging biological threats. It had also given the CDC, NIH, and Department of Defense access to Lilly products and investigational compounds "for testing as potential candidates to target bioterrorism threats," the statement said, without mentioning that this could potentially save Lilly millions in R&D.

The cozy relationship between pharmaceutical companies and the Republican Party was coming under increasing scrutiny. Representatives from the drug lobby, with seemingly bottomless pockets, were making the rounds on Capitol Hill again, pushing for industry pet projects like Medicare reform, senior prescription drug plans, and, of course, protection from vaccine liability. Faced with the threat of multimillion-dollar civil actions over thimerosal, the lobbyists again warned that companies would be hard-pressed to produce bioterror vaccines. To avert disaster, Congress needed to pass the Frist bill.[206]

The drug industry, of course, was offering a big carrot with its veiled-threat stick. Companies lined up to contribute lavishly to GOP candidates for the November midterm elections. Republicans were still smarting from the defection of Vermont senator Jim Jeffords the year before, stripping the party of its majority status in the Senate, and were anxious to win back control. PhRMA wholly supported the effort.

No pharmaceutical company had been more generous with campaign checks than Lilly. Between 2000 and 2002 the company doled out $1.6 million in political contributions, 80 percent of it to Republicans. A good chunk ($226,000) was earmarked for the National Republican Senatorial Campaign Committee, run by Bill Frist.[207] (When Frist authored a book on bioterrorism after the September 11, 2001, attacks, Eli Lilly bought five thousand copies for physicians around the country.)[208]

On June 19, 2002, one week after Sidney Taurel was named to the Homeland Security panel and two days after the GOP unveiled a prescription drug plan crafted largely by industry insiders, Eli Lilly cosponsored a high-rollers GOP fund-raiser at Washington's Mayflower Hotel. George Bush was the headliner. New campaign finance laws would soon take effect, making this one of the last hurrahs of the soft-money era.

"Drug companies in particular have made a rich investment in tonight's event," the *Washington Post* reported the next day.[209] Robert Ingram, of GlaxoSmithKline, had been "chief corporate fundraiser," and his company kicked in at least $250,000. PhRMA, which was also helping underwrite an ad campaign touting the GOP's prescription drug plan, gave a quarter million as well. Pfizer contributed at least $100,000, and Lilly, Bayer, and Merck each paid up to $50,000 to "sponsor" a table.

"The Republicans are smashing fundraising records under the leadership and guidance of Bush and his political team" the *Washington Post* said. The Bush team was "approaching corporations and lobbyists early and often, offering face-time with Cabinet officials and party luminaries." Not surprisingly, every company sponsoring the event had business before Congress. "The juxtaposition of the prescription drug debate on Capitol Hill and drug companies helping underwrite a major fundraiser highlights the tight relationship lawmakers have with groups seeking to influence the work before them," the *Post* said. One official said the GOP was "working hard behind the scenes on behalf of PhRMA."

WILL REDWOOD continued to improve in every facet of his young life. His speech was getting clearer and his vocabulary, while limited, was slowly growing. Lyn continued to credit chelation and the dietary interventions she had been using for slowly bringing her son along the path to normalcy, or at least seminormalcy.

In the summer of 2002, Will had also begun intensive math and reading instruction at the local Sylvan Learning Center. Will himself had asked to go, which pleasantly surprised Lyn. He had seen a commercial for the program on television one day and marched into Lyn's office.

"Mommy," he said, "know what I want?"

Lyn looked up from the computer. "What, honey?"

"I want to go to the Sylvan Learning Center."

"You do? How come?"

"Because," Will said, "Sylvan makes learning fun."

It might have been rote repetition of something heard on TV, Lyn thought. But the fact that Will was having a conversation this complex, with back-and-forth questions and answers, would have been unimaginable just a year or two before. She enrolled him in the program immediately. "If Will doesn't keep practicing his skills," Lyn said to Tommy, "he will lose them."

Still, Will's improvement had been so gradual, Lyn was often unaware of it until moments such as these, much like a parent who doesn't realize how quickly a child has grown until he is bursting out of his clothing.

Will's Iowa test scores were another sign of indisputable progress.

In fact, Will had just completed second grade when he was given the Iowa Test of Basic Skills, a standardized annual exam that tests scholastic achievement in elementary school students. At the end of first grade, Will had scored in the 3rd percentile of children his age. Now, a year later, he had moved up to the 17th percentile, a 560-percent improvement on his scores.

One evening, as Lyn and Will drove home from the grocery store, Lyn noticed a stunning sunset in the western sky. "Look, Will!" she said. "Isn't that sunset *beautiful*?"

Lyn was unprepared for what came next.

"Mommy," Will said, "what is 'beautiful'?"

222 • EVIDENCE OF HARM

Lyn had to fight back tears of joy. Will had never displayed much interest in such abstract concepts as beauty. She was delighted, but unsure how to answer. How does one describe *beauty* to another person? Lyn realized at that moment that she would have to go back and teach Will all of those things that other kids would have learned simply by growing up normal.

But it didn't matter. Lyn was certain of one thing. "We are getting our baby back," she thought.

IF THE DRUG LOBBY were going to buy liability protection, it would need to move quickly. More private and class-action lawsuits were appearing in courts around the country as families realized that they fell outside the VICP three-year statute of limitations.

The sheer volume of litigation that could descend upon Lilly was detailed in the company's hometown newspaper, the *Indianapolis Star*. On July 14 the paper reported that "trial lawyers have met regularly to plan their legal assaults on behalf of autistic children and their parents."[210] The lawsuits posed a costly threat to Lilly. "In the age of product-liability suits yielding millions or even billions of dollars," the paper said, "few cases can compare in jury-awakening pathos to toddlers stricken with autism."

The suits could hardly come at a worse time for Lilly, the *Star* reported. The company already faced losing more than two billion dollars in annual revenues from Prozac, its formerly best-selling drug, whose patent had run out.

In anticipation of the autism lawsuits, Lilly retained the services of Shook, Hardy & Bacon, the same Kansas City law firm it had used during the Prozac wrongful-death lawsuits a decade before. "Lilly's lawyers will fight the charge that thimerosal can cause autism," Lilly spokeswoman Joan S. Todd told the *Star*. "No causal link has been established between thimerosal and adverse reactions in vaccines."

EVEN AS VACCINE MAKERS braced themselves for a legal onslaught in civil court, they faced a second front of litigation in Vaccine Court. The companies technically were not defendants in those cases (because petitioners filed claims against the government), but they were intimately involved in the proceedings. Lawyers for the families were eager to begin discovery. They wanted access to internal company documents on thimerosal and MMR, and all government research into the matter.

But the drug companies (and, it would turn out, the government) did not want the discovery materials to be made available to anyone outside of Vaccine

Court. Such papers in the hands of trial lawyers could be potent in the civil court cases.

The companies also knew that a finding of causation within the VICP would open the pathway to mass civil action. The VICP judges, known as "Special Masters," were distressed by the wave of autism cases sweeping into the program, the likes of which they had never seen before. Vaccine Court was created to adjudicate *rare* cases of injury or death, not the thousands of thimerosal-related petitions making their way into the program.

The Masters' anxiety was sharpened when civil court judges began remanding hundreds of individual and class-action suits into the VICP. By early summer, it became clear that the Vaccine Court's caseload would be unmanageable. On July 2, 2002, the Special Masters, after conferring with plaintiff and government attorneys, issued a ruling on the burgeoning cases, essentially grouping them into one massive proceeding.

Over four hundred cases alleging a relationship between vaccines and autism disorders had been filed in the VICP, more than three hundred of them in the prior six months alone. And with more civil cases being remanded to the VICP, three to five thousand (or possibly more) new cases were likely to be filed in the next several months. "Processing such a large number of cases will stretch thinly the resources of both the court and the bar," the Special Masters said. "It is in the interests of all that the court aggressively but fairly manage this docket to ensure a timely presentation and resolution of the difficult medical and legal issues in these cases."[211]

In order to address the "unusual situation," the court lumped all ASD cases together into a single "Omnibus Autism Proceeding." The Masters laid out a detailed two-year timetable for petitioners to conduct "extensive discovery—documents, studies and raw data from government agencies and possibly vaccine manufacturers"—to build their case. When and if causation was found by the Special Master assigned to the proceeding, "these conclusions would be applied to each individual case."

The court agreed to create an "Autism Master File" on causation issues, "which would be open to inspection by any interested persons, and which would constitute an evidentiary record." It also agreed to have a team of lawyers represent all petitioners in the autism cases. The process would take two years. Discovery would continue until August 2003 and the Omnibus evidentiary hearing was scheduled for March 22, 2004. The Special Master's final decision on causation would be issued on July 3, 2004.

"Unfortunately," the court said, "resolution of the general causation inquiry must await longer than Congress envisioned, but it is clear to all involved that without the extended time frames, petitioners would be unable to

prosecute their claims. In this instance, quick justice would mean no justice."
Score one for the parents.

BY THE SUMMER OF 2002, autism had become a more common subject in the
nation's news. Rising cases were being reported almost everywhere. Even as
the numbers escalated, so did the debate over what the data actually *meant*.
Theories abounded on how to explain the growth while still keeping the
autism model within the realm of genetics. Mark Blaxill, the Boston father,
became Safe Minds' point person against naysayers who insisted on explanations that did not involve an environmental trigger.

Mark had taken on the job of ripping apart a particularly preposterous
theory put forth by Simon Baron-Cohen, the autism researcher from Cambridge University. Baron-Cohen wrote an essay for a Web site called edge.org,
suggesting that the rising case numbers might be attributed to the march of
technology. He called it an "Argument for Autism as a Genetic Epidemic."
Specifically, the professor conjectured that the airplane and computer had altered the mind's "architecture."[212]

The article provided the parents with some much-needed levity, and it
was posted on a number of sites, including FEAT (now called the Schafer
Autism Report).

Autistic people show a variety of symptoms, Baron-Cohen said, but one
commonality is their inability in relating to other people or reading their
body language. And yet, he seemed to confuse full-blown autism with the
milder, higher-functioning form of the disorder, Asperger's syndrome.

Autistics, he wrote, have a "natural flair" for understanding "non-social"
aspects of life. They may be inept at making friends or fitting in with peers,
he said, but they were extraordinarily adept at non-social systems like math,
engineering, computers, or music.

People with autism are usually male, and these men encounter great difficulty in attracting female mates, Baron-Cohen surmised. But then, two "massive changes" hit the planet: the airplane and the computer.

The airplane allowed autistic men to travel. Once in a foreign culture,
Baron-Cohen wrote, their odd behavior might be less detectable. An autistic
man from England might move to, say, Brazil, where his otherness might be
attributed to his being British. Brazilian women might be more willing to pair
with the man than English women were.

As for the computer, it allowed autistic men to make a good living. When
the market for computer-scientists was born and grew, autistic men, regardless
of their social skills, could now take an airliner abroad, secure employment

and wealth, and be able to offer a woman status and money while gaining social acceptance for himself.

This, Baron-Cohen posited, could explain the genetic epidemic of autism, which some had "rashly" attributed to pollution or vaccines. But the evidence for this was slim, he wrote. Instead, because autism runs in genes, his theory went, the upsurge in mating patterns among autistic men produced a new generation of affected children in greater numbers than before.

Baron-Cohen said that society should embrace these "systemizers" who can greatly benefit humanity with their supposed scientific and technological prowess.

Mark was amused, but also disgusted. He could not think of any autistic child who would master the realms of science and technology. Refuting this "theory" would not only be easy, it would be fun. Mark wasted no time banging out a critique, which he sent to edge.org, and posted on the Schafer Autism Report. He called it "Geeks Get Lucky."[213]

"Baron-Cohen argues that social mobility created by air travel has allowed 'geeks on the go' a chance to mate," Mark wrote. "If this were true, then Baron-Cohen would have to explain why other increases in cross-cultural mobility and mating would not have produced similar increases in autism.

"It's hard to make this stuff up. Under most circumstances, one would be tempted to write this off as lunacy from some out-of-touch crackpot. But here is the astonishing part. Baron-Cohen is an autism expert, and a respected academic as well." Although his essay was "pure, malicious nonsense, we must expose nonsense when we see it, especially when it comes from Cambridge professors with international reputations. I suspect he would prefer that those of us he would judge as unfit to mate would simply withdraw to our computer programs. We must not."

Even the silliest ideas can have serious consequences, Mark wrote, hinting at a dark conspiracy that might be lurking behind the geek theory. "Why offer such nonsense in a public forum? Why would such a prestigious researcher make such unsupported claims?" he asked. "I can offer an interpretation, albeit speculative, of his motives."

Suddenly, things didn't seem so funny.

"Let me be blunt. This man is one of the small group of academics who has shaped the science of autism for many years. He has been carrying on studies of the rates of autism in the middle of the largest increase ever seen in a developmental disorder and has failed to detect the changes or to sound the alarm. He has a large number of colleagues who have joined him in this pattern of error. Now, in the face of failure and contradictory evidence, he has resorted to concocting one of the most absurd arguments one could imagine in order to reconcile a genetic model with the inescapable evidence.

"This is bad science. It is malicious propaganda. It is supported by no research and refuted by every shred of available evidence. Yet Baron-Cohen commands respect in the scientific community and his arguments will have a way of creeping into the discussion and gaining respectability as they are whispered in corridors of leading institutions. If it weren't all such a tragedy, we could all share a good chuckle. Instead it makes you want to cry. Where has the integrity gone in autism science?"

A few days later, an apologetic Baron-Cohen e-mailed Mark. He called his essay "casual speculation," without evidence to support it, and thus nothing even close to a theory. They were, he said, "food for thought." Because some were offended, however, Baron-Cohen asked the Web site to pull his essay.

Mark was far from placated. "I recognize that your response is offered in a conciliatory fashion," he wrote back to Baron-Cohen, "but I'm afraid it is an olive branch I cannot accept. As reasonable and well-intentioned as your arguments may seem to you, I can tell you that such arguments are at the very root of the problems. We have a massive public health problem staring us in the face," he continued. "If this were an easily identified, infectious disease threatening our children, we'd have troops in the streets in the face of these rates of disability. But instead, 'experts' like you offer comforting distractions about mating patterns that would take years and years to prove wrong. The sad thing is, I bet a lot of your colleagues take the argument seriously."[214]

ELI LILLY and other drugmakers had reason to be increasingly alarmed over the pending thimerosal litigation, and Senator Bill Frist was ready to go to bat for them once again. In late June, Frist went to the Senate floor to "rally action" on his legislation to reduce "the critical national vaccine shortage."[215] The Advisory Commission for Childhood Vaccines, an HHS panel that advises the agency on improving the Vaccine Court, had just voted in favor of most of the Frist provisions, giving his bill new momentum.

"Today, many parents are being turned away with their children still vulnerable to a range of dangerous and often deadly diseases," Frist announced in his Tennessee drawl, sounding like a family doctor delivering bad news. "Five vaccines that prevent eight childhood diseases have been in short supply in the U.S. since last summer. The longer this shortage continues, the more vulnerable your children will become."

Frist implied that litigious parents were driving vaccine makers out of the business. The few companies left were "confronted with the high risk of liability and little profit motive," he said. "This legal uncertainty has contributed to an exodus of manufacturers from the vaccine market and a subsequent increase in vaccine prices." In some cases, "only one manufacturer is producing some of our most critical vaccines."

Frist said his bill would "restore balance" to the VICP. It would help compensate "those who suffer serious side effects from vaccines," while ensuring that "unwarranted litigation does not further destabilize our vaccine supply." And once again, the senator linked thimerosal litigation to homeland security. "The decision before us is whether to build on the success of vaccines to win the war on terror, and protect us, and our children against biological agents."

Frist's vaccine bill had gone nowhere since it was introduced in March. But on July 23, 2002, he managed to attach it as an amendment to a childhood immunization bill introduced by Hillary Clinton, the junior senator from New York.

That same day, an attorney named Tom Powers, from the Portland firm of Williams Dailey O'Leary Craine & Love, issued an urgent alert to parents on autism lists nationwide.[216]

"The drug companies and thimerosal manufacturers have launched an all-out sneak attack to destroy the legal rights of thimerosal-injured children," Powers warned. "Today in Congress the so-called Frist Bill was set for hearing, debate and vote in a Senate health committee meeting scheduled for tomorrow!" The Frist amendments were "anti-child, anti-justice and are an insult to the families of thimerosal-injured children."

It was "absolutely critical," Powers continued, that committee members "hear from parents who are outraged at this attack on the right to seek justice and fair compensation. Let the Senators hear from you, and do it tonight! We have 18 hours to get messages to the committee in order to make a difference tomorrow."

Sallie Bernard was drafted to write something for Safe Minds. She argued that vaccine court "was never intended to be a substitute for traditional civil remedies, simply to provide a low-cost speedy alternative."[217] The benefits of herd immunity could not be attained "by imposing the costs associated with vaccine injuries on a few children and families." The Frist bill would "destroy traditional civil tort remedies left intact by VICP, without fixing the severe problems that have developed during fifteen years of experience under the well-intentioned, but seriously flawed program."

The vaccine companies already enjoyed a degree of immunity from individual liability unprecedented under American law, Sallie said. But those companies now wanted "complete immunity" from lawsuits filed by parents.

It was "unconscionable," she added, "to slam the door on any relief for perhaps 500,000 families who may face expenses for lifetime care of several million dollars for a seriously injured child."

The Frist bill would "destroy traditional tort remedies by eliminating class actions, imposing an unrealistic short statute of limitations, limiting compensation to a fraction of potential lifetime expenses, extinguishing punitive damages, shifting the burden of proof from manufacturers to parents, and imposing a novel and unreasonably difficult standard of causation."

The threat of tort action was essential to keep industry honest, Sallie said. "Expanded immunity provides perverse incentives for less safe vaccines and will undermine public trust and confidence essential to an effective nationwide program of herd immunity," Sallie predicted. "VICP is badly broken and is long overdue for review and adjustment. Hundreds of thousands of families are counting on Congress to ensure them full and complete accountability and compensation for injuries and costs they were sadly forced to incur allegedly for the overall good of society."

Down in Durham, Laura Bono also jumped into the Frist fray with an emotional letter to the Senate. "The plight we have had dealing with autism (money, stress, medical, educational, therapy) has devastated our immediate family and our relatives," she wrote.[218] "Now Congress is possibly going to deliver another devastating blow by not allowing my family to sue the pharmaceutical companies that caused this by their negligence. To prevent parents from suing on behalf of their vaccine-damaged children is wrong." Drug companies, Laura added, "have taken our children's childhoods and perhaps their future as well." So why were they "going to such lengths to stop us from suing?" she asked. "Because they are in the wrong, the science has caught up with what parents have been saying, and they know they will lose billions of dollars."

In the end, the Frist bill was blocked in committee. Chairman Ted Kennedy had clashed with Frist for days over the issue.[219] Kennedy and the Democrats, however, would soon lose their one-seat majority in the midterm elections.

DR. MARK GEIER is the kind of guy you would want to have dinner with. Quick-minded and affable, with smiling eyes behind wire-framed glasses and a wicked sense of sarcasm, the geneticist and physician never shies away from speaking his mind, especially when the subject is vaccine safety.

Geier is president of the Genetic Centers of America, a private consulting firm in Silver Spring, Maryland. He received a Ph.D. in genetics and an M.D. from George Washington University. Geier was an early critic of the whole-cell pertussis vaccine and is an expert on the biological effects of vaccine-induced infant death. He has published papers in over thirty different peer-reviewed journals, including *Annals of Internal Medicine* and *Rheumatology*, on safety issues concerning hepatitis-B, rubella, pertussis, Lyme disease, rotavirus, anthrax, and smallpox vaccines.

His son, David, followed in his scientific footsteps, founding a medical-legal consultancy called MedCon. David Geier was a graduate student at the National Institutes of Health. Both men had testified before the VICP Vaccine Court on behalf of families. Mark and David do much of their vaccine investigative work out of their home, which is filled with medical documents and other papers.

Lyn met the Geiers in the fall of 2002, at a conference sponsored by the National Vaccine Information Center in Washington. The pair, who sometimes come across as a father-son science tag team, interrupting to finish each other's sentences, had come to the meeting to present their findings from a vaccine safety study.

The two men had obtained access to another database maintained by the government, called the Vaccine Adverse Effects Reporting System, or VAERS. Unlike the Vaccine Safety Datalink, the VAERS system only records problems that are voluntarily reported by doctors or parents. Because it is a "passive" reporting system, it is considered not nearly as reliable as the Vaccine Safety Datalink, which ostensibly records every adverse outcome. But the VAERS database does serve to at least identify, if not prove, associations between certain vaccines and their ill effects.

Mark and David Geier had compared adverse outcomes from the diphtheria-tetanus-pertussis vaccine (DTP) and its newer, safer cousin, the diphtheria-tetanus-acellular-pertussis vaccine (DTaP). DTP contains whole-cell pertussis, while DTaP uses a purified formulation, to reduce side effects like convulsions and high fever.

They had expected to find a higher rate of side effects from DTP than DTaP, but did not. What they did report, however, was a highly significant difference in adverse outcomes between DTaP vaccines that contained thimerosal and those that were preservative-free. This surprised them. For months, parents had been urging them to investigate vaccine mercury as a possible cause of autism and other childhood disorders, but the two men had ignored their pleas, writing off the allegations as little more than the emotional outbursts of distraught parents.

"Our initial reaction was, we didn't believe it," Mark Geier said at the vaccine conference that Lyn attended, "even when parents told us that the rise in autism coincided with a similar increase in the use of thimerosal-containing vaccines." After all, television viewing had also risen significantly during the same period. Was TV just as likely a culprit? Thimerosol made for a ridiculous hypothesis. And besides, there was no way to test it.[220]

But then they realized that there was a way to test it: comparing children who received DTaP vaccine containing mercury with those kids who received the thimerosal-free version.

When the father-son team ran these calculations through the VAERS database, they were startled to find that the relative risk for developing both autism and mental retardation was 6.0 in the thimerosal DTaP group as compared with the mercury-free DTaP group, and the difference was "highly statistically significant," Mark Geier told the conference. The relative risk for speech disorders was 2.2.

The Geiers wrote up their findings and published them in the peer-reviewed journal *Experimental Biology and Medicine,* the official journal of the Society for Experimental Biology and Medicine. Their paper was accepted in December 2002 and printed in June 2003.

After Lyn Redwood contacted the Geiers, they set out to publish a second article on the DTaP data, which was accepted by the *Journal of American Physicians and Surgeons.* The journal, and the American Association of Physicians and Surgeons (AAPS), which publishes it, are considered by many experts to lie on the fringe, if not altogether outside of mainstream medicine. The group is noticeably antiestablishment and perceived to be virulently antivaccine, a characterization that it denies. Many M.D.s, if they have even heard of it, look down their noses at the AAPS, and dismiss it as belonging to the bottom-feeding realm of homeopaths and chiropractors.

Nonetheless, the journal *is* peer reviewed. And there certainly would be no political challenges to getting the Geiers' thimerosal findings printed there. The article was accepted for publication in the spring 2003 issue.

"This study provides strong epidemiological evidence for a link between increasing mercury from thimerosal containing childhood vaccines and neurodevelopment disorders," the two men wrote in their conclusion. "In light of voluminous literature supporting the biologic mechanisms for mercury-induced adverse reactions," and the presence of mercury in vaccines exceeding federal guidelines, they said, "a causal relationship between thimerosal-containing childhood vaccines and neurodevelopment disorders and heart disease appears to be confirmed. . . .

"It is to be hoped that complete removal of thimerosal from all childhood vaccines will help to stem the tragic, apparently iatrogenic epidemic of autism and speech disorders that the United States is now facing."[221]

The Geiers had seen the VAERS database, but they had never seen the Vaccine Safety Datalink database. They knew that the other database existed, and they had tried on their own to gain access to it in the past, always without success. When Lyn told them about the VSD documents that Safe Minds had obtained through FOIA, including the Simpsonwood minutes and the initial Verstraeten analysis showing a relative risk for autism of 2.48, they were more eager than ever to see the VSD data.

In fact, the Geiers had already begun to seek access to the VSD data before meeting Lyn, going back to early August 2002. They had wanted to confirm their previously published VAERS studies (approximately twenty of them), which had looked into adverse outcomes from a number of pediatric and adult vaccines.

But when the Geiers contacted CDC officials about doing such a study, they were met with heavy resistance from the get-go. "They were clearly not happy with our requests," Mark Geier reported to Dave Weldon, whose office had contacted the Geiers about their work. "They want us to come up with every single possible question we might ask of the data, up front, and asked us to make various predictions about what we expect to find." The Geiers spent countless hours to develop a detailed 150-page proposal, but that still wasn't enough to gain access. "CDC is continually putting up additional steps," Mark complained to Weldon. "Now they are requiring fees and creating other new hindrances that seem to make the possibility of ever gaining actual access to the VSD extremely remote."

After weeks of negotiations, with Weldon's office running interference, the CDC said it would accept the Geier proposal. But the father-son team would still have to obtain permission from the Institutional Review Boards of each HMO. When that complex step was accomplished, they would then have to return to the CDC for the ultimate green light.

More than a year would pass before the Geiers would get in to see the data.

10. Homeland Insecurity

NOVEMBER 5, 2002, Election Day, was a marvelous moment to be a Republican. It was a historic victory for President Bush and the GOP. The party had swept through the Senate races, knocking off one Democrat after another. The Republicans hungrily took back the Senate with a 51 to 49 margin, and slightly increased their already wide margin in the House. Not since 1934 had the party in the White House gained seats during a midterm election, and never during a first term. Republican candidates, flush with cash raised in part by Bill Frist, had been masterful in painting some Democrats, including Sen. Max Cleland of Georgia, a disabled veteran, as being soft on the war on terrorism. Bill Frist was an honored guest.

A jubilant George Bush, who crisscrossed the country campaigning for his party, celebrated with an intimate dinner on Election Night at the White House with, among others, Senator Frist.

The drug industry's monetary muscle had helped nudge their preferred party back into total power. Kennedy would be ousted as Health Committee chairman, and Trent Lott would retake the Senate Majority Leader post. The Frist bill, among other drug industry laundry list items, would finally get a full hearing in the Senate.

If drug executives were pleased with the election results, they must have been downright giddy with the other news of the day. On November 6, the *New England Journal of Medicine* released a landmark study on MMR. It was good news for vaccine makers. The investigation, conducted in Denmark, produced the most conclusive evidence to date against any association between autism and the triple vaccine.[222] (The MMR vaccine, of course, contains no thimerosal, but some parents believed the live virus vaccine itself was a cause of autism, while others believed that the MMR shot caused additional gut damage to kids whose immune system was already assaulted by thimerosal-containing vaccines given previously.)

The *New England Journal* report was a sweeping study. Investigators had examined the medical records of every child born in Denmark between 1991 and 1998, including vaccination records and autism diagnoses. Of the 537,303 children in the cohort, 82 percent had received MMR vaccine. The study found 316 children with autism and 422 with a diagnosis of "other autistic-spectrum disorders." But there was no statistically significant difference in the risk for autism outcomes between the vaccinated and unvaccinated children. It was "strong evidence against the hypothesis that MMR vaccination causes autism," the authors said.

Dr. Edward W. Campion, who wrote the editorial that accompanied the paper, was even more positive. "This careful and convincing study shows that there is no association between autism and MMR vaccination," he said. "Other studies have also found no such association." But not even this "objective data" he warned, was likely to put an end to the controversy. "Strongly held beliefs are difficult to change," Campion wrote, adding that the public had already lost "a high degree of trust in the vaccine manufacturers, the government, or the medical establishment," and part of the blame belonged to "controversies such as that over mercury-containing preservatives."

The parents' countercharge was swift and pointed: "The conclusions appear overreaching," Sallie wrote in a letter to the journal. And, they insisted, MMR alone might not be what was fueling the autism epidemic; other vaccines might be involved, and "only biological research, not epidemiology, can answer the question of whether the MMR vaccine plays a role in autism.

"Studies have shown that mercury exposure in utero or during early life—when thimerosal vaccines are given—can cause immune system abnormalities which predispose the child to ongoing viral infections," Sallie wrote. "It is biologically plausible that this immune disruption may have allowed the live measles virus component in MMR to persist in susceptible autistic children, making the symptoms of the disorder worse. This would not be detected through an epidemiology study like the Denmark one."[223]

. . .

THREE DAYS LATER, the *New York Times Magazine* published a feature by Arthur Allen titled "The Not-So-Crackpot Autism Theory." It was a substantive profile of Dr. Neal Halsey, the Johns Hopkins researcher and former participant in the CDC's Advisory Committee on Immunization Practices.

Halsey had been "confronted with the hypothesis that thimerosal had damaged the brains of immunized infants," Allen wrote. Vaccines added to the list "under his watch" had tripled the dose of mercury given to infants.[224] And some thirty million American kids might have been exposed to "levels of mercury that, in theory, could have killed enough brain cells to scramble thinking or hex behavior."

Halsey's first reaction "was simply disbelief, which was the reaction of almost everybody involved in vaccines," he told the magazine. "In most vaccine containers, thimerosal is listed as a mercury derivative, 1/100th of a percent. And what I believed, and what everybody else believed, was that it was truly a trace, a biologically insignificant amount. If vaccine labels had listed mercury content in micrograms, this would have been uncovered years ago. But the fact is, no one did the calculation."

The doctor was accordingly "forced to reckon with the hypothesis that thimerosal had damaged the brains of immunized infants," Allen said, "and may have contributed to the unexplained explosion in the number of cases of autism being diagnosed in children."

Halsey had infuriated many of his fellow vaccinologists, "who couldn't fathom how a doctor who had spent so much energy dismantling the arguments of people who attacked vaccines could now be changing sides," the article claimed. But Halsey was simply looking at the numbers, "and the numbers deeply troubled him."

Not everyone was troubled. Dr. Paul Offit, the pro-vaccine advocate at Children's Hospital of Philadelphia, declared that "full disclosure can be harmful." Removing thimerosal "didn't make vaccines safer, it only made them perceptibly safer."

Halsey freely admitted that the evidence was not yet convincing that thimerosal had caused harm. But, he said, "to keep the vaccine program on a steady keel public-health authorities simply must follow through with the studies and face the consequences without flinching." If damage was found, then Halsey believed there "should be some kind of compensation, though I don't know how. I empathize with families of children with these disorders. How are you going to put dollar values on that?"

Lyn was so thrilled with the *Times Magazine* story she fired off a congratulatory e-mail to Halsey. "Please know that you did the right thing," she wrote. "You'll never know how many children benefited from your input on thimerosal. It's easy to add up the number of children with an infectious disease. It is not so easy to add up the number of children who may not be functioning with their full potential."[225]

A quick reply came back from Halsey, who complained that he had been quoted out of context. "Thanks Lyn," he wrote. "Unfortunately there were a few misquotes in the article and I am sending a letter to the NYT. This is not easy for anyone."[226] His biggest beef was with the article's title and photo caption, which implied that Halsey connected thimerosal to autism, when in fact he had been referring to milder disorders. "The headline, the press release issued prior to publication, and the caption are inappropriate. I do not (and never did) believe that any vaccine causes autism," he wrote to the *Times*.[227] "The sensationalized title sets an inappropriate context for everything in the article. Readers are led to incorrectly believe that statements in the article refer to autism."

Halsey said he had expressed concern "about subtle learning disabilities from exposure to mercury from environmental sources and possibly from thimerosal," but that "should not have been interpreted as support for theories that vaccines cause autism, a far more severe and complex disorder."

Even so, for the parents, the article was a refreshing break in a difficult year. Coming on the heels of the *New England Journal* MMR article and the Republican sweep of Congress, it gave Safe Minds perhaps more legitimacy than anything that had appeared before in the mainstream media.

THE CELEBRATIONS were short-lived. Just three days after the article appeared, on November 13, Lyn got a phone call about the looming Homeland Security Bill of 2002. In a few short hours, the House of Representatives would vote on legislation to consolidate a vast swath of the federal bureaucracy into a single antiterror entity.

Unbeknownst to most members of Congress, however, three riders had been anonymously attached to the massive bill at the last minute. One rider, in language lifted directly from the Frist vaccine bill, classified thimerosal as a *component* of vaccines, and not an additive or *contaminant*, which meant that Eli Lilly would be considered a "vaccine manufacturer" and thus be covered under the VICP.[228]

The net effect would be to dismiss all current and future thimerosal lawsuits filed in civil court. The Redwoods' suit, and hundreds more, would be thrown out the legal window. Potentially tens of thousands of more cases would never be filed at all.

Lyn felt beleaguered and sick to her stomach. She realized what kind of power the lowly parents were up against. But she had an odd sense of vindication, too. Obviously, the Mercury Moms had hit a nerve somewhere. People high up in the political-economic food chain were panicky enough over thimerosal lawsuits to attempt such a brazen move. To Lyn, this underhanded grab at legal immunity smacked of guilt. She smelled scandal, and it gave her hope. Disgusting as the secret rider was to her, she knew that thimerosal would be headline news in short order. The mainstream media, which considered the Safe Minds parents to be fringe antivaccine zealots, had barely touched the story. Now, they would have no choice.

For the vaccine lobby, the rider was an enormous victory, though it wasn't everything that Frist or PhRMA had wanted. Whoever inserted the rider into the Homeland Security bill, for reasons unknown, included the Lilly vaccine ingredient provisions only, and nothing about limiting access to the VICP or preventing families from "opting out."

Lyn Redwood and Laura Bono got the word out to parents nationwide. They desperately tried, but failed to reach Dan Burton before he voted. "I feel so duped once again," Laura told Lyn. "We've been taken in by the very people put into office to protect us and our kids."

When the bill was passed and its rider revealed, a blizzard of indignation swept through the capital. Dan Burton was out for blood. The Homeland Security Act had come within the jurisdiction of his committee, and he was outraged that something had been added to what he called "his bill." (Other committees had partial jurisdiction over the bill, but the measure had originated from Government Reform, and any change to the bill had to be cleared through Burton and his colleagues.) Many Democrats were livid as well. The finger-pointing began immediately, and most fingers pointed at Richard Armey, the folksy Texas Republican and soon-to-retire House Majority Leader.

Well-placed sources quickly began sending tips to Lyn. "The shameful vaccine provisions were sent by e-mail from the White House to Rep. Dick Armey at 10:10 P.M. the night before the vote," one e-mail from Washington said. "Frist's ex-health staffer is employed, (guess where?) in the White House. Go figure."

When Burton confronted Armey about the rider, the Texan told him he had indeed inserted the language. And yes, he acted at the request of the White House. But the next day, Armey denied that the White House had any hand in the action. His chief of staff told reporters on November 15 that the language came from Frist's office.

Frist aides said their boss had nothing to do with it, and Armey later insisted he acted alone. "But several corporate lobbyists said this is not credible," wrote Jonathan Weisman in the *Washington Post*. "Whoever was responsible had to have detailed knowledge of the legal issues, had to know Frist had drafted the larger bill, and had to understand exactly which provision applied to thimerosal because the brand name does not appear in the text." Weisman reported that, according to two sources, an HHS official gave the final okay, "a statement that HHS spokesman Bill Pierce adamantly denied."[229]

Armey, during a November 18 interview with Pat Robertson on the Christian Broadcasting Network, defended his actions. His responsibility in homeland security "was to address the question of a reliable vaccine supply for all of America on the best scientific arguments available," he said. "I frankly did dismiss the arguments of the tort lawyers that are seeking the opportunity for class-action lawsuits. . . .

"It was a necessary thing to put in there," Armey said. "It's something I'm proud I did because we cannot let the tort lawyers define the conditions of science and medicine in America. They'll dumb it down as they've done so many other things."

Robertson joked with the congressman. "Well, you know, I saw a piece on CBS that seemed to act like there was a sinister plot between Eli Lilly and, you know, Mitch Daniels and you, and everybody getting these enormous payoffs. That's not true, is it?"

Armey grinned lazily. "Nah. It's not true."[230]

Lilly executives, when asked, claimed ignorance. CEO Sidney Taurel admitted to being "pleased" with the rider, but insisted that at no time did he ask anyone for favors. Lilly spokesman Edward Sagibel added that the company was "surprised" by the move, but believed it was "a positive step to help assure that manufacturers are protected from lawsuits that are without merit or scientific evidence."[231]

And the White House backed Taurel up, claiming he couldn't have influenced national vaccine policy from his seat on the president's Homeland Security Advisory Council. Frank Cilluffo, a Bush aide and executive director of the council, said that members were asked to recuse themselves from discussions that could affect their particular industries. What he did not mention was that panel members received full access to Homeland Security Chief Tom Ridge. All meetings were off the record.[232]

Taurel's insistence aside, many media accounts of the scandal noted that the drug industry had shelled out more than fourteen million dollars to congressional candidates prior to the November election—nearly 80 percent of it to Republicans.

FOR SAFE MINDS, the paramount question was not the rider's origin, but its future. The Senate was to vote on the Homeland Security bill in a few days.

Senate Democrats Tom Daschle and Joe Lieberman were offering an amendment to remove the riders, but no one thought it would be easy. For one thing, the House had already adjourned. If the Senate were to tinker with the legislation, House members would have to be recalled en masse to a special session to vote on the revamped bill. In the age of Al Qaeda, and with the winds of war bellowing in Iraq, such a delay would be untenable for many lawmakers.

Anyhow, the drug lobbyists were back on Capitol Hill. Lyn learned from her sources that drug lobby reps had paid visits to the offices of at least seven influential senators. The companies were threatening to not make smallpox vaccine if the vaccine rider was removed from the bill, according to several Capitol Hill staffers, journalists, and lawyers.[233]

The controversy, meanwhile, had gained Safe Minds a new and experienced ally. His name was Michael Bender, and he was executive director of the Mercury Policy Project, an advocacy group that promotes policies to eliminate mercury use, reduce the export of and trafficking in mercury, and eliminate mercury exposures. Lyn had known Michael for a couple of years. But because his organization was focused mostly on environmental mercury, the two groups had never officially joined forces until now.

It took a few days for the parties to agree on the proper line of attack. Lyn wanted to go after Congress. "They sold out our kids," she grumbled. "They're more interested in giving immunity to Lilly than finding out why that company misled the public and poisoned our children."

Sallie was guarded about attacking potential allies in Congress. "We'd get more mileage by laying blame solely on the manufacturers," she said. "They are blackmailing the country at a time of impending war, *and* they are selling out children. So let's play that up to the Senate, especially the staffers who are being threatened by PhRMA."

"But Sallie," Lyn protested, "It was lawmakers like Dick Armey who did in fact sell out the kids. But you're right, we do need to go after the drug companies as well, of course."

Attacking industry did not sit well with Mark Blaxill, however. He was not prepared to blame free enterprise for the rider debacle. Many of his company's clients were Fortune 500 firms, and Mark certainly did not view them as "evil." It became a serious point of contention and it threatened to drive a wedge through Safe Minds.

Mark gave his objections in a delicately worded e-mail.[234] "I confess to serious discomfort with some of this," he said. "As you know, I am far more inclined to place blame on those who designed the entire childhood immunization schedule than I am on individual manufacturers."

That said, Mark did believe that, more than any other company, "Eli Lilly deserves special scrutiny due to its direct role in the production and distribution of thimerosal. Lilly's CEO is on the Homeland Security Advisory Council. I am NOT arguing that all is sweetness and light here."

But Mark still worried that Sallie and Lyn's harsh rhetoric crossed the line from being antimercury to being antibusiness. "It offers *ad hominem* criticism of all pharmaceutical companies, without respecting their free-speech rights and obvious interests," he said. "And it presumes that Lilly is guilty without trial. I think we have plenty of ammunition about Lilly's conflict of interest without these attacks.

"I know some of you may believe that corporations are inherently evil and not to be trusted," Mark went on. "I do not share this view. If we cannot walk the fine line more skillfully, this is the kind of position that might require me to resign from the board. I cannot defend these kinds of statements to my colleagues, nor would I wish to."

In the end, Safe Minds, in conjunction with the Mercury Policy Project, crafted a joint statement denouncing the rider and supporting the Lieberman motion to eliminate it. As for the drug companies, the parents attacked them for their threats to stop making bioterror vaccines, and questioned Eli Lilly's openness when it came to acknowledging the toxic effects of thimerosal. But Mark had prevailed. There was no talk of evil corporations poisoning helpless children.

"We are heartened that Senators Lieberman and Daschle are offering an amendment to remove extraneous additions like the thimerosal liability shield from the Homeland Security Act," Sallie said in the statement. "This addition is an example of all that is wrong with a system of using last minute riders to subvert the legislative process."

"Instead of providing immunity," Lyn added, "Congress should be investigating why the FDA and American public were misled by Eli Lilly into believing that their product was safe, when company documents paint a completely different picture."[235]

FOR A COUPLE of weeks in mid-November, the "Lilly rider," as it was now called, was the main topic of chatter within official Washington. Its daring, middle-of-the-night insertion was arguably the first big scandal of the new century. On the Senate floor, in the cable news network studios, and inside the gossipy salons of Georgetown, it seemed everyone was playing the newest parlor game. Up on the Hill, the rider was denounced, defended—and almost defeated. Democrats, still stinging from their humiliation at the polls, were seething at the maneuver. They lashed out at Bush, Daniels, Lilly, Armey, Frist, and whomever else they felt they could pin the deed on.

Henry Waxman was among the first Democrats to come out swinging. On November 15, he faxed a starkly worded letter to Mitch Daniels at the White House.

"The provisions are irrelevant to the Homeland Security bill and have been included without appropriate congressional consideration," Waxman wrote.[236] A number of "reforms" had been proposed for vaccine injury compensation, but when it came to the Homeland Security rider, "only those provisions that provide liability protection to Eli Lilly and other thimerosal manufacturers have been included."

Waxman noted that the Lilly rider was "something that the White House wanted" and reminded Daniels: "As Director of OMB, one of your responsibilities is to coordinate the Administration's position on legislation. For this reason, I am writing to inquire about how these provisions came to be included in the bill."

Waxman then requested a list of "all outside groups or individuals consulted about changes to VICP," including the date, topic, and names of people involved in each contact, plus copies of all documents and records on the subject. "I would also like to know what your role was, if any, in developing this legislation." An answer.

Sen. Debbie Stabenow (D-MI) called the rider "outrageous" and demanded its removal from the bill before the Senate vote. "Don't families and their children merit due process under the law?" she asked in a Senate floor speech.[237] "This bill would severely limit parents' ability to get justice for their children." The rider, she said, protected a company whose CEO was in the top five with respect to compensation in 2001, a company that posted $11.5 billion in revenue in 2001, in an industry "that makes higher profits than any other industry."

"This reminds me of the Immaculate Conception: nobody is responsible," Stabenow told reporters later.[238] "Armey says it was the White House. The White House says it was Frist. All I know is that there are a whole lot of links here, from the very top of OMB to the CEO of Eli Lilly sitting on the Homeland Security Advisory Committee, to Senator Frist. It doesn't take a Ph.D. to make a credible link here."

Joe Lieberman and Tom Daschle made good on their threat to try to repeal the riders. Their amendment would be taken up on Monday, November 18, and the Senate would vote on the full bill the following day.

Frist led the charge to keep the provisions intact. On Monday, he went to the Senate floor to denounce Lieberman's amendment. "It will put the people of our nation at greater risk," Frist warned.[239] "We are talking about homeland security . . . vaccine is the front line for people at risk from anthrax. It is the front line for people at risk from smallpox. That means your children.

That means your spouse. That means your grandparents. That means your family. So we must not do anything—and the Lieberman amendment would do this—to increase the barrier for you to be protected."

In his thirty-minute speech, Frist played fast and loose with the truth.

"The Institute of Medicine has made it very clear," he said, "that there is no established causal relationship between that preservative and autism." Like the institute's Marie McCormick, Frist failed to mention that the IOM also found insufficient evidence to *reject* a causal relationship.

"The provision," he said, did "not prevent patients from suing in court. Instead it merely requires [that] claimants must first go through the compensation program. One can go through that program itself, in a timely way. If someone does not agree with the compensation put forward, they can go to court."

This was an accurate assertion only for families with children whose injury occurred within the last three years. For the Redwoods, Bonos, and thousands of other families, the statement was utterly false. The rider would kill any last shot at redress. Every judge in America would now order them *into* the program before allowing them to file suit elsewhere. But the vast majority of affected families could not get into the program because of the statute of limitations. For them, Frist's assertion that the provisions "do not prevent parents from suing in court" was a lie.

Not all Republicans backed Frist, however. Dan Burton, of course, was up in arms. He faxed a three-page "Dear Colleague" letter to every member of Congress. "These provisions do not belong in the Homeland Security Act," he said. "The scientific debate remains unsolved."[240]

John McCain, the maverick GOP Senator from Arizona, who had made few friends in the White House with his crusade against soft-money campaign contributions, announced that he would vote with the Democrats to remove the Lilly rider and the other two provisions inserted into the bill (one to permit government contracts with U.S. companies that move offshore without paying taxes, and the other to build a "homeland security research center" at Texas A&M University).[241]

It was going to be close. On Tuesday, November 19, the day of the vote on the Lieberman amendment, Lyn and Laura worked the phones like old-time political hacks, frantically trying to call, beep, e-mail, or fax every Senate aide they could think of.

Late in the day, a surprising wrinkle emerged on the Hill. Three moderate Republicans were threatening to vote with Democrats unless they got a promise that the riders would be eliminated from the new law when Congress returned in January. Olympia Snowe and Susan Collins, both of Maine, and Lincoln Chafee of Rhode Island told Vice President Dick Cheney and Trent Lott they would otherwise buck their party.

Lyn was encouraged by the turn of events. She kept working the phone. And she managed to recruit a surprise last-minute ally. Her friend Frank Schmuck, the ex–Air Force Gulf War pilot who had been diagnosed with mercury poisoning, was a buddy of Ross Perot, the feisty billionaire and colorful former presidential candidate. Lyn placed an uncertain call to Perot, not believing she would ever hear back from him. She was startled when Perot called her directly to ask how he could help. Lyn asked him to call Vice President Cheney and several influential senators that Perot knew. He agreed, but told her it was a bit of a long shot. The vote in the Senate was approaching, and Lyn could see that Cheney had arrived on the scene, there to cast a tie-breaking vote, if needed.

"I'll call Dick right away," Perot told her.[242]

Up until the very end of voting, Lyn stayed on the phone, dialing away in her second-floor office. Then news came in that the three moderate GOP senators had gotten the assurances they were seeking from Lott. They would return to the Republican fold.

But it wasn't over just yet. Collins, Snowe, and Chafee were now demanding similar assurances from House Speaker Dennis Hastert, who was on a plane to Turkey. They also wanted a verbal commitment from House Majority Leader Tom DeLay, the archconservative from Texas. "It was kind of a moment of high drama, but we felt very strongly. It was not a done deal," Collins told CNN later.[243] As time for the fifteen-minute vote ran out, the three renegades remained sequestered in the GOP cloakroom, waiting for Hastert's call. The phone finally rang. It was Hastert. He agreed. DeLay also called to say he would "consider" taking up the measure in January. The roll call continued.

Lyn went downstairs to watch. Tommy had dragged himself out of bed after an all-nighter in the ER. He ambled around groggily, a mug of coffee clutched in his hand. Tommy saw the TV, looked at Lyn, and shrugged, as if to say, "Here we go."

Lyn sat on the sofa. Tommy could barely take it. He paced around like a cougar in a cage. Lyn watched the votes come in. Minutes before the voting ended, the three moderates walked onto the floor and cast their "nay" votes. Lieberman failed, 52–47.[244]

The Redwoods were crushed. Lyn slunk back upstairs, unable to look at the TV or at her glum husband, crumpled on the couch. She stared out the window at the silver November mist that obscured the woods beyond. Downstairs on TV, Lyn heard Trent Lott call President Bush aboard Air Force One to deliver the news.

"Mr. President," he said, "you now have the tools you need to protect America!"

Lyn had heard enough. She ran to the balcony and yelled "Holy crap!" "Damn!" Tommy echoed from below.

Lyn watched as Tommy paced around the family room. He stopped abruptly and faced the television. Lyn watched Tommy Redwood, the life-long Republican with the Mississippi drawl, slowly raise his right hand and point a middle finger at the screen. Tommy went back into the bedroom and quietly closed the door behind him.

The entire day passed before they could bring themselves to talk about it. That night in bed, Tommy broke down. "I can't believe they would do this," he said of his party. "You know I've always been a conservative, Lyn. But to see *my* people, who *I* put into office slip this kind of thing in. I feel totally betrayed. It's like finding out there's no Santa."

The next day, the Senate passed the House version of the bill, Lilly rider and all.

Neither the Democrats nor the parents trusted the Republicans to "revisit" the rider in 2003. Once something became law, it was extraordinarily difficult to undo. On the day after the Senate vote, Tom Daschle returned to the floor vowing to fight another day. "This isn't over," Daschle said. "But even if we are successful, I don't know if you can put the pieces back together for these families."[245]

Right after the vote, Lyn's phone began to ring. Bob Herbert, the *New York Times* columnist, wanted her reaction. *Good Morning America* wanted to book Lyn for a live one-on-one with Diane Sawyer.

NOT EVERYONE was outraged at the turn of events. The drug lobby was pleased, for one. The GOP had won back the Senate and held the House. Now they had slipped permanent vaccine liability protection into federal statute. It was time for a little get-together, not only to celebrate the victory, but to devise even more effective ways to capitalize on their ascendant influence in Washington.

On November 20, the day of the Senate vote, drug company executives held a high-powered get-together at the Westfield International Conference Center near Dulles Airport. Among the power players were Robert Essner, president of Wyeth, Peter R. Dolan, chairman of Bristol-Myers Squibb, and Sidney Taurel of Lilly.

"Having spent more than $30 million to help elect their allies to Congress," the *New York Times* reported, "the major drug companies are devising ways to capitalize on their electoral success by securing favorable new legislation."[246] The industry's hand was stronger now "than at any other time in recent years." The lavish amounts of pharmaceutical money flowing into candidates' coffers and the millions more in television ads financed by industry groups were "spent overwhelmingly on behalf of Republicans, who now control both houses of Congress," the paper said. "Drug industry executives who attended the conference, put on by the industry's main lobbying arm, said they were delighted with the election results."

PRESIDENT BUSH signed the Homeland Security Act of 2002 on November 25 at 11:30 A.M. At 8:30 that morning, lawyers for Scott and Laura Bono rushed to the Federal Courthouse in Salisbury, North Carolina, to file suit against Lilly and the vaccine makers. It was unclear if the new law would be retroactive and the Bonos wanted to cover their bases.

Even as Bush put his pen to the act, the national media were still fully consumed with the mysterious origin of the Lilly rider. That same morning, for instance, Bob Herbert titled his *New York Times* column "Whose Hands Are Dirty?" Though thimerosal was no longer added to pediatric vaccines, he said, "a serious controversy continues. Lawsuits have been filed by parents across the country, convinced that their children suffered severe neurological damage from the mercury in vaccines. . . .

"Talking to them," Herbert added, "can be heartbreaking." And then he quoted Lyn Redwood. " 'I have a little boy who was completely normal at birth, walking, talking, smiling, meeting all of his developmental landmarks,' she said. 'Then, shortly after he turned one year old, he lost his ability to speak, to make eye contact.' "

Herbert said the rider had nothing to do with homeland security, and everything to do with Lilly's security. "Maybe it's related to the fact that Mitch Daniels, the White House budget director, is a former Eli Lilly big shot. Or the very convenient fact that just last June President Bush appointed Eli Lilly's chairman, president and CEO, Sidney Taurel, to a coveted seat on the president's Homeland Security Advisory Council. . . .

"There's a real bad smell here," Herbert went on. "Eli Lilly will benefit greatly as both class-action and individual lawsuits are derailed. But there are no fingerprints in sight. No one will own up to a legislative deed that is both cynical and shameful."[247]

IT TOOK A FULL WEEK to make headlines, but on November 19, the same day the Senate defeated the Lieberman amendment, Department of Health and Human Services lawyers had slipped into the federal Vaccine Court to file a protection order in the Autism Omnibus Proceedings. They sought the permanent sealing of all thimerosal discovery materials presented in Vaccine

Court. The move was so stealthy that only one reporter, from Reuters, filed a story at the time.[248]

Under the proposed order drafted by the government, evidence of thimerosal toxicity could not be revealed to anyone but the attorneys arguing cases in front of the Special Master for Autism, George Hastings.[249]

The sharing of discovery documents with family members, the media, or anyone not arguing a case before the Vaccine Court would be subject to sanctions and penalties. More draconian, all government documents relating to thimerosal that had already been released would be rounded up by government lawyers and destroyed. Any evidence presented in the Vaccine Court could never be used in civil court without the written permission of the secretary of health and human services.

By moving to suppress the Lilly files, the Justice Department claimed it was only acting to protect the interests of HHS Secretary Tommy Thompson.

The media again attacked the Bush-Lilly axis. "Republicans in Washington have thrown a one-two punch at trial lawyers and have socked advocates for autistic children in the process," an editorial in *Newsday* said.[250] "If they have their way, pharmaceutical giant Eli Lilly will gain greater protection from lawsuits, while people suing on behalf of autistic children will have a more arduous road to the courthouse. That shouldn't happen."

The protection order would "make future autism claims involving thimerosal more difficult and time-consuming for plaintiffs," the paper said. "The request for secrecy should be denied." Some information, like trade secrets or divorce details, should be kept private. "But scientific studies and information on what Eli Lilly knew and when it knew it should not qualify. If Republicans want to make litigation tougher for autistic children, they should at least have the courage to do it in the open."

Democratic lawmakers were less charitable.

"To be frank, it's as though you first robbed the bank and are now attempting to hide the evidence of the harm," Rep. John Conyers (D-MI) wrote to Tommy Thompson and Attorney General John Ashcroft.[251] "Given this controversy and the concerns for the rights of the families in pending lawsuits concerning thimerosal, I would appreciate it if you would provide me a detailed description of the rationale for your request."

Sen. Patrick Leahy (D-VT) was equally blunt. "Please explain why the protective order sought by the Administration seeks to keep this information secret forever," he asked.[252] "Why does the Administration not want to allow the children allegedly suffering from thimerosal-induced autism and their families to see relevant information from HHS? What is the range of penalties that may be ordered by the Court for violation of the protective order should it be adopted?"

And Leahy wrote, perhaps tongue in cheek: "To the extent that HHS has already produced information that has been shared with children allegedly suffering from thimerosal-induced autism and their families, what would be the penalty for those children or their families violating the protective order?"

ON THANKSGIVING DAY, Albert Enayati picked up a copy of the *Wall Street Journal* and read about the proposed protective order. Another headline caught his eye, too. On November 26, the day after Bush signed the Homeland Security bill, the FDA had approved a new nonstimulant treatment for ADHD. The drug, Strattera, was produced by Eli Lilly, which stood to make billions of dollars from the mushrooming ADHD market. Lilly executives estimated that up to 7 *percent* of all American schoolchildren were affected by the disorder, and 60 percent "carry their symptoms into adulthood," a company release noted.[253] Strattera was also approved for adults. Lilly noted that 4 percent of American adults (eight million people) have ADHD. "Most of them are undiagnosed." Commercials hawking the new drug soon began appearing on television.

To thimerosal activists, the notion of Lilly profiting from the ADHD epidemic was at the least ironic. Conspiracy theorists went further. They returned to the Internet with wild speculation about evil companies whipping up toxic stews for children, possibly on purpose, creating a built-in market for their products.

The thought was too nauseating to consider. Most Safe Minds parents would not allow their paranoid fantasies to drift quite that far into Hollywood horror film territory. But Albert took it personally and was ready to make the leap. "I just read the *Wall Street Journal*," he wrote to Lyn and Sallie on Thanksgiving. "First, Lilly makes money by poisoning our children and causing autism and ADHD," he said. "Then they make money by making medication that does not work. Then, when you try to sue them for their criminal act, they will stop you and you cannot harm them. This is a great business for them, a win-win situation for these SOBs. They are having a nice and peaceful preparation for Thanksgiving and my family was running up and down Route 17, in cold weather, trying to find Payam, who was lost for nearly four hours. We finally found him. I do not think there is a God."

AS IF NOVEMBER hadn't been punishing enough for autism activists, on the last day of the month, things got worse. The British medical journal the *Lancet* published a landmark study showing that infants who received vaccines with thimerosal had mercury blood levels well below federal safety limits.[254] The lead author, Michael E. Pichichero of the University of Rochester, and his team examined 33 infants who got thimerosal-containing vaccines at two or six months, and 15 controls who had mercury-free shots.

None of the thimerosal-exposed children had blood levels that even approached EPA safety limits, the investigators reported. While traces of mercury appeared in initial blood tests, they had completely cleared within thirty days. The investigators also found that children excreted ethylmercury more quickly than previously thought. It did not accumulate from one shot to the next, they said. What's more, children who received thimerosal in vaccines had high levels of mercury in their stools, meaning that it was being quickly eliminated. Pichichero estimated the half-life of ethylmercury in the blood of vaccinated children at just seven days, far short of the forty-five-day half-life of methylmercury from fish.

"We conclude that the thimerosal in routine vaccines poses very little risk to full-term infants," the study declared. But, the authors added, "thimerosal-containing vaccines should not be administered at birth to very low birth-weight premature infants."

It was an extremely important finding from the first published clinical study of thimerosal in vaccines. The *Lancet* article had an enormous impact on the debate, one that lingers to this day. The *New York Times* hailed the study as "small but groundbreaking," and noted that Neal Halsey had called the findings "reassuring."[255]

Pichichero presented himself to the media to promote the safety of thimerosal. In an interview with Dr. Laurie Barclay of MedScape, the online medical news service, he claimed his team had accounted for virtually all vaccine mercury in the exposed children's stools.[256]

"There really is no evidence that there is any mercury unaccounted for which could be accumulating in bone or elsewhere," he said, "although this study was not a toxicity study and did not examine this issue directly." Pichichero said it was all "very reassuring," and that "hypothetical" concerns over thimerosal were not validated.

"The FDA and the AAP should be very pleased with our findings, which speak to the millions of children who have already received vaccines containing thimerosal," he added. "Our findings were also pivotal in the WHO's recommendation that thimerosal will remain in all vaccines provided by them to other countries."

Again the Safe Minds parents geared up for a counteroffensive. Sallie, Lyn, Liz, and Mark began to systematically pick apart just about everything Pichichero had done.

Mark was disgusted. "They are going to hype every piece-of-crap study they manage to get out," he told the group. "They inflate the inferences they draw beyond any reasonable limit, and suppress and dismiss any evidence to the contrary."

Mark worried about implications for the fight ahead. "We still have *zero* hard science that has been published," he fretted. "We'll be back on our heels until that point. The only way to win this debate is to go on the offensive with new science. The only bulwark we have is the mystery of rising rates. But that won't do our kids much good until we get progress on causality."

It was a valid point, but for now the *Lancet* article was begging for a response. In two days it was ready. Safe Minds raised several objections in a letter to the journal.

To begin with, the number of exposed children studied, thirty-three, was too small. "One major shortcoming of a small sample size is the low chance of including infants who are especially sensitive to mercury's effects, or who may have detoxification difficulties," the parents said.[257] "There is wide variability in the population in regard to mercury sensitivity and clearance. Since vaccines are given to virtually all infants, even if 1% retained mercury to a much greater degree than the norm, this would represent a large number of injured children."

The small sample size also "lacked sufficient power to establish safety claims."

What's more, nearly all blood draws missed peak concentrations of mercury. Some were taken a full month after vaccination. "It is evident that earlier peaks existed, because the feces contained high mercury values, and feces reflect earlier blood levels," the letter said. "It is impossible to state what peak values are if they were not measured."

Another problem was the widely ranging, but still considerably low levels of mercury that children in the study were exposed to.

"In a rationally designed study, the dose is kept constant," Safe Minds wrote. "But in Pichichero, two-month-old subjects were injected with 37.5 mcg to 62.5 mcg of ethylmercury, reflecting a 67% difference between the lowest and highest dose. By six months, the typical child in the 1990s would have received 187.5 mcg, or 68% more than the Pichichero group."

Then there were the potential conflicts of interest of Pichichero himself. The author had declared no conflicts in the article. But a quick Internet search proved otherwise. "Pichichero has an acknowledged financial tie to Eli Lilly, the developer of thimerosal and the main target of thimerosal litigation," Safe Minds said. In an article in the American Academy of Family Physicians newsletter of April 2000, they noted, he made the following disclosure: "The author received research grants and/or honoraria from the following pharmaceutical companies: Abbott Laboratories, Inc.; Bristol-Myers Squibb Company; Eli Lilly & Company; Merck & Co.; Pasteur Merieux Connaught;

Pfizer Labs; Roche Laboratories; Roussel-Uclaf; Schering Corporation; Smith Kline Beecham Pharmaceuticals; Upjohn Company; and Wyeth-Lederle."

Apparently Neal Halsey and a colleague had some concerns about the *Lancet* article, even though he earlier called the findings "reassuring." Halsey sent his comments to the journal, which published the letter the following February.[258] Like Safe Minds, he noted that the authors did not measure peak blood concentrations within hours of injection. "If the true half-life of ethylmercury is 7 days, the mercury concentrations in blood measured 7 days after exposure are about half the peak concentrations," he said, "and blood concentrations measured 21 days after exposure are about an eighth of the peak concentrations."

Halsey also observed that the children in the Pichichero study "seem to have come from a population with low background exposure to methylmercury," and so the study did not address concerns over "high blood concentrations of methylmercury from fish consumption, if the effects of ethylmercury are additive to those of methylmercury."

INCREDIBLY, the firestorm over the Homeland Security riders had still not subsided in Washington a full two weeks after the bill's passage. Dick Armey had since recanted his claim of being instructed by the White House to carry out the deed. The buzz went on.

"In a town where knowledge is power, and where there is no shortage of people willing to take credit for even the most minute accomplishment, there has been a sudden outbreak of people playing dumb," wrote political pundit Arianna Huffington in a December 5, 2002, syndicated column. "Official Washington is observing a code of omerta that makes the Sopranos look like the loose-lipped gals on 'The View.' In other words: Nobody's seen nothin'."[259]

On the morning of December 3, ABC's *Good Morning America* dedicated a full ten minutes of air time to the anonymous piece of lawmaking handiwork, and the impact it would have on families with autistic children.

"Well, we have sort of a Washington mystery story this morning, a clause in the Homeland Security Bill," co-host Charles Gibson opened the segment. "Nobody knows who wrote it; nobody's admitting that they wrote it. And it protects just one company."[260]

Diane Sawyer then introduced the guest who would talk about the Lilly rider, someone "who is outraged and says it must be overturned; who at least wants the option to argue her son's case in court."

It was Lyn, appearing via satellite from the network's Atlanta bureau. She appeared calm, dressed in a white blouse with a black vest, and seated in front of scholarly looking bookshelves. At the bottom of the screen, beneath her name, were the words "Blames Vaccines for Son's Autism."

Lyn was nervous but she handled herself professionally. Sawyer asked her how she felt about the Lilly provision. "My initial reaction, Diane, was that of shock," Lyn said. "There had been some legislation last summer introduced by Bill Frist that was very similar to what was added into the bill, but it died in committee with only five sponsors," she continued. "But to have that suddenly appear in the Homeland Security bill when it was not a homeland security issue was very disturbing to us."

As Sawyer's face grimaced with concern, Lyn went on to describe how Will had received 125 times the EPA limit for mercury exposure "in three vaccines given to him in just one day." As she spoke, a photo of Will flashed on the screen. It was an adorable baby picture. Will was smiling and bright-eyed.

"He was completely normal, and suddenly he began to regress," Lyn said. As she described his decline, the screen carried another picture of Will, at this time about two years old. His eyes were glazed over, lifeless, and droopy. His mouth was ajar, with no hint of a smile. Will looked completely out of it. Anyone comparing the two different images would have easily concluded that something terrible had happened to this child.

Sawyer looked kindly. "Are you confident this will be overturned?" she asked.

"It just seems so wrong, I can't imagine that it wouldn't be," Lyn said.

Not all media coverage was so sympathetic. The *Wall Street Journal* bordered on the churlish in blasting anyone opposed to the Lilly rider. On December 5 the paper ran an editorial titled "The Truth about Thimerosal; Democrats and Trial Lawyers Play Politics with Vaccine Liability."[261]

"From the press coverage, you'd think there's no greater question than who put the now-famous thimerosal rider into the Homeland Security Bill," it began. Washington had been so busy "playing political 'Where's Waldo?'" that no one properly explained the "merits" of the rider.

"Protecting thimerosal from runaway legal liability is the right thing to do," the *Journal* said. "Far from ducking behind Capitol pillars, Republicans should be trumpeting their support."

Much to the paper's chagrin, though, that wasn't happening. Trent Lott had offered changes to cover "nervous Republicans," the conservative paper said. "We suggest they talk to Dr. Frist, who could supply a nerve transplant. If Republicans can't explain to parents that thimerosal is about supplying safe vaccines to children, they don't deserve the majority."

Mark was appalled by the editorial. But he also saw a PR silver lining that could be exploited to their benefit "I know it's bad," he told Lyn. "But can you imagine a better enemy than the *Wall Street Journal* editorial page? Before these guys are finished denying the mercury-autism connection, they will have persuaded every uninformed, thoughtful person that the connection is plausible. In a backwards way, it's a big win."

On December 19, 2002, the autism parents and their attorneys savored another victory. The Department of Justice withdrew its motion to seal all documents on thimerosal-related claims in the VICP.[262] Safe Minds and the Mercury Policy Project lauded the withdrawal as "a step in the right direction." But the group still worried that, in the future, the secrecy rule might be applied on a case-by-case basis. They said all information should be publicly available.

"We question the Administration's blatant attempt to hide from the American public documents affecting the health and safety of millions of children," Safe Minds said, "especially when the material in question is as dangerous as mercury."[263]

JUST TWO DAYS before Christmas, and a week after Trent Lott was nudged out as Senate Majority Leader when some poorly chosen remarks he made about Strom Thurmond (the conservative retiring senator who once ran for president on a segregationist platform) became headline news, Bill Frist was elected Majority Leader of the powerful body.

When the new Congress returned in January 2003, Democrats were unwilling to wait for the GOP to "revisit" the Homeland Security bill. Now that Frist was Majority Leader, and Lott's promise to take up the matter was moot, it seemed prudent for Democrats to begin their own initiative. On January 7, Joe Lieberman reintroduced a motion to strike all three of the provisions from the law.[264]

It was time to rally—and lobby—in Washington yet again. By now, Lyn, Liz, and Sallie were getting a little sick of the place. Between them, they had easily made a hundred trips to the capital over the past four years. One hundred trips, and yet here they were, still banging on the doors of power, this time to demand the undoing of something that never should have been done in the first place: the Lilly rider.

Lyn, Liz, and Sallie were fatigued from so many meetings, so many speeches, so many conferences, so many flights. The Mercury Moms were getting burned out.

But reinforcements were stepping in to pick up the flag. In the past year or so, groups of parents, mostly mothers but some fathers, too, had risen up around the country. Energetic, active, and loud, they had banded together to demand the complete elimination of mercury from all medical products, call for research into mercury detoxification, and press for just and reasonable settlements for the damage they felt had been done to their children, in order to pay for a lifetime of care.

Safe Minds welcomed these latest parents into the fold. They were eager to hand off some of the heavy lifting to new recruits. A long war always demands fresh blood.

Laura and Scott Bono, who had been fighting the war for some time, made fine ringleaders. They had joined forces with other rabblerousing Carolina parents. Jo Pike, for one, was a young mother from Marion, South Carolina, whose son Hunter was autistic. Pike had helped start Moms on a Mission for Autism along with Lori McIlwain, an advertising executive from Raleigh, and her husband, Christian. Their son Connor had been diagnosed a few years earlier. Before long, Jo, Lori, and Laura Bono would establish the National Autism Association.

Then there were the Segals, Jeff and Shelley, in Greensboro, North Carolina. Jeff was the neurosurgeon who had testified before Burton's committee in 2002. Jeff had quit his lucrative practice to devote himself to researching the cause and cure of autism, which had hit their son Josh; Shelley, an actress, staged fund-raisers for the cause, including stand-up comedy nights. There was a lot of dark humor in autism.

On January 8, everyone converged on Washington, along with some one hundred parents from around country. On a frosty gray morning under the dull glint of the Capitol dome, they gathered around a small plaza. Posters bore photos of their children and slogans like "Vaccine Injured" or "Victim of Homeland Security." The rally, though well attended by the media, was not widely reported, partly due to a commuter plane crash that day in Charlotte, North Carolina.

Liz, Sallie, Lori McIlwain, and Scott Bono all spoke, as did Debbie Stabenow, who announced her own bill to remove the Lilly rider. Senator Leahy, Rep. Dennis Kucinich (D-OH), and of course, Dan Burton, also spoke.[265] After the rally, the parents, some with autistic kids in tow, fanned out across Capitol Hill for office visits with hometown representatives and the staffs of powerful congressional leaders. For the most part, they were received warmly. Most Democrats pledged their immediate support. Republicans, while sympathetic, were largely noncommittal.

The big prize was a face-to-face meeting with Craig Burton, the top health aide to Sen. Bill Frist. So many parents showed up that space quickly ran out in the meeting room. An overflow crowd accumulated in the halls of the Hart Office Building. They waited outside as Liz, Sallie, and others hammered home their case against Lilly.

It had been a cold, tiring day. The families were worn out. One couple, Dawn and Rodney Roark, had driven all the way from Ohio with their four-year-old son, Noah. Autistic children sometimes lose control in public settings. Noah began shrieking in the hushed white marble hallways. Dawn tried to quiet her son. But a young woman from the Health Committee burst from the GOP staff room, her face twisted in aggravation.

"Hey!" she barked at Dawn Roark. "You need to learn how to control your son."

"I'm sorry," Dawn said, trying to calm Noah. "He's autistic. I'll keep him quiet."

But Noah did not keep quiet. The woman grew angrier. "You're all a bunch of freaks!" she bellowed. "Your son is a freak!" Noah began to cry, and so did Dawn and some of the other mothers. "I'm going to call the Capitol police!" the woman shouted. "We can't have this going on in a place of business."

Minutes later two uniformed officers appeared, perplexed as to how to handle this peculiar scene. The young woman asked them to eject the families and their unruly kid. "You *people*," she sneered, "you're just using your kids to abuse the system to get rich!"[266]

The whole incident, which was caught on videotape by one of the parents, ended when the meeting let out. But the Roarks were horrified that anyone could be treated with such contempt in a congressional office. They tried to find out who the woman was, though the GOP committee staff refused to identify her. They then threatened to send the tape to the media. Fox News Channel had already expressed interest.

Albert Enayati, who witnessed the whole fracas, received an apologetic call from Craig Burton that night. "We want to work with you parents on the Lilly rider issue," he told Albert. But Burton wanted something else: the names of every person in the hallway. And he wanted an assurance that the video would not be shared. Albert said no deal.

Two days later, Republicans made good on their promise to revisit the riders. On the House side, Speaker Dennis Hastert (R-IL) agreed to take up the issue in the new Congress. And under pressure from Senators Snowe, Collins, and Chafee, Frist also agreed to remove the rider.[267] But he made it clear that the subject was not closed. He would bring up his bill again. Only this time, it would include all the original provisions.

Lilly was "disappointed" with the decision, a company statement said. But it acknowledged that the "process by which this legislation was enacted was not desirable" and said that "Lilly fully understands the action taken by the Senate."[268] Lilly still hoped to win similar protections to "incorporate the vaccine ingredient language that was included in the Homeland Security Act."

The drug giant emerged from the scandal "with little more than a public relations black eye," according to an Op-Ed piece in the *Indianapolis Star*.

"Predictably, this careening ride through the halls of Congress has ended in a noisy crash," it said. The company "appeared to have benefited from someone's cynical manipulation of critical national security legislation," but that had backfired. "The legislative sleight-of-hand put egg on Lilly's corporate face. It also heightened the suspicions of those parents who are suing. And it's handed ammunition, at least in a PR sense, to their attorneys."[269]

Apparently, powerful interests were taking notice of the thimerosal controversy. In January 2003 Lyn received two separate e-mails that made her hair stand on end. They brought back bad memories of old fears over tapped phones and shadowy figures watching the parents' every move.

"I want to tell you something that we are hearing," the first e-mail began. "As you know, my husband and I spent several years working in legal fields, both in DC and in New York. It is our network. My husband had lunch with our attorney yesterday, and we received a call from a large, wealthy business owner who is a friend and very connected. Several law firms in DC have been hired to handle the FDA part of the thimerosal issues. We hear that the vaccine business interests are 'Absolutely Furious' (beyond our comprehension, was the term) with what the autistic community has done, and anticipate millions of dollars in lost revenues. I know that in our circle, many concerned citizens are sending information to stockbrokers, asking for reviews of their stocks in Eli Lilly, for example. It is starting to hit them at their house of worship: Money."

A second, more ominous message was shared among all the autism families: "Take prudent safety steps," it said. "I think we should not be naïve, and just be careful. I think a message of prudent safety steps should be shared with all the members of our community, especially the most public and vocal."

IN POLITICS, one of the surest ways for an insurgent candidate to gain traction is to come under heavy fire from an entrenched opponent. Vehement attacks from those in power are an inadvertent form of flattery, because the vitriol demonstrates that the challenge is being taken seriously, that it poses a realistic threat to the status quo.

The same might be said for science. In the spring of 2003, Safe Minds, as well as the Geiers, came under full-frontal assault from the public health establishment.

Pediatrics, the highly influential journal of the American Academy of Pediatrics, led the attack. In March, the journal published a powerful and widely circulated repudiation of Safe Minds' mercury-autism hypothesis. The editorial, titled "Thimerosal and Autism?" was coauthored by one of the country's leading experts on autism and the brain, Dr. Margaret Bauman, associate professor of neurology at Harvard Medical School and a pediatric neurologist at Massachusetts General Hospital.[270] The second author was Dr. Karin B. Nelson, senior investigator at the Neuroepidemiology Branch of the National Institute of Neurological Disorders and Stroke.

"Bernard et al. offered an hypothesis that autism is an expression of mercury toxicity resulting from thimerosal in vaccines," they noted. "They base this hypothesis on their views that the clinical signs of mercury toxicity are similar to the manifestations of autism, that the onset of autism is temporally associated with immunization in some children, that the recent increase in diagnosis of autism parallels exposure to thimerosal, and that there are higher levels of mercury in persons with than without autism."

Then came the point-by-point attack:

Symptoms of autism and mercury poisoning are not *similar.* For example, motor function problems associated with mercury poisoning include ataxia (poor coordination) and dysarthria (slurred speech), and sometimes tremor, muscle pains, and weakness. In autism, however, "the only common motor manifestations are repetitive behaviors such as flapping, circling, or rocking. No other motor findings are common in autism." As for sensory disorders, the most characteristic symptom of mercury poisoning is a bilateral constriction of visual fields and, less often, a compromise of contrast sensitivity. There might also be nervous system abnormalities and pain in the hands and feet. But in autism, "decreased responsiveness to pain is sometimes observed along with hypersensitivity to other sensory stimuli, including sound," they wrote. Autism seemed to "reflect altered sensory processing within the brain rather than peripheral nerve involvement." Other signs of mercury toxicity, like hypertension, skin eruption, and thrombocytopenia (low blood platelets) "are seldom seen in autism."

Timing of vaccination and diagnosis. The two are just as likely to be coincidental as associated, Nelson and Bauman wrote. "Evaluation of causation cannot depend on temporal association as reflected by anecdotal observations of selected instances in which a relatively uncommon outcome such as autism is noted after a common childhood exposure such as immunization," they said. Age of onset of symptoms can be "highly misleading as an indicator that some environmental event has caused or precipitated a disorder." Moreover, some genetic disorders do display a period of seemingly normal development prior to onset of symptoms. In Rett syndrome, for example, symptoms normally began around eighteen months, which happens to be during the vaccination period. In Huntington's chorea, delayed onset can be as long as forty-five years. And these diseases emerge without requiring "an environmental 'second hit.'" Thus, the onset of autism "does not prove (nor disprove) a role for environmental factors in etiology."

Epidemic versus better diagnostics. "There has clearly been a broadening of the criteria for autism, better case-finding, increased awareness by clinicians and by families, and an increase in referrals of children for services," the authors wrote. Whether this could account for all the increased cases "is a matter of contention" to be "properly settled by careful research." But even if there were an actual increase, that did not mean that thimerosal was to blame. After all, the authors noted, the past few decades had seen extraordinary changes in "many environmental exposures and aspects of medical care that could be considered for their biological plausibility as contributors to autism."

Ethyl- versus methylmercury. Methylmercury is better suited to cross the blood-brain barrier and is facilitated by an active transport mechanism, the authors wrote. Ethylmercury lacks such a transport system, and its larger molecular size and faster decomposition rate reduce its ability to enter the brain. That is why higher levels of mercury are found in the blood, though less in the brain, following administration of ethylmercury than methylmercury. "These findings support the observation that the risk of toxicity from ethylmercury is overestimated by comparison with the risk of intoxication from methylmercury," the authors stated.

Mercury levels post vaccination. Bernard et al. claimed that elevated mercury was detected in biological samples of autistic patients "but unfortunately do not provide references," Nelson and Bauman wrote. No paper had been published in the peer-reviewed literature that reported an "abnormal body burden of mercury, or an excess of mercury in hair, urine, or blood." Furthermore, in their literature search, the authors found no evidence that chelation therapy "led to improvement in children with autism."

Brain cell damage. The most consistent finding in the neuropathology of autism is the reduction in a type of brain cell called Purkinje cells, found in the cerebellum. Involvement of another type, called granule cells, has rarely been reported. In contrast, the authors wrote, mercury-exposed brains "have shown significant and consistent damage to the cerebellar granule cell layer with relative preservation of Purkinje cells."

Pink disease. Infants who contracted this disorder presented with symptoms like photophobia, anorexia, skin eruption, and a bright pink color on their hands and feet, which peeled and were painful. These symptoms are rarely, if ever associated with autism. Moreover, the authors claimed that survivors of pink disease were not described as having behavioral disorders "suggestive of autism," as Safe Minds had concluded.

Population studies. There were no studies of mass mercury poisoning that produced signs of increased autism after the fact, Nelson and Bauman wrote, in complete contradiction to what Mark Blaxill found in reports from Fukushima, Japan. "Studies that followed victims of high-dose acute or chronic mercury poisoning resulting from contaminated foods in Iraq, Pakistan, Guatemala, and Ghana have not reported manifestations suggestive of autism," they said. Instead, many survivors had symptoms like ataxia and dysarthria, which again are "seldom seen in autism."

VSD data. The CDC found a "weak but statistically significant" association between exposure to thimerosal and speech delay and attention-deficit/hyperactivity disorder," the authors admitted, but there were "many limitations of this analysis and its ability to identify bias and confounding." The Harvard Pilgrim data did not confirm the findings of the first two HMOs. "Although far from definitive, these studies represent the only direct investigation to date of a possible association of thimerosal exposure with autism," the authors said. "Neither study observed such an association." It was thus "improbable that thimerosal and autism are linked," they concluded. "If thimerosal was an important cause of autism, the incidence of autism might soon begin to decline. One can hope but not expect that that will happen; time will tell."

SAFE MINDS geared up for a formal reply. In the meantime, Sallie issued a preliminary statement the next day. She said the Nelson-Bauman commentary contained "a number of inaccuracies that call into question the legitimacy of the paper's conclusions."[271] For example, the claim that survivors of acrodynia did not have behavioral disorders suggestive of autism was simply untrue. Case descriptions "clearly show that they did," Sallie argued, "such as loss of speech, odd behaviors, and social withdrawal."

Days later, Safe Minds released an official critique of Nelson and Bauman. The response was written by Mark, Lyn, and Sallie. "In their defense of thimerosal, these authors take a narrow view of the original hypothesis, provide no new evidence, and rely on selective citations and flawed reasoning," the parents began. "We provide evidence here to refute the critique and to defend the autism-mercury hypothesis."[272]

Symptoms of autism and mercury poisoning. Despite Nelson and Bauman's assertion, Safe Minds insisted that there are no "typical" symptoms of mercury poisoning. The two authors had constructed a table of six symptoms (reduced from 95 in Bernard et al.) to compare what they called "typical and characteristic manifestations" of mercury poisoning and autism. "The table suggests an absence of overlap in the clinical manifestations of the two conditions," Safe Minds said. But the commentary failed to provide a definition for these "typical and characteristic" symptoms. The omission was not surprising to the parents, since "no 'typical' pattern of mercury poisoning can be or has been described."

No metal better illustrates the diversity of effects caused by different chemical species than mercury. Various combinations of these exposure types resulted in many different disorders, like Minamata disease, pink disease, Mad Hatter's disease, and so forth. "In the specific case of thimerosal-containing vaccines, a new combination of exposures and timing that has contributed to recent increases in autism has been hypothesized," the parents wrote. "Hence the proposition in Bernard *et al.* that this combination describes a 'novel form of mercury poisoning.' "

In fact, the symptoms of Minamata disease and acrodynia "bear little resemblance to the vague manifestations of 'mercurism' (*sic*) that Nelson and Bauman describe," Safe Minds charged. "Each disorder has vivid and unambiguous symptoms, neither set of which resembles the other." By contrast, both Minamata disease and pink disease share many of the autism symptoms cited by Nelson and Bauman, "including mental retardation in Minamata and loss of speech, social withdrawal, sensory defensiveness and 'bizarre positions' in acrodynia." The claim that "typical" symptoms of mercury toxicity and autism are not alike was "inaccurate, misleading and unsupported by evidence."

Brain cell damage. The suggestion that ethylmercury does not readily cross the blood-brain barrier was contradicted by Laszlo Magos, who showed that ethyl- and methylmercury both entered the brain of rats in significant amounts.[273] And though brain levels of ethylmercury were lower than methylmercury, they were not much lower. Wistar rats exposed to ethylmercury had levels that were two-thirds that of methyl-treated rats.

Other studies, not cited by Nelson and Bauman, showed "clear evidence in favor of Purkinje cell involvement in mercury poisoning," Safe Minds said. And in a postmortem study of autistic brains, Bauman herself found "a variable decrease in granule cells throughout the cerebellar hemispheres." Nelson and Bauman had not offered proof for "the lack of involvement of Purkinje cells in mercury exposure nor the lack of involvement of granule cells in autism."

Population studies. Safe Minds restated their conviction that autism rates did indeed increase in Japan following the 1965 mercury disaster in Fukushima prefecture. Autism rates among children in the area born after 1965 showed a sharp increase over rates before 1965, they said. "The inference is clear: the time trends in autism prevalence are consistent with an etiological role for mercury." Nelson and Bauman, they added, used questionable methodology "to dismiss a dramatic increase in autism rates from less than 1 per 10,000 in children born in or before 1965, to over 4 per 10,000 just three years later. The evidence, we submit, speaks for itself here."

Epidemic versus better diagnostics. Nelson and Bauman had offered a "familiar litany of arguments designed to obscure the strong evidence of increasing incidence of autism," Safe Minds said, including diagnostic substitution, greater awareness, and changing diagnostic standards. "None of these hypotheses have been effectively tested and replicated," Safe Minds argued. The incidence of autism had increased tenfold in a decade. "Such order-of-magnitude increases must have environmental roots," Safe Minds said. "Increased mercury exposure is both biologically and epidemiologically plausible as a sole or contributing causal factor. Instead of speculative dismissals of this model, as offered by Nelson and Bauman, we need more evidence-based research. This is what the IOM has recommended and we should get on with it."

Pediatrics refused to print the Safe Minds rebuttal. It did not pass muster with their rigorous peer-review process, something that Nelson and Bauman's commentary was not subjected to. One reviewer's comments were forwarded to Safe Minds with the rejection letter. "I read the manuscript over several times. It is obvious that these authors have a tremendous, emotional fervor for the subject," the unnamed reviewer said.[274] "Furthermore, they accuse Nelson and Bauman of unscholarly behavior and not looking at the facts. I would say that the authors of this commentary are lacking in scholarship and objectivity."

Finally, the parents were "unscholarly" and a menace to public health. "This is a group of dedicated individuals who are determined to push their hypothesis and conclusions on the general public in a society with a free press," the reviewer said. "Unfortunately, I think they can do much more harm than good."

The leaders of the American Academy of Pediatrics clearly felt the same disdain for Mark and David Geier, and for the journal in which they published their findings purporting to show a relative risk of 6.0 for autism in their DTaP analysis.

"Study Fails to Show a Connection between Thimerosal and Autism" was the headline over an unsigned editorial in *Pediatrics* about the Geiers, who were made to sound like dimwits.[275] The bulletin was aimed at "clinicians who may be aware of recent press surrounding an article claiming to show a correlation between thimerosal and autism."

The Geiers had used data from the Vaccine Adverse Event Reporting System (VAERS) "inappropriately," according to the editorial, and their analysis contained "numerous conceptual and scientific flaws, omissions of fact, inaccuracies, and misstatements." The editorial pointed out that VAERS was a "passive" voluntary system and was also vulnerable to "coincidental occurrences or mistakes in filing." Its inherent limits included "incomplete reporting, lack of verification of diagnoses, and lack of data on people who were immunized and did not report problems." (The editorial failed to mention that CDC researchers sometimes used VAERS data to demonstrate the *safety* of certain vaccines.)

The authors had also failed to reveal "how thimerosal exposure was calculated—a critical omission, because much of the data required to estimate mercury exposure are not available in VAERS reports," it said. "It is unclear as to how their data were generated, thus preventing accurate review of their methods and replication of their outcomes." Nor did they describe their statistical methods, making the results "highly unreliable."

And of course, there was no scientific data to link thimerosal "with any pediatric neurologic disorder, including autism." Meanwhile, the "recently published review by Nelson and Bauman cast doubt on the biologic plausibility of symptom similarities between mercury poisoning and autism," something the Geiers failed to note.

Finally, the unnamed editors of *Pediatrics* took a veiled swipe at their colleagues who publish the comparatively radical *Journal of American Physicians and Surgeons*. "Any scientific article that can prove a thimerosal link," they wrote, "must be published in respected and widely read journals" and "apply the highest standards of critical peer review to the results."

"THERE ARE TWO THINGS you don't want to see being made" goes the old adage attributed to German statesman Otto von Bismarck, "sausage and legislation." The Iron Chancellor made the quip in the late 1800s, but he could have been describing the division that racked the American capital in the second half of the Bush administration. The squabble over the Vaccine Injury Compensation Program became an ugly bone of contention.

The Democrats and the GOP had previously agreed to extend the program's statute of limitations to six years, to allow in those children with injuries dating back to 1997. The big deal-breaker was the question of what to do with all the children left over, who were injured before that time. Would there be a "look-back" window for them to enter? If so, how long would the window be open? And how far back would the look-back look? Most contentious of all, if these families were allowed into the VICP through the window, would they be allowed back *out*—with their right to sue in civil court intact?

Such parliamentary minutiae might have seemed mind-numbing to the casual observer, but to the families in question, these fine-print particulars could not have been more important. Even if they were allowed into the VICP, families were not assured of an equitable or timely settlement. Preserving their right to sue in civil court, after VICP, was critical. Why should these children be denied the same full set of rights as those afforded to children injured after 1997? Why relegate them to a second-class tier of justice?

The number of families potentially affected by this question was hardly trivial. At the request of Sen. Hillary Clinton, Mark and David Geier calculated how many American children were reported to the Department of Education each year with autism, developmental delay, and speech disorders.[276]

Between 1988 and 1996, nearly 65,000 children were reported with autism, about 40,000 with developmental disorders, and some 1.45 million with speech delay, the Geiers found. Obviously, not all families would file a claim. But even a fraction of these numbers would be enough to wipe out the entire VICP in a matter of months.

In March 2003, Senate Majority Leader Bill Frist resurrected his controversial VICP reform bill. The announcement unleashed a series of motions and countermotions, backroom deals, and prickly late-night negotiations that, in the end, all died in committee. It was a tortuous four-week route to nowhere.

On March 11, Majority Leader Frist attached his VICP reform bill to "Project Bioshield" (the Biodefense Improvement and Treatment for America Act).[277] It was basically the same bill he had introduced the year before, including the Lilly liability protections that had been cut and pasted into the Homeland Security debacle in November. It extended the statute of limitations to six years, but did not provide for a "look-back" window.

Safe Minds and other autism groups launched a counterattack two days later. Laura Bono, who had recently started a new group with Lori McIlwain and Jo Pike called the Right to Fight Mercury Damage Campaign, was key to the effort. Their goal was to stop the Frist legislation and pass a more parent-friendly VICP reform bill, one that would offer the same rights to all families, regardless of their date of injury. As part of the campaign, thousands of parents were sent "action alerts," asking them to call or fax Frist and the rest of the Health Committee, voicing their opposition to the Frist bill.

On March 19, the parents held a rally in Washington, the same day they placed a full-page ad slamming Frist in *Roll Call,* a Capitol Hill daily that is considered required reading among Congressional staff.[278]

"Our children have been injured and Senator Bill Frist is once again trying to take away their rights by supporting drug companies," the headline blared. "Tell Senator Frist to Keep His Corporation-Protecting Legislation Away from America's Children." In the main text, they wrote that "vaccine-injured children are suffering with little medical coverage to come to their aid. Families are being forced to take drastic measures to pay for treatments . . . some have even sold their homes. Many are left with no options at all."

They accused Frist of using "groundless threats of vaccine-makers throwing in the towel" as justification for his bill. "We don't buy it. Neither should you. The vaccine-induced autism epidemic is very real and needs to be addressed by our government with unbiased research, not poorly-designed studies carried out by doctors on the drug companies' payroll."

Later that morning, Bill Frist backed down and withdrew the provisions from the Bioshield bill.[279] He began conferring with Dan Burton, Ted Kennedy, and Sen. Chris Dodd (D-CT), and with groups like Cure Autism Now (CAN) to craft a more palatable bill. They devised a compromise that would open a "look-back" window going back ten years to allow people into the program—but there would be no "opt out" to go to civil court. The window would be opened only when and if autism was added to the Vaccine Court's official "table" of compensable injuries. But legal experts told the parents that chances of this happening were next to zero. Since 1995, conditions had only been deleted from the table; nothing had ever been added. "This agreement is nothing but fluff and promises based on things that will never happen," Laura told the other parents.

The proposed window in Frist's bill was ample enough to include the Redwoods, but not Jackson Bono, who was older than Will, placing him outside even a ten-year window.

Many parents thought it was a terrible idea. But groups like Cure Autism Now, signed on to the compromise.[280] It appalled Lyn and the Bonos, and left Sallie, who was a member of both CAN and Safe Minds, in an uncomfortable position.

Raymond Gallup, a parent and the founder of the Autism Autoimmunity Project, posted a blistering attack on several Web sites, suggesting that donations from drug companies had co-opted mainstream autism organizations. "Cure Autism Now should be called Cure Autism Never," he sneered, "since they don't want to fund research or help parents that have vaccine-damaged children."[281]

Infighting intensified within the autism community and emotions over the compromise bill grew rawer. Albert Enayati blasted CAN president Jon Shestack in a widely shared e-mail. "You have absolutely no right to endorse legislation that every damn autism organization does not support," Albert said.[282] "Where were you when I was calling CAN, begging them to look at thimerosal, and the only support I got was to 'Go to hell'? Where was CAN when we went to rallies? Where was CAN during the hearings? Where were you, Jon?"

Shestack fired right back. He said that CAN "got Frist to make huge concessions" in the negotiations and insisted that CAN "always had an open mind about vaccine research." True, the foundation accepted donations from drug companies, he said, but added, "CAN is not bought by or sold to anyone."[283]

"But neither do we make donors take a purity test," Shestack said. "I would take money from Saddam Hussein if we could spend it on autism research, and so would you." That night, coincidentally, the U.S. military began its "shock and awe" bombardment of Baghdad, and President Bush's long-anticipated major offensive against Saddam Hussein was under way.

Parents such as Lyn, Liz, the Bonos, Jo Pike, and Lori McIlwain refused to back down. McIlwain sensed that Frist was becoming politically vulnerable on the issue. "He knows he's running out of chances, so he's throwing us a bone and we're supposed to reciprocate by throwing him our blessing," she told Laura Bono. "Let's get real. If he were truly in the driver's seat, he wouldn't need a letter from CAN. Instead of reaching a compromise with a defeatist attitude, my gut is saying to take that vulnerability and get him the hell away from our kids for good."

The parents stood their ground. "We will have no part in negotiating away the rights of all our children," Laura said on a conference call. "This is just like dealing with the devil, folks."

After days of intense back and forth, the entire process broke down. On April 1, Frist walked out of the negotiations and returned to his original bill, the one without any "look-back" window at all. It was a measure that even many Republicans failed to support.

"Just because you are unaware that a government compensation program exists, doesn't mean you sit around if you have been injured by a product," he said.[284] "You would sue the manufacturer or the doctor, and would be immediately informed that you must first file a claim in the compensation program. What is the point of having a deadline if Congress is going to periodically say the deadline doesn't matter?"

On April 8, Bill Frist and Sen. Judd Gregg (R-NH) held a joint press conference to promote their own vaccine bill, the Improved Vaccine Affordability and Availability Act of 2003. Frist denounced all thimerosal lawsuits as "unnecessary and expensive," and Gregg warned that "our vaccine industry has been essentially wiped out by fear of liability."[285] He cautioned that if manufacturers were sued "frivolously," they might not subsequently produce vaccines against smallpox, anthrax, or the latest threat: SARS.

One might have left the press conference surmising that vaccine makers were barely getting by. But Mark Benjamin, an investigative writer for UPI who was covering the thimerosal controversy, reported otherwise. Vaccines were once "a sleepy backwater of the global healthcare industry," he wrote, but they now outpaced drugs in terms of sales growth. In the 1990s, the vaccine market had 14 percent annual growth, while drug sales grew at just 8 percent. The global vaccine market had reached $6.5 billion and was expected to top $10 billion by 2010, Benjamin said.[286]

On the night of April 8, negotiations continued between Frist, Kennedy, and Dodd, with the participation of NVIC. Kennedy was said to be furious at Dodd for allowing the legislation to get that far. Kennedy staffers reported that their boss finally got Frist to agree in the wee hours of the morning to a full look-back to 1986, and would allow children to apply for compensation if a table change was made connecting thimerosal with a casual relation to vaccine injuries. Once such an injury was placed on the table, any family could return to the VICP even if they had been turned down before.

The next day, April 9, the newly concocted Frist bill met a sudden and unexpected death when some vaccine makers opposed the measure as being too lenient on families.

"Majority leader Bill Frist and other lawmakers arrived at work today expecting the Senate Committee to adopt the measure," the *New York Times* reported.[287] Instead, when the meeting began, congressional aides watched, stunned, as lobbyists for several vaccine manufacturers huddled anxiously with the staff of Senator Gregg. Moments later, Mr. Gregg announced that the meeting, called a "mark up" in Senate parlance, would be postponed for lack of a quorum.

Lawmakers were startled by Gregg's rebuke of Frist. Gregg told the *Times* that he saw no reason to "rush" the bill, when some companies had "concerns." Merck and Wyeth had opposed the measure and forced Gregg to pull it. "We are concerned with any changes that would add significantly to the already great burden of civil litigation against vaccine research companies such as ours," Ian Spatz, vice president for public policy at Merck, told the *Times*. A Democratic aide later told the Associated Press that Merck and Wyeth felt the compromise was "too generous to families," and wanted a stricter statute of limitations.[288] But Lilly and Aventis supported the measure. "Lilly is facing several lawsuits that would be moved to the vaccine fund under this bill," the aide said.

. . .

TERM LIMITS had ended Dan Burton's run as chairman of the Government Reform Committee in 2002. When his replacement, Rep. Tom Davis (R-VA), took over, pharmaceutical companies lobbied hard to block Burton from heading any of the seven subcommittees under Government Reform's jurisdiction.[289] But Burton managed to carve out a role for himself as chair of the Subcommittee on Human Rights and Wellness.

By spring of 2003, Burton and his committee staff—including Liz Birt—had completed their report on the three-year investigation into vaccines and autism. Liz herself had reviewed thousands of pages of documents, and participated in interviews between committee staff and officials from the FDA and CDC.

The committee's chief of staff, Kevin Binger, had planned on leaving for another job but agreed to stay on for another two months until the report was finished. The entire team was highly dedicated to this project. Binger and lead investigator Beth Clay would burn the midnight oil for weeks to ensure the accuracy of every statement and recommendation within the weighty document. Reports and transcripts were read and reread by each staff member involved in the investigation to ensure that nothing was missed.

As the report was finalized, an exhausted Beth Clay would submit her notice of resignation from the subcommittee, citing her need as a single mother to spend time with her four teenage children while they were still at home. But she, Kevin Binger, Liz Birt, and the others felt satisfied that the report was about as complete as it could be.

Unfortunately, the committee staff chose an inauspicious time and place to unveil the document, a Saturday afternoon in Chicago, which guaranteed that the major media would ignore it.

On May 3 Burton traveled to Chicago to present his report at the annual Autism One Conference, a three-day symposium on autism research and treatments, being held at Loyola University. A few local TV stations showed up, but it was an anticlimactic coda to three years of heavy lifting. "Fifteen years ago, one in every 10,000 children in America was autistic," said Burton, who was joined onstage by Boyd Haley, Mark Geier, Lyn Redwood, and others. "Today, that may be as high as one in every 150 children. We have an epidemic on our hands. If this trend continues at a constant rate, the number of autistic children could reach four million Americans in the next decade."[290]

Burton said that conflicts of interest were clouding the federal investigation into the alleged malfeasance covered in the committee report. "Is there collusion between the pharmaceutical companies and our health agencies?" he asked. "The appearance in many cases is that there is."

Lyn hailed the Burton report as solid evidence of government-industry corruption and called for a full congressional investigation into how thimerosal "was allowed to continue to be utilized in vaccine preparations for years, without ever having any safety studies. We want to know why the FDA and American public were misled by Eli Lilly that thimerosal was safe and effective when their internal documents paint a completely different picture. We must ensure that this totally avoidable public health tragedy never happens again," she said. "Those responsible must be exposed and held accountable."

The eighty-four-page report, "Mercury in Medicine: Taking Unnecessary Risks," retraced the history of thimerosal use over the decades, outlined the various government exposure levels and warnings issued on mercury toxicity (including from seafood), compared the rise in autism cases with increased exposure to thimerosal in vaccines over time, and detailed how Eli Lilly knew, but did not reveal, the dangers of their product. The report addressed "growing questions on whether mercury in childhood vaccines is related to autism spectrum disorders."[291]

Mostly, it was a harsh indictment of what the authors felt was bureaucratic inertia and neglect of the public interest by federal agencies. Among the charges were:

- Ethylmercury's toxicity was neglected by manufacturers and regulators.
- Thimerosal manufacturers accumulated evidence of toxicity but did not share it.
- The FDA's actions to remove mercury from OTC products should have prompted a review of mercury in vaccines.
- Vaccine makers never conducted adequate testing of thimerosal, nor did the FDA require it.
- The FDA and CDC failed to be vigilant as new vaccines containing thimerosal were added to the immunization schedule.
- The CDC is conflicted in its duties to monitor the safety of vaccines while also purchasing vaccines for resale and promoting immunization.
- Studies conducted or funded by the CDC that dispute any correlation between autism and vaccines have been of poor design, underpowered, and fatally flawed.

"Many FDA officials have stubbornly denied that thimerosal may cause adverse reactions," the report went on. "Ironically, the FDA's unwillingness to address this issue more forcefully, and remove thimerosal from vaccines earlier, may have done more long-term damage to the public's trust in vaccines than confronting the problem head-on." And anyway, the committee "did in fact find evidence that thimerosal posed a risk," the report stated. "The possible risk for harm from either low dose chronic or one time high level exposure to thimerosal is not 'theoretical,' but very real and documented."

Despite the mounting evidence, in 2001 the CDC had refused to express a preference for thimerosal-free vaccines. That decision was "particularly troubling," the report said. With the exception of the influenza vaccine, all major childhood vaccines were being made without thimerosal at the time, so there was little threat of shortages. "Their failure to state a preference was an abdication of their responsibility," the report stated. "As a result, thimerosal-containing vaccines that remained in stock in doctors' offices continued to be used. In fact, we have no proof that, in 2003, some children are not still receiving thimerosal-preserved vaccines that have lingered in medical offices or clinics."

The report offered many recommendations, including:

1. Full access to the VSD database for independent researchers
2. A more integrated federal approach to mercury research
3. Greater collaboration between agencies on public health and heavy metals
4. A White House conference on autism to "assemble the best scientific minds"
5. VICP reform to extend the statute of limitations to six years and open a look-back window
6. A ban on federal funds for purchasing medical products that contain mercury
7. An NIH order to give priority to research into mercury exposure and autism, ADD, Gulf War syndrome, and Alzheimer's disease

"Thimerosal used as a preservative in vaccines is likely related to the autism epidemic," the report concluded. "This epidemic in all probability may have been prevented or curtailed had the FDA not been asleep at the switch," it said. "Our public health agencies' failure to act is indicative of institutional malfeasance for self-protection and misplaced protectionism of the pharmaceutical industry."

FAMILIES SEEKING COMPENSATION for what they believed had caused their children's autism were treading water in choppy seas. The Frist bill was in limbo. The Autism Omnibus proceedings within the VICP were moving at a much slower pace than anticipated. In fact, the big causation hearing, originally scheduled for March 2004, had been postponed indefinitely. Lawyers for the families complained of governmental foot-dragging in the release of discovery materials, including the VSD data, which they had requested.

Meanwhile, a few cases that had languished in Vaccine Court for more than 240 days were now, under court rules, eligible to opt out of the VICP and file private lawsuits in civil court. A few such cases were pending in Maryland, Mississippi, and Louisiana. But apart from these few exceptions, the wheels of justice were barely moving at all.

In July 2003, some parents and attorneys began to rethink their legal strategy and came up with what they thought was a rather brilliant plan. It might take years for individual cases to work their way through the system (whether in the VICP or civil court), they reckoned. But there was another way to seek justice.

The idea was first launched by a group of parents in Kansas—headed by Bobbie Manning, an autism activist mother with an affected son named Michael, and Linda Weinmaster, whose son Adam is also autistic. They decided to seek the help of state attorneys general to file suit against vaccine makers. The states were facing budget-busting costs for the care and education of autistic children. Perhaps, the parents thought, the attorneys general could be convinced to pursue compensatory damages, not unlike when the states sued big tobacco a few years earlier, resulting in a $246 billion national settlement.

On July 17, Manning, Weinmaster, and a small group of parents, along with Mark and David Geier, who flew in for the day, met with Kansas Attorney General Phill Kline at his Topeka office. They presented all the latest studies coming out to support the mercury-autism hypothesis, including Amy Holmes's baby-hair study, Jeff Bradstreet's chelation study, Boyd Haley's neurotoxicity work, and of course, the Geiers' finding of a 6.0 relative risk for autism and mental retardation for children who received thimerosal-containing DTaP vaccine, compared with those who had mercury-free shots.[292]

The meeting was slated to last one hour, but it went on for three. Attorney General Kline told reporters afterward that he was "interested in the information" and wanted to discuss it further with his assistants before deciding what course to take.

Weinmaster was happy with the meeting. "They said it was well worth their time. That's pretty positive," the mother told a local paper. "We want the kids taken care of when we're gone, and we don't want any more kids damaged."[293] Mark Geier hit a characteristically dramatic note. "This is the biggest cover-up in medical history," he told the paper. "It's bigger than 9-11 and AIDS and no one knows about it." Health care costs for autistic children would reach two trillion dollars over the course of their lives, including ten billion dollars in Kansas, he said. "If this is allowed to continue, you will not recognize our society in 20 years. We'll be like a Third World nation."

An Eli Lilly spokesman, asked about the attorney general's meeting, told the paper that there was "no scientific, credible, causal link established between thimerosal and autism. We need to let the science guide us," he said. "We don't support politicians and trial lawyers demagoging the issue."

Emboldened by the meeting in Kansas, parents like Laura Bono, Jo Pike, and Lori McIlwain began to organize a state-by-state effort to get attorneys general nationwide on board. "Forward this letter to anyone and everyone, but make sure to send a hard copy to your state's Attorney General," they wrote to parents. "It explains why states should sue to recover costs for children unnecessarily injured by poorly manufactured vaccines." Some 93 percent of autistic children will be institutionalized as adults, not even capable of living in group homes. It would be incredibly expensive to the states. One huge advantage of this approach would be the delivery of discovery materials obtained by the attorneys general to parents seeking their own compensation against the companies.

As for potential defendants, the list was lengthy. The "obvious" defendants were vaccine makers, thimerosal manufacturers, and Eli Lilly. But more parties could easily be named. There were the committees and their members that provided advice to the FDA on the approval of vaccines.

Over the next several months, parents and the Geiers would arrange similar meetings with their own attorneys general in California, Iowa, Minnesota, Missouri, Nebraska, New York, North Carolina, South Carolina, Virginia, and Wisconsin.

11. "Proof" on Both Sides

NEARLY TWO YEARS had passed since the Institute of Medicine had found insufficient evidence to accept or reject a link between thimerosal and autism, and called for more research on the issue. Until now, the only major study to address the question was the Verstraeten VSD analysis, with its inconsistent findings.

That began to change in mid-2003, with the successive publication of three separate large-scale population studies, all offering compelling evidence against the thimerosal hypothesis—sufficient, potentially, to dismiss the idea once and for all. All three studies involved Denmark.

The first report, funded by the CDC, ran in the August 25, 2003, issue of the *American Journal of Preventive Medicine* under the title "Autism and Thimerosal-Containing Vaccines: Lack of Consistent Evidence for an Association."[294] The article's lead author was Dr. Paul Stehr-Green, from the Department of Epidemiology at the University of Washington's School of Public Health and Community Medicine, and the participant at Simpsonwood in 2000 who wrote the internally conflicting summary. Stehr-Green was also a paid consultant to the CDC.

The authors compared thimerosal exposures and autism rates among children in Denmark, Sweden, and California. In all three, the incidence of autismlike disorders began to rise around 1985–1989, and then accelerated

into the 1990s. In California, thimerosal use in childhood vaccines had continued until around 2001. Sweden and Denmark, on the other hand, had
eliminated the preservative from pediatric shots in 1992. Yet their case numbers continued to go up, according to the study. If thimerosal had been causing autism, the rates should have dropped following its removal.

For the section on California, the authors referred to the calculations that
Mark Blaxill had presented to the IOM, showing a time correlation between
rising exposure levels and rising case numbers. The authors even reproduced
Mark's chart in the article (without permission). But their motive was hardly
to flatter the Boston father. They suggested that his California autism figures
had been exaggerated.

"As with most ecologic analyses, these data had several limitations," the
authors wrote, adding that the definition of autism used by the California
Department of Developmental Services was somewhat "vague" and difficult
to verify. The increase could have been due to greater awareness and changes
in diagnostic criteria, the authors said. During the period in question, California began to include subcategories of autistic-related illnesses, such as pervasive developmental disorder (PDD). "These subcategories of PDD accounted
for the largest increases in the reported California cases reflected in the data
used," the authors said. (This assertion, Mark would later argue, was untrue.
He said the California statistics had always included only full-blown cases of
autism, and not PDD. If anything, the diagnostic criteria for "classic" autism
had become narrower over the years.)

In Sweden, autism rates continued to climb after thimerosal was removed
from pediatric vaccines in 1993, according to the report. But the study only
counted autism cases diagnosed in a hospital setting. Autism is almost always
diagnosed in doctors' offices or clinics, not in hospitals. Few parents rush
their child to an emergency room if they stop talking.

Looking only at Swedish inpatient cases, the autism numbers rose and fell
during the study period of 1980–1997 but showed an upward trend over time.
Case rates went from 5 or 6 cases "per 100,000 person-years" (or 10,000 ten-
years-olds) before 1985 to a peak of 9.2 per 100,000 person-years in 1993.

"This was generally similar to the trend in California during the same time
period," the study noted, even though few vaccines containing thimerosal
were ever used in Sweden. Swedish children who received the three recommended doses of thimerosal-containing DTP or DT prior to 1992 would have
received a 75-microgram cumulative dose of ethylmercury by age two.

In Denmark, case rates also went up after thimerosal was removed, in
1992, but the trend was linear, and breathtaking. Before 1992, Danish children had received up to 125 micrograms of mercury by age ten months.
Autism cases, meanwhile, remained more or less steady, at about 10 new

FIGURE 8. Graphical ecologic analysis comparing average cumulative ethylmercury dose received from vaccines and the incidence rate (per 100,000 person-years) of autism cases in children aged 2 to 10 years diagnosed during 1987–1999 in inpatient settings in Sweden, by birth-year cohort from 1980 to 1996. (Data not available for year 1981.)

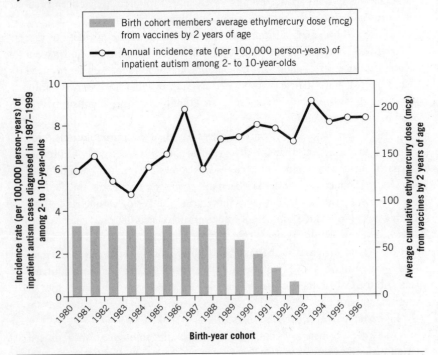

Source: Paul Stehr-Green, et al., "Autism and Thimerosal-Containing Vaccines: Lack of Consistent Evidence for an Association," reprinted with permission from the *American Journal of Preventive Medicine*, 25, no. 2 (August 2003): 101–6.

cases a year. But by 2000, long after thimerosal was eliminated, annual case numbers were up to 181.

The Danish results were riddled with even more problems than the Swedish ones, however. Even the authors admitted that they "may have spuriously increased the apparent number of autism cases." As in Sweden, they had counted only inpatient cases, at least from 1983 to 1994. Then in 1995, for reasons that went unexplained, the researchers began including outpatient cases as well. In that same year, the total number of children reported with autism more than doubled over the year before: from about 40 cases in 1994 to 100 cases in 1995.

"Changes over time in the rates of diagnosis of autism-like disorders in inpatient versus outpatient settings may have affected the ascertainment of

FIGURE 9. Graphical ecologic analysis comparing the average cumulative ethylmercury dose received from vaccines by birth-year cohort from 1981 to 1998, and the annual number of incident cases of autism in children aged 2 to 10 years diagnosed in Denmark from 1983 to 2000.

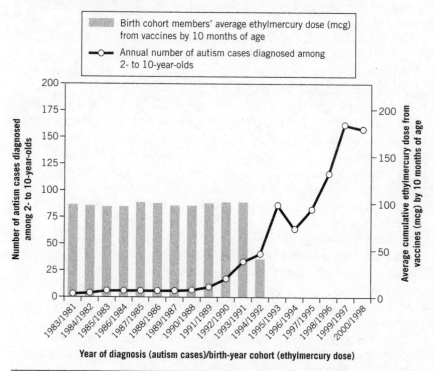

Source: Paul Stehr-Green, et al., "Autism and Thimerosal-Containing Vaccines: Lack of Consistent Evidence for an Association," reprinted with permission from the *American Journal of Preventive Medicine*, 25, no. 2 (August 2003): 101–6.

cases," the authors said, in what the Mercury Moms thought was the understatement of the year.

A second flaw was that prior to 1992, the data did not include cases diagnosed in a busy clinic in Copenhagen, where 20 percent of all Danish cases were diagnosed. By adding in these previously excluded cases, the authors found a spike in rates in 1992, the same year that mercury was removed from vaccines.

A third change in methodology occurred midway through the study. In 1993, Denmark had updated its psychiatric diagnostic codes and adopted new diagnoses for autism-related disorders. Government workers conducted training seminars with clinicians in order to promote the new coding system.

274 · EVIDENCE OF HARM

This campaign "may have stimulated reporting of autism cases (as well as other health outcomes)."

Population studies involving large groups, instead of individuals, as the unit of analysis are inherently limited in their ability to prove or disprove causation, the article conceded. "Such studies can be useful in exploring possible associations, [and] searching for areas of possible further study," it said. "However, the greatest difficulty in interpreting ecologic studies is that of adequately controlling confounding factors due to unavailability of data and/or methodological limitations."

Despite these limitations, the authors said that the results from Scandinavia provided "compelling evidence in sharp contrast to the alleged association observed in California." They said the "body of existing data" was inconsistent with the hypothesis that thimerosal-containing vaccines were "responsible for the apparent increases in the rates of autism." It seemed more plausible that other factors were affecting these changes, "such as those mentioned above: an increased recognition of the disorder, and/or other as-yet-unidentified environmental or genetic factors."

Mark Blaxill was primed to attack. "This one's going to be easy," he told Sallie and Lyn on a call in late July. "Of course, that doesn't mean people will listen." Everyone knew that the study would command international attention, and leave the impression that the thimerosal issue had been settled for good.

Before their response was finalized, however, another version of the same study appeared in the journal *Pediatrics* one week later, on September 2, 2003. Titled "Thimerosal and the Occurrence of Autism: Negative Ecological Evidence from Danish Population-Based Data," it also concluded that "ecological data do not support a correlation between thimerosal-containing vaccines and the incidence of autism."[295]

As in the previous study, the authors conceded that adding outpatient cases into the study after 1995 "may exaggerate the incidence rates, simply because a number of patients [diagnosed] before 1995 were recorded for the first time, and thereby counted as new cases in the incidence rates." In order to "elucidate the contribution of the outpatient registration to the change in incidence," the authors went back and looked at inpatient cases only. Among this minority of cases, they said, "There was no trend toward an increase in the incidence of autism during the period when thimerosal was used."

This time, Safe Minds was ready with a prepared statement, which they issued to the media the same day the *Pediatrics* article appeared.

"Vaccine Health Officials Manipulate Autism Records to Quell Rising Fears over Mercury in Vaccines," the statement's headline said.[296] The *Pediatrics* report "clearly manipulates the incidence of autism in an attempt to clear thimerosal-containing vaccines of any role in the etiology of the disease." The increase that was found was "falsely created by the author's use of techniques which artificially boosted the number of cases identified."

The biggest flaw, of course, was the exclusion of outpatient cases prior to 1995. Safe Minds said that the large MMR study conducted in Denmark and published in the *New England Journal of Medicine* in 2002 showed that outpatient cases outnumbered inpatient cases there by a 13.5-to-1 ratio. Outpatient cases represented 93 percent of all autism cases nationwide. The parents also criticized the study for adding in the Copenhagen clinic midway, and claimed that the change in national diagnostic codes also contributed to the upswing.

Finally, the study was conducted by researchers with inherent conflicts of interest, Safe Minds alleged. "This study appears to be a clumsy attempt to provide support for policy choices in which the authors and their collaborators are involved," Lyn wrote. "Two of the authors of the study work for the Danish manufacturer of thimerosal vaccines. This conflict of interest was not disclosed by *Pediatrics* and the journal itself receives significant advertising revenues from vaccine manufacturers."

Even if autism rates were shown to be rising in Denmark, they were still extremely low both before *and* after thimerosal was removed, Mark Blaxill observed in a separate statement.[297] Prior to 1992, the *Pediatrics* study recorded a prevalence rate of just 1 per 10,000, among the lowest rates reported in the world. This also contradicted a previously published survey of autism in Denmark, which showed an autism rate of over 4 per 10,000 as far back as the 1950s.[298]

"Normally, authors cite relevant studies in their introductory or discussion sections," Mark said. But the authors "failed to mention this study, as they failed to comment on the unusually low autism rates for the earlier years of their study period."

By the end of the decade, with thimerosal removed, the Danish rate had "risen" to 4 to 6 per 10,000, according to the *Pediatrics* article. This was about the same level as that found in the United States before the increase in thimerosal exposure tripled in the early nineties. And it fell far below U.S. rates at the end of the decade, which were around 60 per 10,000.

"While emphasizing their illusory increase, the authors never mention that their rates are actually quite low" compared to those in the United States, Mark wrote. "The authors fail to provide the most basic statistics that might enable a full comparison with other reports. These crucial omissions suggest a clear bias toward elevating the perception of Danish autism rates later in their study period."

In sum, Mark said, public officials and vaccine makers "once again, rather than seriously evaluating the autism-mercury hypothesis and carrying out the research agenda specified by the IOM, have instead chosen to issue another piece of propaganda masquerading as science—with the only possible outcome being that legitimate research and discussion might be suppressed."

The mainstream media portrayed the Danish study as definitive. A front page headline in the *New York Times* declared: "Study Casts Doubt on Theory of Vaccines' Link to Autism."[299] It quoted Dr. Robert Davis as saying the evidence was "clear-cut."

"If you remove cars from highways, you'll see a marked decrease in auto-related deaths," Davis said. "If thimerosal was a strong driver of autism rates, and you remove it from vaccines, you should have seen some sort of decline—and they didn't."

Other vaccine experts also praised the findings. Neal Halsey called the report "helpful and important," the *Times* reported, and Dr. William Schaffner, chairman of the Department of Preventive Medicine at Vanderbilt University in Nashville, said the study added to "the whole mosaic of studies that have addressed this. Each is imperfect, but they all add up to this theme: thimerosal is not the culprit."

The *Times* article did incorporate criticism from Safe Minds, which said that the researchers "artificially boosted the number of cases by adding outpatients and those at a large Copenhagen clinic to earlier inpatient figures." They also said that two scientists in the study worked for the Danish vaccine manufacturer, "suggesting a conflict of interest."

But Dr. Kreesten Meldgaard Madsen of the Danish Epidemiology Science Center, who led the study, replied that in Denmark "a diagnosis of autism must be made by a psychiatrist and registered with the health system, which categorizes any patient who even visits a hospital for a test as an 'inpatient.'" (Of course, this still did not mean they had been diagnosed as inpatients.)

And, Madsen said, Danish vaccines are not made by private companies but by a nonprofit government agency, the State Serum Institute, which he compared to the CDC.

ON OCTOBER 1, 2003, the third Danish study came out against the thimerosal theorists, this time in the *Journal of the American Medical Association*.[300] This third study was quite different from the other two. The investigators, led by Anders Hviid, of the Danish Epidemiology Science Center, had looked at the medical records of all children born in Denmark between 1990 and 1996, or nearly 470,000 kids.

In Denmark, the only thimerosal-containing childhood vaccine had been for pertussis (three injections in the first ten months of life with a total of 75 micrograms of ethylmercury). But in March 1992, the last batch of this shot was released from the Statens Serum Institut, and only thimerosal-free versions were produced after that. In this way, they could compare kids who got 75 micrograms of mercury before mid-1992 with those who received zero micrograms from mid-1992 on.

They found little difference between the two groups in terms of autism.

The authors had identified 440 autism cases and 787 cases of "other autistic-spectrum disorders." But the risk of an adverse outcome was almost the same. In fact, kids in the thimerosal group had a relative risk of 0.85 for autism, compared with the mercury-free group. This meant they were 15 percent less likely to get autism, suggesting that mercury exposure in very young infants might actually have a small protective effect. The relative risk for "other autistic-spectrum disorders" was 1.12 for the mercury-exposed kids. Neither result was considered statistically significant. Likewise, the authors found no significant evidence of a "dose-response association" (where the risk rises with each increase in exposure). "The results do not support a causal relationship between childhood vaccination with thimerosal-containing vaccines and development of autistic-spectrum disorders," they concluded.

For Safe Minds, challenging this study was going to be more delicate, and difficult. They simply did not have the necessary backup information, such as that they had obtained with the American VSD study. But Mark Blaxill and Sallie responded anyway.

The two had identified a flaw that they believed resulted in a substantial loss of autism case records from the Danish registry, which would essentially render the findings invalid. "The registry allows 10-25% of diagnosed autism cases to be lost from its records each year," Sallie wrote in a letter to *JAMA*. "The effect of this loss is such that the records will disappear from older age groups to a much greater degree than from younger age groups in any given registry year."[301]

As a result, older children were underrepresented in the cohort, even though they were the ones who received thimerosal-containing vaccines before 1992.

Hviid and his Danish colleagues flatly denied this in their own letter to *JAMA*. "In response to Ms Bernard, we do not agree that autism cases are lost retrospectively from the Danish Psychiatric Central Register," they wrote. "The registry records all contacts to psychiatric departments and has been used extensively for psychiatric epidemiological research in Denmark," they added.[302]

"We contacted the Danish Psychiatric Central Register to verify the nature of the data obtained by Ms Bernard," the authors continued. "The Danish

Psychiatric Central Register verified that these data do not represent prevalences of autism but are simply the numbers of cases with a contact to a psychiatric department in a given year. However, not all cases in the population are seen in a psychiatric department every year. Nevertheless, those without any follow-up contact with psychiatric departments after diagnosis can also be identified in the register. We used such data in our prospective follow-up study. Contrary to Bernard's claims, all individuals who were diagnosed with autism were included in our analysis."

There were other problems with the Hviid study, Mark and Sallie contended. For instance, the researchers had not broken down reported cases of autism by birth year, the way Mark had done to arrive at the California calculations. There is often a difference between the number of children diagnosed with autism from any given birth cohort and the number of autism cases reported in any given calendar year. Analyzing the data according to birth cohort would paint a far more accurate picture, Mark believed.

"Safe Minds reanalyzed the Denmark registry data and used an alternative method to avoid the record removal bias," the letter to *JAMA* said. They looked at same-age children—5- to 9-year-olds—but from different registry years: 1992, when all of the children received thimerosal-containing pertussis vaccines; and 2002, when none of the children received thimerosal. "After adjusting for the lack of outpatient records in the 1992 registry, the analysis found a 2.3 higher number of autism cases among the 1992 thimerosal-exposed group relative to the 2002 non-exposed group," Safe Minds said.

Mark had also calculated the autism incidence rate among all Danish children who received mercury in their pertussis vaccines, and found that it was 20 per 10,000 births. But when he calculated the rate among all children vaccinated after thimerosal was removed, the rate had dropped to just 6 to 7 per 10,000. (It should be noted that the thimerosal-exposed children would have been older, and perhaps more likely to have received an autism diagnosis than the younger nonexposed children.)

"In the Hviid study in JAMA we can clearly see how the data was misinterpreted so a conclusion could be drawn to clear thimerosal from any role in autism," Lyn was quoted in the statement. "This misinterpretation is not surprising given the authors' employment with the maker of vaccines in Denmark, Statens Serum Institut. This conflict of interest should have been stated by JAMA."

The parents then called for a "complete analysis of the Denmark autism registry data set by independent, unbiased epidemiologists who have no involvement in vaccine development, production, promotion, or administration."

. . .

MARK AND DAVID GEIER had been wrangling with the CDC for nearly a year over their attempts to secure access to the VSD data. They had gone to some lengths to obtain approval from each Institutional Review Board at the HMOs. And the Geiers haggled over every aspect of the data: what amount they could see, and when.

The impasse lasted well into the summer, despite repeated conference calls between the warring parties, mediated by Rep. Dave Weldon's deputy chief of staff Stuart Burns. The Geiers had submitted all their IRB approvals to the National Immunization Program for review in June. Assuming their paperwork was complete, they expected to be assigned a date for their visit to the CDC computer center. But the process was not quite over yet.

CDC officials told the Geiers they would need to request specific data sets in advance, in order for the agency to prepare and transfer the information onto the computer that would be assigned to them. But the Geiers had assumed that they would have free access to all the data, at their fingertips and without preset limitations. They argued that they needed to see the data first before deciding which groups of children they wanted to select for analysis.

"This is absurd," Mark Geier told the CDC officials during a three-way call with Stuart Burns. "Most researchers look over all of the data first, before deciding which questions they want to try to answer. You're asking us to search blindly for answers *before* we have the questions. Please, don't exclude any data. We want as much information as possible."[303]

But the officials were adamant. A few weeks later, the Geiers came back with their specific requests. First, they asked for the data sets used in nine separate VSD studies previously done by the CDC, including the Verstraeten thimerosal investigation. These data sets were critical to confirming or disputing what Verstraeten had found.

But the Verstraeten data was off limits because the study had not been published.

"They are still changing it in response to the peer-review process," Mark Geier complained to Weldon. This seemed odd to him, given that the study had already been submitted to the journal *Pediatrics* and was scheduled for publication in the fall. "What kind of study is it where you change the data in response to peer-review comments?" he asked. "The data is what the data is. You don't go back and change it when people make suggestions—how can you change it?" Weldon agreed that it did seem suspicious.

The Geiers had also requested other data sets to analyze. Their top priority was to examine DTaP vaccines with and without thimerosal. They wanted to see if they could find the same 6.0 relative risk for autism they had identified in the VAERS data.

In late July, the CDC informed the Geiers that the requested data sets had been assembled. After paying a processing fee of $3,200, the Geiers were given two dates in August to come and run their studies. But there was another, entirely unexpected wrinkle.

Just two days before their appointment, a CDC technician called to make sure they were fluent in the programming language SAS, which is used in the VSD database. The Geiers had never heard of it before.

"You must not be epidemiologists," the technician said. "They all speak SAS."

If that were true, it was news to the Geiers. There was no sense going in now to look at the data. They needed to find an SAS programmer first. Reluctantly, they canceled the appointment.

It took weeks to find someone who could run SAS, was available to work, and who could travel to Maryland on the appointed days. Eventually Stuart Burns of Dave Weldon's office referred the Geiers to a Dallas technician named Vale Krenik, who had an autistic son. A former computer programmer, he was happy to help. But Krenik was not familiar with SAS either. He volunteered to teach himself the program. He ordered and paid for the training materials and spent long hours in his free time learning it.

Finally, the Geiers were ready. Their dates were rescheduled for October 9 and 10, 2003. Krenik flew in from Dallas (also on his own dime) and the three men headed out to the Research Data Center of the CDC's National Center for Health Statistics, in Hyattsville. The center is housed in a nondescript office building behind a shopping center in the middle-class suburban town.

Because the CDC was now deeply involved with monitoring the nation for signs of bioterrorism, security was tight. After passing through a phalanx of guards and metal detectors—and being searched for cell phones, tape recorders, pens, and paper—the men were led into the lobby. There they were greeted by a pleasant-looking woman who introduced herself as their "monitor." She escorted them to the elevator and up several floors, where long corridors stretched in each direction. They walked to a small white-walled room with nothing in it but a desk, a few chairs, and an aging computer terminal.[304]

The computer screen was already turned on. But it was completely blank, save for a small, blinking prompt at the bottom. Vale Krenik wanted to know how to get to the SAS interface. The interface provides a more user-friendly way of sorting and managing the data. But he needed the interface software. Without it, running the program would be like trying to operate a PC in DOS mode, writing code at the C: prompt without benefit of Windows' point-and-click navigation.

"Where's the interface?" Vale asked uneasily. "How do I access it?"

The monitor said she did not know. She agreed to call in some other technicians. Many hours later, the staff admitted they could not find any copies of the software. "This is the computer you were assigned to," one of them said. "If the interface was not loaded onto it already, there's nothing we can do. You're on your own." And with that, they left the room. The three men stared at the blinking screen, clueless about how to proceed.

"How on earth can this be happening?" Mark muttered, shaking his head. "Once again, they got us." Silence filled the room. There would be no number crunching today. The men stared at the screen.

"Wait a minute." It was the female monitor. She rose from her chair, peered out into the hallway, and closed the door. She sat down and took a deep breath.

"Do not tell *anyone* this," she said in a low voice. "But I can help you."

The woman explained that she had an "affected child" in her family. Nervously, she sat at the terminal and began banging away in computer code.

The woman told them that the CDC keeps a full-time team of three SAS programmers to run the VSD numbers. She said it was absurd to expect that an outsider, working on his own without help and without interface software, could possibly decipher the complex commands needed to operate the program.

She showed Krenik how to find the data sets for children who had received at least three DTaP shots. The Geiers worried that they would not find any children who had received thimerosal-free versions of the vaccine. At the time the data was collected, there was only one thimerosal-free DTaP vaccine, from GlaxoSmithKline. It had not been on the market for long. The Geiers had no idea if any of the HMOs used that version. But at the end of the day, they were happy to discover that tens of thousands of children had indeed received the Glaxo vaccine, while tens of thousands more received a thimerosal-containing version. They had two groups to compare—they could study their question.

It took most of the next day to sort through the records to determine which children had received which vaccines. Each thimerosal-containing DTaP shot contained 25 micrograms of ethylmercury, so children would have been exposed to anywhere from 0 to 100 micrograms, depending on the number and type of DTaP they received (on top of any exposure from other vaccines).

The woman helped them again. They discovered that all but one of the autism diagnoses fell within the higher exposure combinations. The risk for autism increased significantly with each additional 25 micrograms of mercury. When they finally calculated the relative risk for autism at each exposure level, the Geiers were shocked to find that children who received three mercury-containing DTaP shots had an increased risk of autism nearly twenty-seven times that of children who got three preservative-free vaccines.

The woman did not seem surprised. She told the Geiers that she had been running VSD data on thimerosal for quite some time. She knew these numbers inside out.

"I'm telling you, they know," she said conspiratorially. "There's a big problem."

The Geiers stopped dead and listened. The woman explained that the CDC was constantly monitoring the database for up-to-the-minute signs of a bioterror attack. The "rapid sampling" method would indicate, for example, if clusters of unusual symptoms were suddenly being reported in a certain location. She was assigned to look at the most recent data, checking to see what the rates for autism were doing. She was asked to determine if the numbers of diagnoses had begun to decline, especially in the younger children. If so, this would implicate thimerosal, which began to be phased out in 2000.

"The autism numbers are going down," she said. "We're watching them drop."

A FEW DAYS after their trip to the computer center, Mark Geier paid a keyed-up visit to Dave Weldon's Capitol Hill office. He showed Weldon and Stuart Burns the results from Hyattsville. The methodology looked sound.

And, Stuart informed the Geiers, he had recently learned that the intermediate data sets constructed by Verstraeten (the ones containing the original raw data) were "no longer maintained by the CDC." It was a mystery as to what had happened to them.

Weldon was livid. "This has to be published," he said. "It's very important. You should try to get this into JAMA." Mark Geier was skeptical that the Journal of the American Medical Association would accept such an indictment of thimerosal. But Weldon felt the gravity of the findings was such that JAMA would give it full consideration.

Then Mark Geier recounted the odd tale about the woman at the computer center. "She helped us analyze the data. It was totally against the rules," he explained. "It's probably going to cost her that job."

Weldon was alarmed. He had always placed the utmost confidence in the CDC, but now it was beginning to falter. If this potential whistle-blower was telling the truth, then all bets were off. Stuart Burns made contact with the woman to inquire about the Geiers' experience and the faulty data sets. But the woman told him she could not cooperate.

"I have a career ahead of me at the CDC," she had explained earlier to the Geiers. "Going public with this information would end that. It could make my life miserable," she said. "They could prevent me from getting another job, or blackball me from future research grants."

That anyone would willingly conceal information so important from the public just to protect their career was, Weldon thought, appalling.

In the meantime, the Geiers sent their VSD findings to Dr. Walter Spitzer, the eminent epidemiologist from Montreal. He agreed that the data looked solid, and also urged that it be submitted to *JAMA*. Mark and David Geier wrote up their report in a matter of days. In their submission letter to *JAMA,* they mentioned that Spitzer, Weldon, and Dan Burton had all endorsed the work.

A few days later, the CDC finally published its own long-awaited report on the VSD thimerosal study.

THOMAS VERSTRAETEN and the VSD team had spent four years analyzing the massive HMO database for signs of an association between thimerosal and neurological disorders. Four years of tinkering with the numbers had yielded at least three different generations of results: the classified Verstraeten report of February 2000, the allegedly watered-down version presented at both Simpsonwood and the June 2000 meeting of the Advisory Committee on Immunization Practices, and the third version, presented at the Institute of Medicine meeting in July 2001, which showed even further reductions and eliminations of relative risks.

Now, in the fall of 2003, the CDC was going to issue its fourth and final version, in the November issue of *Pediatrics.* By this time, they had stopped looking at autism as an outcome altogether. Meanwhile, the risk for ADHD had evaporated completely, and the risks for tics and language delay had fallen to near insignificance. In fact, an increased relative risk for tics (1.98) was found at just one HMO (Northern California Kaiser), while an increased risk for language delay (1.13) was seen only at Group Health Cooperative. When the investigators completed Phase II, the Harvard Pilgrim follow-up study, they found no risk for any of the disorders at all.[305]

"No consistent significant associations were found between thimerosal-containing vaccines and neurodevelopmental outcomes," the authors concluded. "Conflicting results were found at different HMOs for certain outcomes." Further studies were needed to "resolve the conflicting findings."

This time, the parents were prepared well in advance with their reply. Safe Minds was among the first groups to speak out. They had obtained a copy of the final report a week ahead of its release. Stuart Burns, at Dave Weldon's office, suggested they hire a Washington PR consultant to make sure their voice of dissent was heard in the flurry of press coverage that was sure to ensue.

With financial backing from Sallie, Safe Minds retained Cheri Jacobus, a publicist and GOP political consultant with wide connections in Washington. Jacobus, an articulate woman with light blond hair and powder-blue eyes, is a regular on the cable news talk shows, mostly Fox, where she extols the leadership of George W. Bush and the GOP.

Sallie, Lyn, and Mark dissected the *Pediatrics* report quickly, looking for any new signs of apparent manipulation.

"This new study is a piece of work," Mark wrote in an e-mail to Sallie, Lyn, Laura, Lori McIlwain, and Stuart Burns. "There are some creative new ways to cheat."

One thing the researchers had done in the final version was to break up data from the largest HMO, Northern California Kaiser, into data from its individual clinics. This "stratification" would "mess up the thimerosal correlations" at the HMO with the best "statistical fit," Mark explained. In this way, the researchers eliminated any "consistent statistically significant risk" of ADHD or speech disorders that might be found within the Northern California Kaiser system as a whole. "My jaw drops every time I see these guys go to work," Mark marveled.

In the final version, the VSD team had also eliminated the combined umbrella of "neurological developmental disorders," or NDDs. By breaking that general outcome into individual categories like ADHD, speech delay, and tics, they were able to reduce or eliminate the relative risks and statistical significance of nearly every outcome. Mark outlined the evolution of the major findings across the four study "generations":[306]

Lyn also identified ways that the number of outcomes in each category may have been reduced, she said. This had occurred in the report's third generation, as reported by Verstraeten at the 2001 Institute of Medicine meeting. Lyn went to the IOM Web site and played the entire audio recording of his remarks. She found something she had previously missed.

The researchers had conducted a side analysis: a chart audit in which they pulled the medical records of children with speech and language delay, ADHD, and autism and checked to confirm the veracity of each diagnosis. "They decided to include only those cases that had been confirmed by a behavioral specialist. If the behavioral specialist had been outside of the HMO, the diagnosis would not be included on their HMO chart," Lyn claimed. This gave the authors the opportunity to "cherry pick" cases out of the original data set. "They made the numbers change quite a bit," she told the group.

Among the ADD/ADHD cases, only 40 percent were confirmed in the charts by a behavioral specialist, and thus 60 percent were excluded, Lyn said. For speech and language delay, 50 percent were confirmed and 50 percent were excluded. For autism, 80 percent were confirmed.[307]

FIGURE 10. Downward trends in calculated relative risks for autism and other disorders across four generations of analysis by the CDC.

	Generation 1	Generation 2		Generation 3	Generation 4
	Phase 1 February 29, 2000	Phase 1 June 2000	Phase 2 Harvard Pilgrim	IOM Report July 2001	Pediatrica November 2003
Autism risk	2.48 (n.s)	1.69 (n.s.)	not done	n.s.	n.s.
Neurological developmental disorders risk (NDDs)	1.59	1.64 1.007 per mcg dose-response ($p<0.01$)	not done	"results not consistent between HMOs A and B"	not reported
Speech/language delay risk	n.s.	1.008 per mcg dose-response ($p=0.0004$)	n.s.	"results not consistent between phases"	"chance alone" would yield some positive associations

n.s.: not significant

Source: Safe Minds, "An Analysis and Critique of the CDC's Handling of the Thimerosal Exposure Assessment Based on Vaccine Safety Datalink (VSD) Information," October 2003.

"This means that approximately half of the outcomes were excluded from the data because they were not confirmed," Lyn said. "This is huge. It must be brought out."

There were other lines of attack as well. The article had failed to disclose that Verstraeten worked for a vaccine manufacturer at the time of publication. "This means that the data was manipulated even after Verstraeten was working for GlaxoSmithKline," Lyn surmised.

And of course, there was that same question of age. "Nowhere do they mention the average age of the children, nor do they give any age breakouts of the data," Lyn said. "The paper is mute on this inherent weakness, and no effort was made to address it."

There was also the questionable practice of changing the exclusion criteria midway through the study. "Verstraeten initially tried to have the cleanest possible data for analysis," Lyn said. When the authors added back in children "at risk" for adverse outcomes, regardless of their thimerosal exposure, it further "muddied the waters" by producing more outcomes in the lower exposure categories, resulting in an overall lowering of relative risks.

There was also the questionable record-keeping practices at Harvard Pilgrim, and the fact that Massachusetts had placed the HMO in state

286 • EVIDENCE OF HARM

receivership in 2000. What's more, the diagnostic coding practices differed greatly between Harvard Pilgrim and the two West Coast HMOs. The West Coast groups used ICD-9 codes, whereas HP used something called "Co-Star coding." It was a totally different system that depends more on symptoms than on hard diagnoses, Lyn said. It wasn't surprising that Harvard Pilgrim was inconsistent with the other HMOs: "They are comparing apples to watermelons."

The researchers were successful in "making the findings from their early investigation in 2000 completely disappear," Lyn said. "They altered entrance criteria, reclassified children with outcomes through chart audits, and made numerous statistical manipulations of the database."

Safe Minds, with the help of Cheri Jacobus, managed to get their written reactions into the hands of top national health reporters a day before the study's publication. They included a forty-six-page critique produced by Mark that detailed how investigators altered the data sets across the four generations, reducing relative risk and statistical significance.

The CDC's approach demonstrated a "pervasive pattern of bias and conscious manipulation of samples, statistics and findings to produce a negative finding," Mark wrote. And yet, "despite significant problems" with study design and data quality, and "contrary to public statements" made by the CDC, the analyses still supported a causal relationship between thimerosal exposure and childhood developmental disorders.

To demonstrate this, Mark compared the vaccine compliance rate at each HMO with the percentage of children diagnosed with NDDs or speech delay. Generally speaking, the higher the vaccination rate, the more likely the kids were to get sick:

These numbers did not bode well for society at large. At the highest exposure levels, NDD outcome rates reached 5 percent, though this was likely understated, given the young age of the study population. "Assuming that high levels of thimerosal exposure prevailed in the entire decade of the 1990s," Mark said, "then roughly 40 million children born during the decade were at risk of harm from thimerosal exposure." If NDD rates exceeded 5 percent, then over 2 million children could have been harmed.

Safe Minds issued a press release alongside the critique. It was shorter, sharper, and more political. "CDC Manipulated Data in Study on Link between Children's Vaccines and Autism, CDC's Earlier Results Showing Significant Link Covered Up—Exposed by Freedom of Information Act Documents," the headline said.[308]

The group chose to highlight two of the most blatant problems. First, there was Verstraeten's undeclared conflict of interest. After he began work at

FIGURE 11. Increase in percentages of adverse outcomes associated with rising vaccination compliance rates at three HMOs.

	HMO B	HMO A	HMO C
Actual HMO	Northern California Kaiser	Group Health Cooperative	Harvard Pilgrim
Population size	114,965	15,929	17,547
Full compliance rate at three months	15%	60%	65%
NDD rate (%)	1.3%	6.7%	not done
Speech delay rate (%)	2.6%	3.9%	4.5%

Source: Safe Minds, "An Analysis and Critique of the CDC's Handling of the Thimerosal Exposure Assessment Based on Vaccine Safety Datalink (VSD) Information," October 2003.

GlaxoSmithKline, "the data, sampling and methodology of the study were altered, so that results would point to enough inconsistencies to cast doubt that mercury in vaccines causes autism," they alleged. Verstraeten had not been named as a GSK employee in the study and was "misidentified as an employee of the CDC," it said.

As for the Harvard Pilgrim issue, aside from the low autism numbers reported in Massachusetts and the HMO's inconsistent diagnostic codes, Harvard Pilgrim owned computers with "little compatibility to communicate effectively with one another" and "incapable of consolidating the data accurately," according to the *Journal of Law, Medicine and Ethics,* Safe Minds said.

The controversy was enough to unite autism groups still feuding over the Frist bill. Established groups like Cure Autism Now and the Autism Society of America joined with more unconventional organizations like Safe Minds and the Autism Research Institute to issue a demand for opening up the VSD to outside researchers.

"The current practice of restricting access to the database to a limited group of possibly biased individuals is not acceptable," the newly reformed coalition declared. Their statement added that the *Pediatrics* report "cannot be accepted as final."

CDC rules had made the approval process long and arduous. Those who did gain access (the Geiers) could only "utilize a limited portion of the VSD data set, and their examination of the data is subject to constant monitoring by CDC staff." Even so, the Geiers had found "significant and large increases in relative risk for autism and speech/language disorder from thimerosal exposure in DTaP vaccines."

The autism groups were not the only ones to sound the alarms. Dave Weldon placed a call to Dr. Julie L. Gerberding, the recently appointed director of the CDC, to complain. He followed up the call with a widely circulated letter of admonishment.[309]

"I have reviewed the article and have serious reservations about the four-year evolution and conclusions of this study," Weldon said. "I have read various e-mails from Dr. Verstraeten and coauthors. I have reviewed the transcripts of a discussion at Simpsonwood. I found a disturbing pattern which merits a thorough, open, timely and independent review by researchers outside of the CDC, HHS, the vaccine industry, and others with a conflict of interest in vaccine related issues (including many in University settings who may have conflicts)."

Rather than making a good faith effort to determine if thimerosal had harmed some children, Weldon said, "there may have been a selective use of the data to make the associations in the earliest study disappear."

"I cannot say it was the authors' intent to eliminate the earlier findings of an association. Nonetheless, the elimination of this association is exactly what happened and the manner in which this was achieved raises speculation," Weldon said. The Simpsonwood transcripts "clearly indicated how easily the authors could manipulate the data and have reasonable sounding justifications for many of their decisions."

Mark and David Geier had been approved for access to the VSD, but the "treatment that these well-published researchers have received from the CDC thus far has been abysmal and embarrassing," Weldon stated. The congressman was curious to know if Verstraeten, an outside researcher for more than two years after he left for GlaxoSmithKline, was required to go through the same process.

THE PREEMPTIVE ATTACK on the VSD study proved to be effective. The challenges from Weldon, Safe Minds, and others found their way into nearly every article on the study. Reuters, for example, began by saying that "no significant link between thimerosal and neurological problems" had been found. "But," the second paragraph countered, "critics charged that the study had been manipulated to protect the federal government and vaccine manufacturers from embarrassment and potential lawsuits."[310]

It was a big leap forward for the parents. Never had their objections been placed so prominently in news reports on thimerosal. "Public health activists, including those who work with autism sufferers," the Reuters story continued, "said that neurological disorders had been found at significantly higher rates in the original analysis of the study in 2000, but had been watered down in the final version."

The Associated Press confronted the CDC with allegations the parents had sent out in advance. According to the Associated Press, Frank DeStefano "acknowledged that the early results suggested stronger links with some disorders, though not autism, but denied that there had been pressure or a cover-up. He said the final data reflect a more thorough recent analysis."[311]

The Associated Press also investigated the parents' complaint that Verstraeten had been employed by GlaxoSmithKline for the past two years of the study, and reported that "Verstraeten, who left the CDC in July 2001, did not respond to an e-mail request seeking a response, and company spokeswoman Nancy Pekarek said he did not wish to discuss the results." Pekarek provided a statement in which Verstraeten said that "since leaving the CDC he was only an adviser as the study was finalized and prepared for publication."

Perhaps the most gratifying coverage came from a long article by Kelly Patricia O'Meara in the magazine *Insight on the News,* a conservative weekly spin-off of the right-wing *Washington Times.*[312]

O'Meara interviewed Dave Weldon at length and quoted him as saying that the CDC staff "didn't recognize the amount of mercury they were giving kids, and now they're in the process of investigating themselves." Those same CDC staff members "bounce to and from the drug companies. I think it all is very, very murky and very suspicious."

Mark Geier was even blunter. "This is fraud," he told O'Meara. "The CDC and the FDA know what is happening. They just can't admit it because it is one of the worst things ever to have happened to this United States. If a terrorist had done this, we wouldn't attack them, we'd nuke them. We're talking about one in eight children in the U.S. that currently are in special education, and that number is going to change to about one in five. What percentage of our young population can we destroy before we realize how serious this is?"

Despite the complaints, the CDC stood by the study, CDC spokesman Von Roebuck told the magazine. "We pretty much looked into that [manipulation of data] in the sense of how the information was presented, and we do stand behind it." Yes, the CDC knew Verstraeten now worked at Glaxo-SmithKline, he said. "The one thing that we would want to happen differently is that would have been known before. But the work that Dr. Verstraeten did was for the CDC at the time the work was produced—the work that he did for the study was done when he worked for the CDC."

On television (where pharmaceutical ad dollars represent a huge segment of revenues), the controversy did not get as much coverage—with one very big exception. Steve Wilson, an Emmy Award–winning, well-salted investigative reporter for Detroit's WXYZ-TV News, aired a three-part series on thimerosal and autism when the CDC data came out.

It was an impressive piece of reporting, even if Wilson occasionally ventured to the border of sensationalism.

"The mercury we're talking about inside this vial is so highly toxic we were warned not to even open it to show you the beige powder called thimerosal," he said at one point, holding a small glass jar with a red label.

Wilson interviewed Dr. Benjamin Schwartz, M.D., the acting director of the CDC's National Immunization Program, who denied the allegations that thimerosal was harmful. "All of the scientific data that we have suggests no link between exposure to thimerosal and health problems such as autism in children."

Then the camera cut to Mark Geier. "You gotta understand this is the biggest doctor-caused catastrophe that has ever happened," he said. "The American Academy of Pediatrics who attacked us—they just don't want anyone to know the horrendous thing they allowed to happen."

"It took us filing all these documents you see here to be able to have any chance of seeing the data at all," said David Geier, pointing to a stack of paper.

When the Geiers finally did get in to see it, "we discovered that children were twenty-seven times more likely to get autism," he said.

"Twenty-seven *times*?" Wilson asked in disbelief.

"If they took vaccines with thimerosal versus thimerosal-free vaccines, yes."

Back at the CDC, Dr. Schwartz visibly sneered at the Geiers' work. "Those statements are just not true," he said.

"But, but, this is your own data!" Wilson blurted.

"It does not concern me in the absence of a scientific peer review that would indicate that this analysis is accepted by the scientific community," Schwartz sniffed.

Wilson also noted that the Geiers had published an earlier research paper (from the VAERS database) in the "peer-reviewed" *Journal of American Physicians and Surgeons*. But Dr. Gary Freed, M.D., director of the Division of General Pediatrics at the University of Michigan, said he had never heard of it. "It's not a mainstream or well-respected pediatric or medical journal," he said.

Wilson disputed that. "The journal *is* respected by many," he said off-screen, "and it uses the same double-blinded peer review as others that are more widely quoted."

Wilson continued: "Our investigation reveals many, if not most, health-care professionals and even state health officials have made up their minds that mercury in vaccines poses no real risk, without personally reviewing the studies suggesting it might. . . .

"Despite the mounds of evidence, doctors like Dr. David Johnson [of the Michigan Department of Health] and a Simpson-Wood attendee maintain, 'It is crystal clear that there is no connection between Thimerosal in vaccines and things like autism.' Even though Dr. Johnson admits to never having studied the Geier research, nor that of Dr. Boyd Haley at the University of Kentucky, nor others who published troubling conclusions to the contrary. . . .

"Wouldn't it be better if you actually, as Michigan's adviser to parents, took the time to *read* these studies, which have caused many to conclude that there is a link," he asked Johnson, a tall man with cropped gray hair, a trim silver beard, and wire-frame glasses.

"Certainly," Johnson replied, smiling nervously.

"So," Wilson demanded, "why haven't you done so?"

Johnson looked trapped, but kept smiling. "Many competing interests," he said.[313]

QUESTIONS OVER the VSD analysis did not go away. Dr. Neal Halsey, the vaccine expert/advocate from Johns Hopkins, published a letter in the December 17 issue of *Pediatrics,* along with some colleagues, in which they second-guessed much of Verstraeten's methodology and called for further analysis of the data.[314]

Halsey and colleagues noted that the published results differed from those presented at the Institute of Medicine. In the 2001 IOM version, there had been a statistically significant, dose-escalating association between thimerosal and the umbrella code of "neurodevelopmental delay." This aggregate diagnosis had been eliminated in the final version. But the critics contended that it had been a "reasonable" form of analysis, given the wide variety of diagnostic codes for children with developmental delay, and because mercury toxicity was associated with "multiple effects on neurological development."

By dividing the umbrella category into separate diagnoses, the authors "may have substantially reduced the power to find important relationships," Halsey and colleagues said. Moreover, selection criteria in the final study "appear to have been more lax" than in the IOM version.

The critics did not stop there. Like Lyn, Halsey et al. questioned the use of chart reviews to eliminate diagnoses made by regular doctors. "Were diagnoses that were not made by a specialist excluded from analyses?" they asked, noting that primary care physicians "are capable of diagnosing ADD without input from a sub-specialist."

And like Mark Blaxill, they questioned the wisdom of comparing data from a large HMO (Northern California Kaiser) with two much smaller ones (Group Health Cooperative and Harvard Pilgrim).

Halsey and his coauthors called for an independent organization, "perhaps the IOM," to convene a panel of experts to review the data and "conduct additional analyses if indicated." Public confidence in vaccines would be enhanced "if there was greater independence in vaccine safety assessments from the highly successful program to promote immunizations."

IN LATE 2003, the IOM's Immunization Safety Committee announced it would hold another meeting on autism and its possible connection to both thimerosal and MMR. The meeting was scheduled at the request of the CDC, which was eager to present the Verstraeten findings and the Danish study, among other CDC-supported work.

Parent groups and their attorneys were sure that the CDC's rush to return to the IOM reflected its desire to disprove the thimerosal theory before any causation hearings got under way in civil courts or the Vaccine Court. The parents fretted that IOM members might be influenced by the government to retract their prior statement of biological plausibility, or worse, determine that there was now evidence to reject causation.

Evidence to support an association, however, was still coming in all the time. It was imperative, the parents knew, to furnish the IOM with as much data as possible to support their side.

The body of clinical, laboratory, and epidemiological evidence was impressive. Bradstreet and Holmes had shown how mercury accumulates in autistic children compared with controls. Haley had demonstrated how thimerosal kills neurons, especially in the presence of testosterone or aluminum. Baskin had shown how ethylmercury eats away at brain cells. Blaxill had correlated increased mercury exposure with autism rates in California. And the Geiers had reviewed data from the VSD and VAERS and found dramatically elevated risks for autism among children in the higher exposure groups.

Still, two very big pieces of the thimerosal puzzle remained largely unsolved. What was the apparent genetic predisposition that rendered some kids less able than others to shed mercury and more susceptible to its toxicity? And what was the biochemical process that actually led from mercury exposure to the physical and mental symptoms of autistic kids?

The group had learned that a handful of scientists working independently around the country were racing to help solve these all-important questions. What began to emerge from their investigations implicated specific genetic mutations, which impaired the production of certain enzymes, sulfates, and amino acids essential for proper nerve functioning. Mercury, along with other heavy metals, further impeded that production; children with one or more of the genetic mutations would therefore be even more vulnerable to neurological disorders when exposed to mercury, according to the theory.

Parent groups and the DAN! think tank members had been zeroing in on what seemed to be a weakness in cellular "methylation" (see below) and detoxification capacity that would make the autistic children more sensitive to common environmental toxins than normal children. Suddenly, several isolated pieces of the puzzle were starting to snap into place. A remarkable convergence of clinical and scientific evidence provided strong support for parental observations and conviction that interventions such as methyl B-12 injections could improve cognition and attention.

The research came from three separate quarters.

First, Richard Deth, a pharmacology professor at Northeastern University, and colleagues from the University of Nebraska, Tufts, and Johns Hopkins University, discovered that two substances—insulin-like growth factor 1 (IGF-1) and dopamine—were needed for the proper functioning of a chemical reaction called methylation.

Methylation occurs billions of times a day within cells throughout the human body. The term refers to the transfer of a "methyl group" (composed of one carbon atom and three hydrogen atoms) from one molecule to another.

Why is methylation important? Because every cell in the body contains the same DNA strands, the same genes. In other words, every cell has the potential to do the exact same things. For the most part, methylation of DNA is what tells the cells to perform the functions specific to that type of cell. Methyl groups essentially shut down the genes in DNA that aren't supposed to be active. Methylation is critical to normal DNA function and gene expression. Methylation is also needed to produce certain membrane phospholipids—the essential fatty acids required for proper nerve development, including the myelin sheath.

Deth found that toxins such as ethanol, heavy metals like mercury, aluminum, and lead, and thimerosal block the pathway of IGF-1 and dopamine to activate methylation of DNA and phospholipids inside cells cultured in the laboratory.[315]

"Since each of these agents has been linked to developmental disorders," Deth wrote in his study, "our findings suggest that impaired methylation, particularly impaired DNA methylation in response to growth factors, may

be an important molecular mechanism leading to developmental disorders."
Of the toxins studied, thimerosal was by far the greatest inhibitor of DNA
methylation.

At the same time, Marvin Boris, a private physician, and Allan Goldblatt,
a researcher, from Long Island, New York, had begun to test autistic patients
for a common genetic variant in an enzyme that is also important for normal
methylation reactions. Mutations in this enzyme, methylenetetrahydrofolate
reductase or MTHFR, had been shown to occur at an increased frequency in
other neurobehavioral diseases. To their surprise, the pair of researchers
found that 22 percent of the autistic children had this variation compared to
12 percent in the general population. Because this mutation (also known as a
"single nucleotide polymorphism," or SNP) in MTHFR is also present in
many normal people, it cannot be considered to be a "cause" of autism, but
it could offer important clues to the metabolic pathway that may be genetically abnormal in autism.[316]

It turned out that the MTHFR enzyme was essential for the same metabolic pathway that Deth was finding to be inhibited by thimerosal.

The same year, Jill James, a professor of pediatrics at the University of
Arkansas for Medical Sciences, began analyzing plasma from autistic and control children and discovered that the levels of certain substances used in metabolism (called "metabolites") in the autistic samples were severely abnormal.

Remarkably, the abnormal metabolites were in the same methylation
pathway as Deth's enzyme and Boris and Goldblatt's MTHFR mutation. The
low levels of essential metabolites in this pathway provided scientific evidence
that autistic children had reduced methylation capacity and a reduced ability
to detoxify heavy metals such as thimerosal, according to the researchers.[317]

For example, James found that autistic children had low levels of the
amino acids methionine and cysteine, which are essential precursors for the
synthesis of glutathione, the sulfur-based "mercury capturer" thiol protein
and a major antioxidant. This, perhaps, provided the missing link to the mystery: glutathione is the molecule that binds mercury and carries it out of the
body in the urine and feces. Without adequate levels of glutathione, autistic
children cannot excrete mercury normally and "this potent neurotoxin would
tend to accumulate preferentially in the brain, kidney, and gut," James said.

In an attempt to determine whether the abnormal metabolic profile could
have a genetic basis, James had independently begun to test for the same
polymorphism (genetic variant) that Boris and Goldblatt were studying. Although her MTHFR data was not as strong as that of Boris and Goldblatt,
she discovered several other polymorphisms in the methylation and glutathione or "transulfuration" pathway that were significantly more frequent
in autistic children than in her control population.

James made another observation that could help explain why autism affects boys more than girls. Estrogen enhances the transsulfuration pathway and increases glutathione antioxidant capacity in females, she said. The female hormone was also shown to increase glutathione levels in animals. "The evidence suggests that both cellular methylation capacity and antioxidant activity are higher in females than males," James wrote. "The increased rate of methionine transsulfuration and glutathione antioxidant activity in females may have a protective effect against the development of autism."

Taken together, the independent discoveries of Deth, Boris and Goldblatt, and James had for the first time provided a cohesive genetic and metabolic explanation for why children with autism may be more vulnerable to mercury—and why they may be less able to excrete the mercury in vaccines.

Now that a metabolic and genetic weakness had been identified, these researchers said, the next logical question was whether a targeted nutritional intervention strategy could fix it. In fact, the question had already been explored by a physician with a large autism practice in Edison, New Jersey, Dr. Jim Neubrander.

Even prior to any of the Deth-James scientific discoveries, Dr. Neubrander had been electrifying autism conference audiences with his discovery that subcutaneous injections of high doses of methyl B-12 could dramatically improve speech, cognitive function, and social interaction in many autistic children who had lost or never had those abilities.[318]

The subsequent presentations of Deth and James at the 2003 Defeat Autism Now! conference offered up a scientific explanation for why methyl B-12 should be so effective. James provided metabolic evidence that the children had reduced methylation capacity and increased oxidative stress due to low cysteine and glutathione levels. Deth had previously reported that thimerosal could inactivate an enzyme required for methylation and glutathione synthesis. Boris, Goldblatt, and James found genetic polymorphisms that would suppress these pathways, and Neubrander found that methyl B-12 could improve clinical symptoms.

Jill James pronounced Neubrander's methyl B-12 treatment as "scientifically validated" when she reported that nutritional intervention with trimethylglycine, folinic acid, and methyl B-12 completely normalized cysteine and glutathione levels in the autistic children she studied. The scattered pieces of the puzzle could now be fit into a clearer picture that provided a plausible explanation for why autistic children would be more sensitive to thimerosal and why nutritional intervention could result in clinical and metabolic improvement. This unforeseen convergence of ideas and evidence provided a strong basis for further research and refinement of intervention strategies, the researchers argued.

"Many more scientists with different types of expertise are becoming in-volved—indeed, it will take an army of scientists and clinicians to broaden the understanding of the etiology and treatment of autism," James said. "Now it is only a matter of time—the parents are not alone anymore."

Much of the Deth-James-Boris-Goldblatt science was presented in October 2003 at the DAN! conference, but there was a big problem: none of the work had yet been published, and the IOM meeting was just weeks away. Moreover, none of the scientists investigating the MTHFR-methylation connection had been invited to present their findings at the IOM.

Jeff Bradstreet, on the other hand, was scheduled to testify. Asked to submit his presentation in writing prior to the February 9 meeting, he chose to include a summary of the various studies investigating the MTHFR link.

"The data come from a consortium of clinicians and research scientists working together and representing numerous institutions, all sharing their ideas and efforts through regular 'think tanks,'" he wrote to the IOM. "When considered with data collected from other independent scientists, the previously murky picture of vaccine related neurodevelopmental injury is now clear and compelling."[319]

Bradstreet said that his group, the International Child Development Resource Center, had tested patients and controls for concentrations of plasma cysteine and sulfate. "We are observing, despite using a different lab and completely distinct populations, the same sulfation issues as James reports," he wrote. "James observed 22% lower cysteine from normal and we observed a 21% difference. This demonstrates remarkable consistency within two distinct data sets."

Bradstreet said that his data, and those of James, supported Bill Walsh's observations on metallothionein—namely, that defective functioning of MT proteins "may represent a primary cause of autism." But, he wrote, "The defect is not limited to metallothionein. The more complete picture is that of decreased methionine transsulfuration, which would simultaneously adversely effect methylation and sulfation, with resultant disruption in numerous critical biochemical pathways."

THE YEAR SEEMED to be ending on an up note for the parents. They had fought Bill Frist, whose bill was dead for now. They had helped the Geiers gain access to the VSD, and emerge with their provocative results. And they had managed to get their voice into most, if not all the media coverage on the Verstraeten VSD study. Safe Minds helped to make the report controversial—rather than the last word—and it felt like a victory.

It had been a phenomenal year for Will Redwood, Lyn thought as she secretly wrapped the kids' Christmas presents upstairs in her room (now in fourth grade, Will still believed in Santa Claus). This year, Will had clearly written out his Christmas list in neat letters and properly spaced words, rather than the chaotic lists of the past year, when all the words ran together.

Progress for Will, of course, was what Lyn craved. But his cognitive improvements came with challenges. When Will started third grade, in the fall of 2003, Lyn had gotten him placed in a high-performing private school, and he was having a tough time keeping up. The teacher would tell everyone to get out their schoolwork, and by the time Will retrieved his papers and pencils and homework, the class had moved on.

In June of 2003, when Will had taken his Iowa tests at the end of third grade, Lyn thought she had been sent the wrong child's scores. Will, who could not even speak a few years back, was now in the 51st percentile—a perfectly average little boy. To Lyn, he was starting to seem more like a child with perhaps severe ADHD than one with autism.

Lyn had read the work of Richard Deth and Jill James, whose research showed that vitamin B-12 was needed to ensure that children with a genetic mutation and/or heavy metal exposure produced the enzymes and amino acids that facilitated proper nerve function. She was now convinced that two years of keeping Will on high-dose vitamin B-12 therapy, combined with chelation, was the reason for his measured progress. Now, she wanted to try adding folinic acid to the mix.

Lyn and Tommy had also started Will on the ADHD drug Adderall, which seemed to help him focus at school (though the drug's speedy side effects cause him to eat less and lose weight). Even so, while Will's classmates were earning As and Bs on their tests, Will was coming home with Cs and Ds.

"Mom?" he asked one day after school. "What's wrong with me?"

Lyn looked at Will, who was sitting with her on the deck, watching a large hawk circle silently in the sky. How do you tell your child, she thought, that he was poisoned by modern American technology? Lyn figured that Will was old enough to be told.

"Honey, you were exposed to too much mercury as a little boy," she said.

Lyn wondered if Will understood what this meant; she wasn't sure. A week later, in October, the Redwoods drove up to North Carolina for an autism fund-raiser. They stayed with the Bonos, and Will went with them. Will had never met Jackson Bono before. But when he saw the older boy, he instantly recognized Jackson as autistic. Later, Will went up to Laura Bono and asked: "How much mercury did Jackson get?"

When Lyn heard about this, she knew that Will had understood everything.

. . .

LIZ BIRT was also enthusiastic about the findings of Deth and James. In December, 2003 she took Matthew to a DAN! doctor in the Chicago suburbs by the name of Anju Usman, a kind woman with a gentle bedside manner. Usman did a full workup of Matt's blood and discovered that, sure enough, his levels of cysteine, glutathione, and other sulfates were alarmingly low—the same characteristics that Jill James had found in the autistic children she studied.

"There is very little sulfation in Matthew," the doctor told Liz. "His entire metabolic system has gone haywire, the whole pathway has been wiped out." She recommended giving him regular nutritional supplements including oral vitamin B-12.

Liz wanted to try all new treatments right away, but Matthew was too sick. His stools had become pale yellow again, meaning that he was absorbing and digesting his food improperly. And his behavior was becoming even more erratic and aggressive. He was attacking other kids at school, pulling their hair or hurling his shoes at them. Matthew had also started to assault his mom. One day he bit her arm with such ferocity, his teeth broke the skin and a welt rose up like a purple goose egg. The excruciating wound became infected and took weeks to heal.

Liz was scared. She called a doctor she had become friendly with in Long Island, New York, Arthur Krigsman, who was treating autistic kids with severe gut problems. Krigsman was typically booked months in advance, but agreed to make time for Matthew. Liz told him they would be there right after the New Year.

ON DECEMBER 29, 2003, the *Wall Street Journal* ran yet another editorial of invective against the antithimerosal cartel, titled "The Politics of Autism: Lawsuits and Emotion vs. Science and Childhood Vaccines."

"This is a story of politics and lawyers trumping science and medicine," the editorial began.

"Like night follows day," the dispute brought in the tort lawyers, the piece continued. Vaccine makers were supposed to be protected from lawsuits by the VICP, but the lawyers were finding "loopholes to file billion-dollar suits that threaten to punish the few companies that still make vaccines." The suits were without merit, the paper contended, insisting that "study after study" failed to show the connection and citing Pichichero, Nelson and Bauman, and Denmark.

The paper singled out Safe Minds for being "especially active in blaming vaccines" along with their powerful ally Dan Burton. "But their understand-able passion shouldn't be allowed to trump undeniable evidence and damage childhood immunizations that are essential to public health." The column ended by calling on Congress to take up the Frist bill when it reconvened in January.[320]

The editorial unleashed a wave of protest from parents, Safe Minds in-cluded. The group fired back in a letter circulated on the Internet, though never printed in the paper.

"Instead of this being a 'story of politics and lawyers trumping science and medicine' as alleged, it would be more accurately described as a story of how the pharmaceutical industry uses the media and politics to accomplish its goals," they wrote.[321] "Why does the Wall Street Journal feel it necessary to pick on families of children with autism and a small research advocacy group, Safe Minds? The answer is simple, money."

The paper was flooded with venomous and sometimes threatening calls, letters, and e-mails from parents around the country. The uproar received lit-tle notice in the United States, but was covered by the British press, which has followed the vaccine-autism controversy more closely.

"For days, e-mails burned and telephones rang at the offices in downtown Manhattan with diatribes directed at staff on the main opinion page," Charles Laurence wrote in the *Telegraph*. "In the end, the department's sec-retary unplugged her telephone and the writer, whose name had leaked out, went home for his own safety."[322]

To be sure, there were plenty of people who shared the *Journal*'s views. Many of them posted their complaints against the thimerosal theorists on sites all over the Internet. "Safe Minds wants money wasted on attempting to prove a causal connection where all evidence points to there being none," wrote one critic on talkaboutparenting.com. "The WSJ is protecting the tax-payers' money from these fear mongers."[323]

One man, who identified himself as Peter Bowditch, spared few insults in expressing his contempt. "Safe Minds is one of the most disgusting, egre-gious and dishonest anti-vaccination liar sites I have ever come across," he wrote. "It is a site which exists for the purpose of frightening parents into en-dangering their children's lives, using the threat of autism."

12. Showdown

ONTROVERSY over the VSD study continued to roil into 2004. On January 3, the nonpartisan *National Journal* published a meticulous account of the entire contretemps by Neil Munro, a respected Washington journalist.

"A CDC official who helped write the study accepted the critics' charge that it contained many children too young to be diagnosed as autistic," Munro wrote.[324]

" 'This is true,' said scientist Frank DeStefano," the article said. It was the first public admission of error by a VSD team member that the parents could recall.

Munro also quoted Mark Blaxill, who alleged that CDC officials "reduced by roughly 45 percent the number of children in the study who were age four or older. Because autism is normally diagnosed only after age four, the CDC's method greatly reduced the number of children in the study who could be found with autism."

The CDC claimed that older children were excluded because their health records were incomplete, Munro said. But DeStefano declined to say why the agency "did not exclude a comparable proportion of the younger children, to balance out the age groups."

In the piece, Mark Blaxill also accused the CDC of disguising autism rates by counting early symptoms of autism as other illnesses. "The inclusion of many children too young to be definitely diagnosed with autism would result in autistic children being mislabeled with other ailments, such as speech or language delays," the article said.

"It is true," DeStefano admitted, once again. The study could have mislabeled young autistic children with other disorders. But he insisted this was only an "initial evaluation." The CDC was preparing a follow-up study of 300 autistic children and 900 other children, for publication in 2006.

Meanwhile, Mark and David Geier were trying to go public with the results they had obtained from their trips to Hyattsville, namely a relative risk for autism of 27 among kids who received the highest exposure levels to thimerosal in the DTaP vaccines, compared with children who received no thimerosal in their DTaP. They drafted two separate papers for submission.

The first was a broad overview of the neurological damage they had attributed to a number of vaccines over the years, including thimerosal-containing DTaP. They submitted the article to a journal called *Expert Review of Vaccines*. The commissioning editor told them that the article got "stellar" reviews and the authors were asked to make suggested revisions before acceptance. But just as they were expecting to receive the galley proofs, they learned that the piece had been killed.

The Geiers were shocked. Mark Geier had been publishing since the 1960s and nothing like this had ever happened to him before.

The move upset Dave Weldon. He asked his deputy chief of staff Stuart Burns to call *Expert Review of Vaccines* and demand an explanation. Burns was told that the editorial board had met to review the article and deemed it "unacceptable."[325]

The second article was a straightforward presentation of the DTaP data the Geiers had extracted from the Vaccine Safety Datalink. This was the data that Dave Weldon had urged the Geiers to submit to *JAMA*. After months of waiting, it was rejected by JAMA in January 2004.

The Geiers did manage to place a lengthy letter berating the VSD analysis in the January 9 (online) issue of *Pediatrics*. They decried Verstraeten's apparent conflict of interest and attacked the CDC's methodology.[326]

"A number of very serious issues have been raised as to whether thimerosal causes neurodevelopmental disorders," they wrote. "We respectfully request that Verstraeten *et al* consider withdrawing this study." It was essential to admit to "past errors" and conduct open investigations, the Geiers concluded, "in order to restore the badly damaged confidence in our much needed vaccine program."

As it turned out, the same issue of *Pediatrics* carried a letter from Frank DeStefano, Philip Rhodes, and Robert Davis, responding to the criticism from their esteemed colleague Neal Halsey.

Halsey had asked why the VSD team eliminated the umbrella NDD category from the final report. Most of the children in this category were diagnosed with speech or language delay, the team wrote. So they had already been analyzed according to these outcomes. The minority of NDD outcomes were comprised of "several heterogeneous conditions," the trio wrote. "We were advised by some reviewers to delete this category."[327]

In terms of the selection criteria, which Halsey suggested had been expanded between versions, the authors denied that they were "more lax for the published report than for the IOM presentation." In fact, they said the criteria were more stringent for the published report, without offering details.

Then, in a possible contradiction to what Verstraeten had said at the IOM meeting, the authors denied counting only those diagnoses made by specialists, and not general practitioners, as well as "cherry picking" the data during chart review, as alleged by Safe Minds.

"We did not validate all the diagnoses by reviewing charts," they said. "We performed chart review validation for a sub-sample of speech delay, ADD, and autism diagnoses to gauge the validity of these diagnoses. The chart-review findings for these three conditions, however, were not used in the analysis."

The authors claimed they did not "mean to discount" the positive association found at Northern California Kaiser between thimerosal and language delays, just because no association was found at Harvard Pilgrim. But that was just what they did.

The VSD team wrote that they were conducting a rigorous follow-up study of the computerized data. It would include children from the same HMOs, who would be evaluated in person for neurodevelopmental effects, according to their different levels of thimerosal exposure. They were also to undergo an extensive standardized battery of neuropsychological tests, including complete evaluation of speech and language function. The examiners would not be informed of the children's thimerosal exposure level. "We believe that the follow-up study will provide more reliable data for drawing causal inferences than the analysis based on limited computerized diagnostic codes," they wrote.

The authors welcomed additional scrutiny of their study, but questioned "the value of such a review at this time." After all, they noted, it had been reviewed by the CDC, by "external experts," by an IOM committee, and by reviewers at *Pediatrics*. In effect, there was no room for improvement.

"We do not think that any analysis would be able to fully overcome the inherent limitations of computerized health services data," they asserted. The in-person study was scheduled for completion in 2004. It was unlikely that "an independent re-analysis of the computerized HMO data could be completed much before the more definitive results from the follow-up study."

JANUARY 2004 saw some of the coldest weather ever logged in the Northeast. New York temperatures broke all kinds of records as wind chills plummeted to 20 below or more. It was a miserable place and time for a sick child, but Liz was desperate. She and Matthew flew to Long Island to see Dr. Krigsman. It was a ghastly trip. The night Liz returned, she confided her misery to her parent/comrades:[328]

> As many of you already know Matthew's health has been deteriorating. This week after a particularly painful day at school where he spent 45 minutes lying on the floor sobbing and kicking his head back, I called a "saint" to help—Arthur Krigsman. We were so fortunate that Arthur had a cancellation and could see Matthew on Wednesday. After a lot of work, including a 3:00 A.M. visit to Arthur's office on Thursday morning for a nose tube insertion of a laxative, *in a friggin' snowstorm,* Matthew finally "pooped." He was scoped by Arthur on Thursday and it appears that this disease has progressed. Matthew has swelling and ridges in his esophagus (I wonder why he hits his chest); he has an abscess in his colon; his stomach color is pale and his terminal ileum is grossly inflamed. In short, it ALL SUCKS. Sorry, I said it. The "good" news is that we may be able to relieve his pain with steroids and a new GI medication.
>
> Tonight the ride home was anything but easy. When we arrived in Chicago, Matthew started sobbing uncontrollably. He was clutching his stomach and pounding his chest for almost one hour. I was in baggage claim alone with him doing what I could as a mother and thinking "What in the hell is next?" How much misery can a little boy take? Of course many people stopped to help, but there was nothing to do—and that is my frustration. After 6 years there is nothing we can do but try to get on with our lives and fight against incredibly bad odds to save these children—maybe not to have a "normal" life but to have a life free of pain. I look at my son and I admire him so much. He is a beautiful child and endures it all with a sense of humor and mischief. He is completely charming and all of the nurses fell in love with him. He even smiled at Arthur despite the fact that he was coming at him with hoses all of the time. Perhaps this is the best legacy

our children can leave us: to remember the good in people in spite of the pain of each day.

Matthew like so many of our children should have been playing baseball, soccer, doing Boy Scouts and sleepovers, and that is the pain for me; it is a loss of a life that was full of potential and he and we were robbed of that by a system that is set up to fail.

Well, the game is almost over for them and I for one want to watch the fall, at least for a sense of retribution for the immense suffering that this policy has caused. I love all of you and thank you for your prayers and friendship. Believe me, those prayers help at times like this. Love, Liz.

In mid-January, Safe Minds and its allies had become so distrustful about the timing of the IOM meeting that they tried to have it postponed. Sallie and Lyn had been negotiating with IOM committee staff on the agenda, and felt that their side was being squeezed out of the proceedings.

Moreover, none of the new research by Deth, James, or other researchers had been published, and none of those researchers had been invited to present. The parents were convinced that the proceedings were being rushed at the request of the CDC, which wanted a negative finding of causation before any court case got under way.

"The premature scheduling of the upcoming IOM meeting at the request of a government agency for the sole purpose of a liability issue is in direct violation of the Institute of Medicine's charter," Lyn wrote in a letter to the committee on January 15. "Currently, numerous investigations are underway that would offer much additional science to the debate," she said. "Holding a hearing at this time, with little new data, is a waste of taxpayer dollars."[329]

Lyn was surprised that the meeting was scheduled at all, given that in October 2001 the Institute of Medicine had issued a very thorough and comprehensive report on thimerosal. The broad-based research agenda proposed by the IOM in their 2001 report had yet to be implemented, and little new data was available that would necessitate a hearing at this time, she said.

When Safe Minds inquired as to why the meeting was scheduled now, they were told it came at the request of the CDC, "in light of the fact that these issues would be heard later in the year as part of the vaccine compensation program assessment of autism cases," Lyn wrote. When the IOM was asked if the meeting could be rescheduled at a later date when more information was available, "you responded that the decision would have to be made by CDC. You also commented that the Institute of Medicine is under contract with CDC to hold the hearing; therefore they must do as the CDC requests."

A week later, Rep. Dave Weldon sent his own letter to CDC director

Gerberding. He said the premature meeting date, "which you have the ability to change," was in "the best interests of no one who is seeking the truth about a possible association between vaccines and neurodevelopmental disorders."[330] Weldon said that "recent actions and statements" by CDC officials, along with the timing and agenda for the IOM meeting, "raise serious questions about the purpose, value and objectives of this meeting. Presently, the National Immunization Program is engaged in what amounts to an investigation of their own actions, which does not create an air of confidence."

The VSD study also raised "serious concerns about the objectivity of the NIP's top vaccine safety officials," whom Weldon claimed were "the very ones driving the IOM meeting and agenda." Some critics, he noted, "have leveled serious charges that perhaps officials within the NIP manipulated data to 'disprove' a theory they find objectionable." His review of Simpsonwood, the various incarnations of the VSD study, and internal e-mails obtained through FOIA "appear to give support to this claim."

Weldon suggested that some officials were "more interested in a public relations campaign than getting to the truth about thimerosal," causing him to lose faith in the CDC's ability to run an honest internal evaluation. "Given these concerns, the CDC's contributions to the IOM discussion would be viewed as suspect and non-objective."

Finally, Weldon complained about the agenda for the meeting. Only one hour had been earmarked for discussion of the MMR vaccine. And the time set aside for thimerosal was "heavily biased against those who have raised these concerns and will not allow for a fair and balanced discussion of the literature." Weldon again asked that the IOM meeting be postponed. "Given the slow pace of research and lack of federal support for this research, conducting this meeting prior to late 2004 to early 2005 is premature."

In the end, the IOM committee refused to postpone its meeting. But after a number of terse conference calls with Weldon, the parents managed to secure more spots for their side to testify.

MARK AND DAVID GEIER were resolute in getting back in to reexamine the VSD database. Weldon's office had run interference between the Geiers and the CDC for weeks, trying to arrange the dates. The Geiers had requested access for an entire week, beginning on January 7, 2004. That request was denied. Instead, CDC officials offered a smattering of dates: one day one week, two days another week, and so on. This would require flying their programmer in from Texas at great expense.

After receiving Weldon's letter, CDC director Dr. Julie Gerberding called the congressman to discuss his objections. Weldon asked Gerberding to ensure that her staff would be more responsive to the Geiers. She agreed.

There were only two consecutive days available, however, according to the CDC: January 29 and 30. The Geiers accepted. But their return to the computer center was hardly triumphant. This time, the helpful woman was gone, and two blank-faced men were appointed as their monitors. When the Geiers ran their programs, the results were printed out in a separate, secured room. When they went to collect the printouts, the staff person with the keys to the room could not be found. Three hours went by before they could check their results.

But by then, the results had been tampered with, they alleged. They accused the monitor of whiting out most of the findings that were in the data tables that were printed out. David Geier called Weldon's office, and Stuart Burns called CDC headquarters in Atlanta and asked them to intervene. "I want you to grant the Geiers the same quality of access they had in October," Stuart said, "and which they expected to have today." But the CDC brass never called David back. "We're just wasting time," he told his father. "We're not getting any usable data, and we have no access to our printouts. The whole thing is melting down."[331]

In the end the unsound computer they were working on couldn't handle the strain of the day. In the late afternoon, it crashed completely. The session was over, and the Geiers ended up with nothing.

THE WEEK leading up to the IOM meeting in Washington was punishing. Lyn and Sallie were exhausted from fighting with committee staff over who would be able to speak for their side (no slot was offered to Safe Minds). Fresher faces like Jo Pike and Lori McIlwain, along with Scott and Laura Bono, prepared weighty press kits summarizing all the research to date showing an association between thimerosal and autism. The stakes were enormously high. Everyone knew it: the gathering was going to be a showdown.

Perhaps it was no coincidence that mercury made prominent headlines that week. EPA scientists reported that 1 in 6 American children, or some 630,000 kids, were being born with unsafe levels of mercury, levels that could produce learning, attention and memory disorders. This was double the previous estimate of 315,000.[332]

One reason, according to EPA researcher Kathryn Mahaffey, was that recent studies showed mercury levels in umbilical cord blood were 70 percent higher than in maternal blood. Scientists had always assumed that mother and fetus had equal levels.

Then came a report out of the Harvard School of Public Health, where a team of researchers led by Philippe Grandjean conducted follow-up studies on mothers and children exposed to methylmercury from whale meat in the Faroe Islands. They found that not only prenatal exposure but also *postnatal* exposure irreversibly damaged brain function. Each type of exposure seemed to affect different targets in the brain. This had significant implications for thimerosal, which is typically given after birth.[333]

Grandjean and his team had also found brain signaling delays among affected Faroese children in the follow-up study. As maternal and child mercury levels increased, irregularities became more pronounced. Heart function was also diminished. Children with the highest mercury levels in their blood were less able to maintain a normal heart rate, needed to supply oxygen to the body.

Finally, on February 5, Northeastern University released the methylation study by Richard Deth and colleagues—a full two months before its scheduled publication in *Molecular Psychiatry*. Their complex, novel work was virtually ignored by the American press (with a few exceptions, including a small article in *USA Today*).

In Canada, however, it was banner news. "Vaccine Additive Linked to Brain Damage in Children; Mercury-Based Preservative Tied to Autism, ADHD, U.S. Researchers Say," a typical headline read in the *Vancouver Sun*.[334] "After assuring parents that additives in vaccines don't cause brain damage, scientists have found what they believe could be a 'smoking gun' linking these additives to autism and attention-deficit hyperactivity disorder in children," the lead paragraph said.

It left Lyn, Liz, and Sallie reeling. They had never seen words like that in a mainstream American newspaper.

But many Canadian doctors were unimpressed. "What they are doing in the test tube may or may not have any relationship to what happens in the body," Dr. Ronald Gold, professor emeritus of pediatrics at the University of Toronto, told reporter Sharon Kirkey of CanWest News Service.[335] Of course, he was right. But the study bolstered the parents' case—at least from a public relations point of view—and opened a path for further research.

ON FEBRUARY 8, the night before the IOM showdown, about forty parents gathered in the Washington office of Jim Moody, the attorney who had advised Safe Minds since its inception. Lyn, Liz, and Sallie were there, along with Scott and Laura Bono, Jo Pike, Lori McIlwain, and Albert Enayati. Researchers presenting the next day included Boyd Haley, Jeff Bradstreet, and

Mark and David Geier. Most talk centered around the MTHFR gene. Jeff Bradstreet had nicknamed it the more pronounceable "mother-father gene." The Mercury Moms, however, called it the "motherfucker gene."

Spirits were guardedly high as the group took over the rear section of a restaurant overlooking the Potomac River. The guest of honor: Richard Deth, who had come down from Boston to attend the meeting. Everyone was in a fighting mood. They knew that the other side would present a mountain of epidemiological evidence to refute the thimerosal link. And there was no time scheduled for refuting what the CDC and others put forth.

But the parents and their collaborators thought they had at least a chance. They did not have large population studies, it was true, but they did have an interesting assortment of biological evidence, much of it extracted directly from their own kids. At the very least, they hoped to convince the IOM to maintain its finding of plausibility.

THE NATIONAL ACADEMIES, which include the IOM, are headquartered in an ornately neoclassical marble and tile building near the west end of the Mall, right across from the State Department in Foggy Bottom. The day-long meeting was staged in the surprisingly gaudy auditorium, a circa-1970 cavernous space lined with white concrete arches, just off the majestic vaulted and domed Great Hall.

The long day began at 8:00 A.M. and was combative and exhausting for all sides. The tension at times was palpable. The room was populated with pharmaceutical lawyers and PR reps, health bureaucrats and government researchers, CDC officials in their crisp military-style uniforms and private scientists, some neatly groomed and others rumpled, from both sides of the fence. Then there were the parents, perhaps sixty or more, hanging intently on to every word, or erupting into spontaneous applause rarely heard at medical meetings. Sometimes it felt more like a political debate than a scientific inquiry.

Part of the committee's mission was to conduct a two-pronged assessment of vaccine safety. There was a *causality* assessment, based on epidemiological data from large population studies and case reports. Then there was the evaluation of *biological mechanisms*, using samples collected from laboratory, animal, and human studies.

As it turned out, nearly all the evidence presented against the thimerosal theory was based on population studies (epidemiology), while arguments supporting the theory (except for some of the Geiers' work) used biological data collected from labs and clinics, often based on the blood, hair, and urine of autistic children.

What emerged was an extraordinarily murky and contradictory picture.

Epidemiological studies are extremely useful because their large numbers and high statistical power can detect even subtle differences in outcomes between groups in varying exposure categories. But epidemiological analysis is notoriously susceptible to misinterpretation, and even manipulation. Two sets of researchers can extract diametrically opposed results from the same data.

In order to demonstrate causation, therefore, epidemiological evidence must be backed up by consistent biological evidence. Immunology, toxicology, pathology, virology, and other disciplines must be brought to bear. But these types of studies are also subject to limitations—and criticism. Improper handling of specimens, contaminated work environments, and inconsistent or inferior lab work are often cited when biological research comes under fire. And results from in vitro studies performed in the lab sometimes bear no resemblance to what actually happens inside the body.

And so the day inexorably devolved into a muddled confrontation between the epidemiologists, who generally disputed the causality question, and the toxicologists and clinicians, who supported it.

Chairwoman Marie McCormick called the meeting to order as the fourteen-member committee filed into the first two rows of the auditorium, their backs to the audience. McCormick said that this would be the ninth in a series of meetings on "the hypothesized relationship between an adverse event and a vaccine." The committee had made no conclusions, and it would be "a mistake for anyone to leave here today thinking otherwise." The report would be issued in three months, pending review and revision.[336]

Much of the morning was given over to the epidemiologists, and it was a near slam dunk for the CDC side, with two exceptions. The first was Dave Weldon, who delivered the opening remarks and offered a barrage of criticism.

"I am very disturbed," he began, speaking in slow, quiet cadences, "by the continued number of reports I receive from researchers regarding their experiences. It is past time that individuals are persecuted for asking questions about vaccine safety."

Weldon said many researchers looking into the subject had encountered apathy from government officials, difficulty in getting papers published, and the loss of grants. "Others report overt discouragement, intimidation and threats, and have abandoned this field of research," he said. "Some have had their clinical privileges revoked and others have been hounded out of their institutions."

Weldon said that the "atmosphere of intimidation even surrounds today's hearing." He had received numerous complaints alleging that the event was "not a further attempt to get at the facts but rather a desire to sweep these issues under the rug."

Then Weldon blasted the government for its shabby treatment of Mark and David Geier. Their experience, "and what we have discovered subsequently," further undermined his confidence in the CDC's ability to monitor vaccine safety.

"The CDC erected excessive barriers and has imposed severe limits on access to the data," Weldon alleged, saying that:

- Researchers were not provided data collected beyond December 2000, impeding the chance for independent research on the effects of the removal of thimerosal.
- The IRB approval process forced researchers to seek approval from as many as seven IRBs—each with its own requirements.
- The CDC placed strict limits on what data was available, access to the complete database was virtually impossible, and data was made available on an inadequate PC.
- Raw data sets used by the CDC to conduct their studies were not made available to independent researchers. Only altered data sets were provided; "thus the CDC's work cannot be evaluated by outside researchers."

Weldon said that it took more than a year to secure access for the Geiers. And once they did get in, "it was quickly discovered that if you sort the VSD looking at the children who received thimerosal-free DTaP versus those who received thimerosal-containing DTaP, there is a dramatic, statistically significant increase in autism."

Weldon said that CDC director Gerberding assured him she would devote "additional time personally to this issue" and that she believed the research should not end with this meeting. She indicated her "desire to see this research continue and emphasized that we should let the truth prevail, regardless of the consequences."

After Weldon finished, to thunderous applause from half the room, most of the morning session was scheduled for research that refuted a thimerosal-autism connection. It was not clear whether the IOM staff realized that the first presenter, Dr. Mady Hornig, would start the session with powerful and graphic biological evidence of increased harm from mercury exposure in genetically predispositioned animals.

Dr. Hornig was an associate professor of epidemiology at Columbia University. Her work focused on how infection, immune disturbances, and neurotoxins lead to neurodevelopmental disorders and nervous system dysfunction. Young, bright, and personable with a mop of black curly hair, Hornig received sixty thousand dollars from Safe Minds, among other grants, to help study the effect of thimerosal on genetically sensitive mice.

Hornig discussed her animal research, including the effect of environmental insults on infant animals, and how their disease type differs radically from that of adult rats exposed to the same substances. "One cannot necessarily translate what is done in an adult system to what is relevant for a neonatal organism," she said.

Hornig and colleagues studied infant rats infected with Borna disease virus, not because autistic children have that virus, but because "it is a good model for understanding developmental sensitivity." Adult rats showed a very different response than newborn animals, even though they were infected with the same virus. Disease manifestations were based on the maturity of the immune and nervous systems.

In the adult rats infected with Borna, Hornig's colleagues found heightened "startle responses," involuntary motor movements, and encephalitis (swelling of the brain). But in the infant rats, there was hyperactivity and a range of social disturbances to play behavior, she said, "reminiscent of the disorder that we know as autism."

For example, the young infected animals were unable to right themselves in the proper way. Instead of turning over from their backs in corkscrew fashion (where the upper torso turns first, followed by the rest of the body), they could only turn over "en bloc," by rocking over their entire body at once. In humans, normal infants right themselves in a corkscrew, while many autistic babies turn over "en bloc," Hornig said.

The infected neonatal rats also developed social communication problems. When separated from their mothers, they emitted an "abnormal waveform," an unusual increase in calls. "We believe these calls fail to elicit the mother's normal maternal response, certainly, evidence of social communicative disturbance."

Hornig also reported that damage to Purkinje brain cells, whose destruction is reportedly associated with autism, appeared in the infected rats as well. The rats also showed altered brain chemistries that often appear in autistic children following autopsy.

"So what do we learn from this model?" Hornig asked. "We know that genes, environment, and timing all interact with one another. We know that there is a wide variety of infectious agents that have very similar effects, and probably other xenobiotic [foreign] agents that have similar effects." Rats with certain genetic mutations, she added, differed in their susceptibity to Borna virus from those without the mutations.

"This brings us to the mouse strain–dependent model of ethylmercury neurotoxicity," Hornig said. "The sensitivity in mice predicts neurotoxic effects following postnatal thimerosal. We hypothesize that it would not be just any individual that would have these effects, but rather those that had a specific genetic vulnerability that created a mercury-related sensitivity." Eighteen percent of the human population has skin sensitivity to thimerosal, she noted. Population differences also occur in natural levels of glutathione and metallothionein.

Hornig's team replicated the childhood immunization schedule in mice, devising a microgram-per-kilogram dose at day 7, day 9, day 11, and day 15, which roughly mirrored the human schedule in terms of relative developmental milestones. Day 7, which roughly reflected the two-month dose in humans, was chosen to "come close to the end of most migrational events in brain," Hornig explained.

"We looked at mouse strains that were known to have differential sensitivity," she said. One strain was sensitive to mercury, and the other two had less sensitivity. Once exposed, the sensitive mice showed significant delay in weight gain. There was also "behavioral impoverishment" with highly significant effects in the sensitive strain.

Even more alarming, some 40 percent of the mice at six months became "self-mutilatory," frantically grooming themselves or biting on their tails compulsively. "One animal, who wildly self-grooms, not only takes care of his partner, but he also grooms his partner," she said, putting up a photo of two mice. "He has groomed through the skull, and eventually destroys his partner," Hornig said. Every parent of an autistic kid in the room could be seen grimacing in dark recognition of such destructive behavior.

Hornig also found severe brain disturbances in the sensitive mice that were not found in the less sensitive strains. The sensitive mice had enlarged brains, which have been noted in autistic children by some researchers, including Margaret Bauman.

"We know that host-response genes are really critical in determining sensitivity to mercury-induced autoimmune disturbances in this animal model," Hornig concluded. "Postnatal xenobiotic challenges are at least possible in these types of settings. Of course, we need to determine the relevance of animal models for human neural development."

The rest of the morning produced little more than a string of broadsides against the vaccine hypothesis. First up was Dr. Kumanan Wilson, of the Toronto General Research Institute, who reviewed much, if not all of the published medical literature on the connection between MMR and autism. His report roundly refuted any association. Wilson was followed by Frank DeStefano, who presented data showing that children vaccinated with MMR at eighteen months were no more likely to develop autism than children vaccinated with MMR at thirty-six months.

Then came Dr. Elizabeth Miller, Head of the Immunisation Division of the UK's Public Health Laboratory Service. Miller, who spoke with an educated British accent and could charitably be described as aloof, chided the American doctors for attaining lower vaccination rates than in the UK. It endeared her to no one.

Miller's presentation was unanticipated by the parents. The data she presented was yet another epidemiological affront to the thimerosal hypothesis. The new and still unpublished study was sponsored by the World Health Organization, which wanted to determine whether it was safe to continue using thimerosal in the developing world. The British team examined medical records of some 100,000 children, which were collected into a database quite similar to that of the VSD.

The only thimerosal-containing vaccine in the UK is DTP. Beginning in 1991, the country accelerated the DTP series from three, five, and ten months to two, three, and four months. Still, the total mercury burden for British children at six months of age (75 micrograms) was less than half that of U.S. children who received the full schedule of immunizations by the same age (187.5 micrograms).

Researchers found that children who received all three doses of DTP were no more at risk of developmental disorders than children who received two, one, or zero doses. In fact, the British team discovered, vaccination with thimerosal-containing DTP seemed to have a somewhat "protective" effect on children. Fully vaccinated children had a risk of autism of 0.94 (or 6 percent less likely) compared with unvaccinated children. Other outcomes with apparently reduced risks among vaccinated children included ADD (0.82, or 18 percent less likely) and "unspecified delay" (.084, or 16 percent less likely).

The conclusion, Miller announced, was that the study did not show "any evidence of increased risk, as in the preliminary analyses of the VSD study, and no reason for WHO to accelerate changes in [developing] countries to thimerosal-free vaccines, particularly as withdrawal of thimerosal-containing vaccines may have very substantial health risks for those populations."

It was a serious blow. And now the data would be entered into the official IOM record without so much as a whimper of dissent. Half the room, one could sense, was pleased. The other half looked glum.

Lyn, Sallie, and Liz all frowned and slowly shook their heads. They knew that more was to follow in the punishing hours ahead, including the Denmark and VSD studies, before their side could present the evidence it had amassed.

Robert Davis, the pediatrics professor from the University of Washington, made the formal presentation of the VSD study as published in *Pediatrics*. He walked the audience through the most recent data. Much to the surprise of the parents, Davis brought up the previous incarnations of the VSD study, including the initial unreleased report that Safe Minds had obtained through FOIA.

It was the first official public explanation of what had transpired over the four generations of analyses.

"Our initial findings were somewhat worrisome," Davis conceded, noting that the team found an "increased risk of nearly 2.5 times among children who received 62.5 micrograms ethylmercury at three months, versus 37.5 micrograms of exposure." Although the finding did not meet the criteria for statistical significance, "it certainly was cause for concern on my part and on other's parts, and internally."

This finding was precisely why the researchers wanted to collect more data before making a final determination. "We wanted to continue to accrue data, assuming that, if this were a real finding, we wanted to know about it," Davis explained. "The finding, if anything, should obtain statistical significance if we were able to add more cases as they accrued in the data set."

The updated data sets included an extended follow-up period, which allowed additional autism cases to be identified. During this period, the exclusion criteria were also "modified," Davis said, "based on scientific input from yourselves, from the CDC, from VSD investigators and others."

When the team presented their data at Simpsonwood and the ACIP in June 2000, "we had, at this point, more than twice as many cases," Davis said, without explaining how the caseload managed to double in just six months since the initial report, which was done in February 2000. Nor did he explain why the highest relative risk for autism had fallen from 2.48 to 1.69 in the intervening period. One year later, when the same team presented the same study to the IOM committee, the highest group had a relative risk of 1.52. Again, Davis offered no reason for this decline.

Davis then launched into an unexpected and preemptive strike against the Geiers, who were scheduled to present their own VSD findings a bit later in the day. "There have been some recent outside analyses of VSD data," he said. "They were asking whether, among children that got a minimum of either three consecutive thimerosal-containing DTaPs or three consecutive thimerosal-free DTaPs, there was a difference in the number of autism cases in the two groups.

"That is a very nice hypothesis, and it certainly is one that can be addressed."

The outside investigators claimed to have found "large differences, more than 20 times higher," Davis said. "This, of course, was very concerning to us. Had we missed a signal that was present in our data that we, in fact, should have seen?"

To find out, Davis and colleagues tried to replicate the Geier analysis using the same data. They limited their analysis to children born after 1997, since only these children had the chance of receiving a thimerosal-free DTaP shot. The group looked at all children receiving DTaP between 1997 and 2000, and broke them down into five exposure categories: 0, 25, 50, 75, and 100 micrograms, depending on which vaccines they had received.

Among these children, there were 76 cases of autism, he said. "And we find what the investigators found, which is that there are, in fact, very large differences" in overall risks depending on exposure. Davis put up a slide showing a striking trend.

EXPOSURE	RISK
–0 μg	(reference)
–25 μg	4.81
–50 μg	4.75
–75 μg	6.72
–100+ μg	18.43

The parents were puzzled. What was Davis up to? Was he really going to confirm the same findings claimed by the Geiers? That seemed unlikely. And it turned out not to be the case. "There is, however, a substantial issue, problem, other shoe that has to drop here," Davis said with a dramatic flourish. "It had to do with age. Children in the lower exposure categories were much younger than those in the higher categories, because they were far more likely to get all thimerosal-free vaccines than the older kids."

EXPOSURE	MEDIAN AGE AT LAST FOLLOW-UP
–0 μg	1.03
–25 μg	1.91
–50 μg	1.82
–75 μg	2.20
–100+ μg	2.92

Why was this important? "If you remember our study of autism," Davis said, "the median diagnosis date of autism is 4.4 years. Children with 100 μg of exposure had 2.2 years of available follow-up." These children "had up to three times more opportunity to be diagnosed with autism. In other words, age at last follow-up has the opportunity in these data to act as a confounder."

Lyn was stunned by what she was hearing. "Can you believe this?" she said to Sallie and Liz. "Davis is using the exact same too-young-to-be-diagnosed argument against the Geiers' study that we used against the CDC!"

If Davis was aware of the irony, he wasn't saying so. He continued to pummel the Geiers. "We reanalyzed these data, matching cases to controls on month and year of birth, which will equalize the group according to the length of follow-up and the ability to be diagnosed with autism," Davis said. "Now we see no statistical association."

EXPOSURE	RISK
−0 μg	(reference)
−25 μg	1.10
−50 μg	0.93
−75 μg	0.75
−100+ μg	1.21

"In all situations, it looks as if they are simply random snapshots of the data taken from the same bell-shaped curve," Davis concluded. "In other words, there is no evidence here of an increased risk for autism in this analysis." Davis never said it, but the obvious inference was that the Geiers had made the same mistake (or deliberate manipulation) in their findings. It was an allegation that the Geiers would fiercely refute.

In the question-and-answer session, a committee member asked Davis a simple but potentially loaded question: "Do you expect to find any association between thimerosal and autism?"

Davis seemed to vacillate from certainty to neutrality. "I don't," he replied quickly, but then added: "I think we are going to learn a lot about autism, and I think we are going to learn a lot about environmental influences. I actually have no honest-to-God feeling about it one way or another. I haven't even attempted to formulate an expectation prior to launching the study, one way or another."

Liz looked at Lyn and Sallie and laughed silently, as if to say, "Yeah, right."

Next up was Anders Peter Hviid, from the State Serum Institute in Copenhagen, to present the data from Denmark that had been published in *JAMA*. The study showed that pertussis vaccination with or without thimerosal made no statistically significant difference in autism outcomes.

"The results we obtained are not compatible with the hypothesis of causal association between thimerosal-containing vaccines and autism or other autistic spectrum disorder," he announced in a halting Scandinavian accent.

Hviid was not prepared for the grilling he was about to receive. Boyd Haley was first to the microphone. "What I am wondering is if we are really comparing two similar incidences," he said in his Kentucky voice. "The rate of autism per 10,000 in Denmark compared to the United States and Britain, could you tell me what those are?"

The Danish doctor seemed not to understand. "Come again?" he said.

"I would like to know," Haley repeated, "what is the rate per 10,000 of autistic children born in Denmark versus the United States and Britain?"

It was more than a trivial question. Total exposures in Denmark had been a fraction of those in the United States. One might expect to see a lower rate of autism as well (which indeed was the case, with about 3 to 6 per 10,000 in Denmark and 40 to 60 per 10,000 in the United States). "I don't have the numbers from the U.S. or Britain," Hviid replied. "In our cohort, you can calculate the crude incidence rates from this table here and from—"

"I *know* I can," Haley interrupted, with uncharacteristically unsouthern brusqueness. "But I would expect you to know that. I mean, it's what is printed in all the papers—"

Haley was stopped by Dr. McCormick, who runs a tight meeting. "I think he has answered your question," she said, cutting Haley off.

The last presentation before the break was Mark and David Geier. The Geiers, it is fair to say, suffered from their own overpreparation. Their Power-Point presentation consisted of 101 slides, far too many to get through in the twenty minutes allotted. The overload of information they tried to convey was barely contained in a twelve-hundred-page document submitted to the committee in advance. Instead, they ended up flipping quickly through slides, stopping here or there to explain things, then moving on. They played tag team, handing off comments to one another in a presentation that may have hindered their credibility.

David Geier opened by stating that when he and his father were first approached about thimerosal, "we were among the most highly skeptical people of all." Indeed, when the IOM held its last hearing on the subject, "we didn't have any evidence, we didn't believe in what was being said at all, and we were, and still are, strongly pro-vaccine."

The two men then ran through the epidemiology they themselves had done, including their studies from VAERS (where they found a relative risk of 6.0) and, of course, from the VSD.

"Most recently, we have gone to the Vaccine Safety Datalink," David said, preparing to blunt the argument made by Davis. "Issues have been raised about that. We present this in direct response to what was said."

David said the relative risk of 27 was found among children who had received all four of their DTaP shots, and not three, as Davis had said. "Lo and behold, when you do this—and by making it four doses, we are talking about children that are eighteen months to two years old," which was older than kids in the Davis data set, "these children had time to have a diagnosis of autism. You find similar stark results as those we found from VAERS. By requiring four doses of vaccine, DTaP is given two, four, six, fifteen to eighteen months, we are extending the period of immunization out far enough that we are into the time of diagnosis."

And, Mark Geier added, "the chart that was shown [by Davis] to show that we were wrong, showed one dose of DTaP, when we excluded those children. In order to get into our study, and we are trying to do more studies, but we are being interfered with, you had to have taken four doses of DTaP. So to show up there that they are under a year [in the Davis numbers] I don't know how they did it, but it is not how we did it."

Mark Geier's face hardened in anger. "This is not a scientific issue, this is about as proven an issue as you are ever going to see," he said, feeding off the rising applause from parents in the audience. "What is occurring here is a cover-up, under the guise of protecting the vaccine program. And I am for the vaccine program. If you keep covering it up, you are not going to have a vaccine program."

As he closed, Mark left the panel with a powerful final thought. Namely, if thimerosal had not caused the apparent spike in autism cases, then what was it?

"If the committee determines, despite what I think is the overwhelming evidence that thimerosal is strongly contributing to this epidemic, that either they are not sure or there isn't an effect, I would suggest that you recommend spending $10 billion or $20 billion to go find out what you think is causing this epidemic."

But nobody was rushing to do that. "The reason, I purport to you, is that it is well known to the authorities." If thimerosal was found not to be the culprit, "then this society is going to be in big trouble. We cannot have a generation of people damaged the way this is happening. Our answer is that we are going to build homes for these people? We had better prevent it from happening anymore."

The room, or half of it anyway, exploded into applause, whistles, and cheers, lasting for minutes.

For the parents, things started to appear brighter from that point on. The next speaker was H. Vasken Aposhian, professor of molecular and cellular biology and pharmacology at the University of Arizona. With his ring of salt-white hair wrapping around the back of his bald head like a skirt, Aposhian looked like a Hollywood version of a mad professor. But his words were sound.

"I am here to present a toxicologist's view of thimerosal in autism," Aposhian opened. "Three years ago, I didn't even know what autism was. Because of a number of reasons, primarily political reasons, I was asked to learn about autism, and have become fairly familiar with the subject."

Aposhian postulated that autism is caused by what he termed an "efflux disorder." He offered an example of another efflux disorder called Wilson's disease, a movement disorder caused by an inherited metabolic disease. It has very definite central nervous system symptoms, due to a genetic mutation. Wilson's disease was first described in the late 1800s, but only in the past three years was the genetic mutation identified.

Scientists now know it was caused by a mutation in the ATP7B gene, Aposhian said. "ATP7B is a copper transport protein. The signs and symptoms of Wilson's disease are the accumulation of copper in the tissues. The ATP7B copper transport protein is expressed primarily in the liver, and it is deficient and lacking in Wilson's disease." The disorder causes liver and central nervous system copper accumulation to the point of toxicity. Wilson's disease is one of the rare treatable genetic disorders. "Not very many genetic disorders can be treated," he noted. "In this case, there is a group of chelating agents that have been used very successfully, they have kept people alive."

Aposhian projected some slides based on the Amy Holmes baby hair study, showing that autistic kids were found with significantly lower mercury hair levels than controls. "One can always criticize an experiment," he admitted. "This experiment could be criticized that it wasn't done in a research environment, the hair was sent off to a commercial lab. There are many things one could say." But he pointed out it was a "very, very important" study. And Aposhian startled everyone in the room, parents included, when he announced: "It has now been confirmed."

Days before, Aposhian had come across a paper on baby hair by researchers at the Massachusetts Institute of Technology. "This paper is from three nuclear scientists who went out and got the hair, did the analysis at MIT, using neutron activation analysis," he said. The results confirmed what Holmes had found. "There is no question the results were the same, remarkably close."

The two papers strongly indicated that autistic children "lack an effective mercury efflux system," he said. Typical individuals benefit from a natural efflux system that binds glutathione molecules with mercury, removing it from tissue and into the blood and hair follicles. "In the autistic child, you are going to see a block," Aposhian said. "The mercury supposedly cannot leave the tissue to get into the blood."

If autism were a mercury efflux disorder, the professor said, it would be quite easy to determine definitively. He would simply analyze tissue. Aposhian had called colleagues around the world looking for tissue from autistic individuals to examine for mercury accumulation. "I was shocked to learn that no one has such data," he said. "It is really amazing to me as a scientist that no one has taken the tissue from autistic children to see whether mercury is accumulating there, especially since the idea of mercury being high in children with autism has been around for some time."

Aposhian was well aware of the legal implications, he said. "If I were a CEO of a company that made thimerosal, I would want to know. If I were the parent of an autistic child, I would want to know if there is a lot of mercury in the tissue of autistic children. If there is, then there is no question that they have a mercury efflux disorder."

The thimerosal theory "has become more plausible," he concluded. "I think after studying it very, very carefully, I believe it has become more plausible than when your committee first discussed the subject. Thimerosal appears to add organic mercury to the mercury burden of children with mercury efflux disorder."

No one had expected to hear anything like this. It was a powerful presentation. Committee member Dr. Bayer asked Aposhian about any clinical or epidemiological evidence "that lends credence to the theory you have put forward."

"I am going to call some people and get some tissue from autistic children, and analyze it," he answered. "I think that will be the key question. It has nothing to do with epidemiology. Epidemiology, as I'm sure you know, has been wrong many times. Epidemiology just shows a correlation or not. It does not show cause and effect."

Bayer seemed offended. "So-called bench science has been wrong, too."

"Of course," Aposhian replied. "We are the first to admit it. I want to make it clear that this is a hypothesis. We have gone with as much hard experimental evidence as I think we have. What really tipped me, I must say, was the MIT study. That tipped me enough to have much more confidence in the single experiments that were done before."

David Baskin, who was no longer officially associated with Safe Minds, gave his data on brain cell death triggered by exposure to even miniscule amounts of thimerosal. For a number of years, Baskin's lab at Baylor University had looked at various methods of measuring "apoptosis," a form of self-induced cell death. There are various methods: a test for the enzyme caspace-3, which is activated in apoptosis; a test looking at membrane permeability with dye; and a newer, more sensitive test that looks at changes in a critical cell component called mitochondria. Researchers can also examine cells with light and an electron microscope, to assess them visually.

Baskin and colleagues cultured brain cells and incubated them with thimerosal. After six hours, cellular damage was noted as well as activation of caspace-3, which, he said, indicated apoptosis. The team found the lowest toxic concentration at six hours was just two micromolars of mercury, or two-billionths of a gram.

After twenty-four hours, the lowest toxic dose dropped to about one micromole, showing increased sensitivity with longer exposure. Baskin was able to document DNA damage, nuclear membrane damage, and caspase-3 activation in these cells.

Then he projected slides of the dye test, clearly showing that, as cell membranes were damaged, they were invaded by a dark blue dye as the membrane was perforated. These were cells from adults, however, which would be less susceptible to damage than cells from infants.

Baskin's team studied immune cells from autistic children's blood, and compared them to blood from unaffected siblings to see if there was a difference.

They treated cells at different doses for twenty-four hours. The normal children exhibited no statistically significant increase in caspace-3, but the autistic child did.

Baskin emphasized that his work was preliminary, and not ready for publication.

He then turned to the researcher sitting in a back row in the auditorium, Richard Deth. Baskin quipped that Deth would "probably cringe" from the oversimplification of his work, but he lauded the Northeastern University professor's work on methionine, methionine synthase, synthase and methylatin.

Baskin noted that all gene regulation is based on methylation. Gene activity is silenced with the addition of methyl groups to DNA, while activity is stimulated when methyl groups are removed. Therefore, someone who was deficient in methionine synthase would have decreased methylation. The result would be that all those genes that were silenced would become activated. Recent studies indicated that autistic children have low levels of methionine and methionine synthase, Baskin noted. And, he said, decreased methionine synthase also decreases levels of glutathione. He insisted that none of this is speculative: it was well documented by reputable research.

The next speaker was Dr. Polly Sager, assistant director for international research at the National Institute of Allergy and Infectious Diseases, a branch of the NIH better known for its work in HIV/AIDS, anthrax, and other deadly disorders.

Dr. Sager presented findings from a government-funded study of primates (macaques) born and raised at the University of Washington. Infant apes were divided into two groups. One group received vaccines with 20 micrograms of ethylmercury at birth, one week, two weeks, and three weeks. The other group was given equal doses of methylmercury, consumed orally.

The young apes were "sacrificed," and blood and brain samples were sent to researchers at the University of Rochester for analysis by Dr. Tom Clarkson, one of the world's foremost authorities on mercury toxicity. Clarkson found that the initial absorption and distribution of both methyl- and ethylmercury were similar. However, ethylmercury was eliminated from the blood much more quickly (half-life: nine days) than methylmercury (half-life: twenty-five days). And he found that ethylmercury "washed out" of the brain in eighteen days, while it took fifty-nine days for the methylmercury to clear. Blood accumulation in the ethylmercury group was minimal, while the methylmercury continued to accumulate throughout the exposure period.

On the other hand, Clarkson did discover that the brain-to-blood mercury ratio was much higher in the ethylmercury group than in the methylmercury group: 5.1 times more mercury in their brain than in their blood, versus 3.4 times more in the brain. Even so, Sager said this failed to make up for the "much shorter half-life and much greater clearance of thimerosal-derived mercury from the systemic circulation."

This time, Lyn was first to the microphone. Given that there was a higher brain-to-blood ratio in the ethylmercury group, she asked, "Could it be the fact that ethylmercury more rapidly seems to change over to inorganic mercury, which would account for more accumulation in the brain?"

Dr. Sager did not know. "That certainly is one possible explanation," she said.

After Sager, it was Boyd Haley's turn to present his toxicology studies, where neurons exposed to thimerosal and testosterone died the most quickly of all. He also presented data on the baby hair study. Initiated by Amy Holmes and coauthored by Boyd and Mark Blaxill, the paper had been published in the *International Journal of Toxicology*. Normal children had a mean hair mercury level of 3.7 parts per million, and some ranged as high as 19 ppm. But autistic children had levels at or below 1 ppm.

The next slide was "the most telling" he said. As cases became more severe, hair mercury dropped. "There is in my opinion an inability to excrete mercury that is paramount in this disease," Haley said, adding that "males will get this disease or become affected with autism even if they are better excretors than females."

As one moves across the graph, the number of female cases drops. "Invariably they are below the line, indicating that they have to be much poorer excretors to become autistic than the boys," Haley said. "When we get to the end, there was only one female in the group, so this does have a gender property as well as a biochemical property."

As the day dragged slowly to a close, Jeffrey Bradstreet gave his review of virtually all the new data accumulated since he had spoken before the committee in July 2001. He presented his chelation study showing that autistic kids treated with chelation had excreted nearly six times more mercury than vaccinated controls. And he walked the committee through the complicated work of Deth, James, and Boris and Goldblatt and the complexities of MTHFR, the methionine cycle, methylation, and the transulfuration pathway.

FIGURE 12. Birth hair mercury levels of nonautistic versus autistic children.

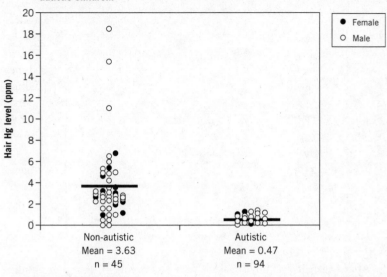

Source: Amy S. Holmes, Mark F. Blaxill, and Boyd E. Haley, "Reduced Levels of Mercury in First Baby Haircuts of Autistic Children," *International Journal of Toxicology*, 22 (2003):277–85.

Bradstreet also presented evidence of persistent viral infection. "We found measles virus in the G.I. tract of kids with autism," he said. "It was typed to the vaccine strain. That told me we needed to look at the cerebral spinal fluid (CFS)."

His group looked at three boys (including Matthew Birt) with autistic regression following MMR, and enterocolitis confirmed by endoscopy. Two of the three boys had measles virus in their blood, and all three had virus in the cerebrospinal fluid. Spinal taps from three control children being treated for another disease showed zero virus.

Bradstreet and others eventually did spinal taps on twenty-eight autistic children, and found that 70 percent of them had measles virus RNA in their spinal fluid. They also examined the spinal fluid of about forty control children (who were being treated for leukemia) and found that only one of them had measles virus.

A half hour remained in the meeting, and this was allotted to public comment. Dr. McCormick reminded everyone that the committee had to leave at 6:00 P.M. and not a minute later. Public comment would be held to its limit.

It was the emotional pinnacle of a killing day. One by one, parents rose from their chairs to tell the committee about their children, about the high

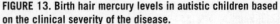

FIGURE 13. Birth hair mercury levels in autistic children based on the clinical severity of the disease.

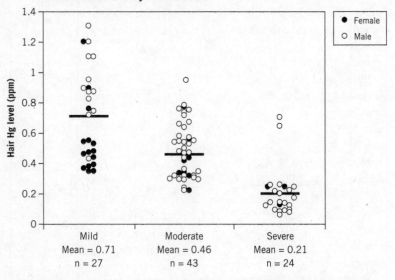

Source: Amy S. Holmes, Mark F. Blaxill, and Boyd E. Haley, "Reduced Levels of Mercury in First Baby Haircuts of Autistic Children," *International Journal of Toxicology*, 22 (2003):277–85.

levels of mercury and measles virus they had found, and the promise of chelation and other interventions helping to bring their kids, and themselves, from the brink of despair.

"I was told when my son was three that he would probably be dead by five," Scott Bono said haltingly. "So much for that doctor's opinion. We have been chelating for three years. Jackson Bono passed the seventh grade standard course of study test for the state of North Carolina. . . .

"I want my son to be working. Most of all, I just want my son to fall in love, to have a friend." He looked unblinkingly at the panel and continued. "*You* hold the public trust. The greatest threat to the trust in our public immunization program lies with the people who profit most from it. They are the greatest threat right now. You are looked up to and looked to for scientific advice, reason, and logic. It is thousands of children who may not ever go to that human condition that each of you already have. You have fallen in love, you have had a friend. That's all I want."

Liz Birt was more blunt in her message. She brought in full-color copies of the results of her son's most recent colonoscopy and endoscopy. "Three weeks ago, I received a call from the school nurse that she was going to have to call an ambulance because my son was in pain on the floor for two hours, grabbing his stomach and pounding on his chest," she told the hushed auditorium. "So I called the GI and my son was scoped. His disease has progressed to the point that he has terrible esophagitis, lesions in his bowel, his colon is diseased, and it is a progressive meltdown of his G.I. tract. He also has measles virus in his spinal fluid.

"I do believe there is a subset of children at risk for this type of thing," Liz continued, trying not to lose it. "I think thimerosal plays a role in that it skews the immune system and makes their bodies so they can't accept a live virus. I have laboratory documents documenting all of this. I live with this every day. I think the epidemiology won't answer this question. It is going to be the science looking at these children individually to see what caused this, and how to fix it."

Then, in the waning moments of the afternoon came a gripping sermon delivered by Lisa Sykes, pastor of the Christ United Methodist Church in Richmond, Virginia, and the mother of an autistic boy, Wesley. Sykes spoke in an almost theatrical, meditative southern drawl, and her testimony flowed like words from a lost O'Neill play.

Sykes had brought a blowup of her son's chelation reports, plotted on a graph and held aloft by three moms. "The graph shows mercury dumps," she said. "After we got all this mercury out of my child, who is now eight years old, he is finally starting to learn.

"I am not anti-vaccine," Sykes drawled. "I have got a passion right now to be intently and doggedly anti-thimerosal until this does not happen to other children. We have gotten rid of infectious disease and have exchanged it for lifelong and widespread developmental disorders that our children may never recover from. We are decimating an entire branch of the genetic family tree. . . .

"I have lost one," she continued. By now many parents were sobbing. "I have a healthy younger son. You can more easily put a gun to my head and pull the trigger than you could inject thimerosal into that baby!"

The day concluded with tears and applause from half the room. The other half looked grim and perturbed.

THERE WERE no "winners" coming out of IOM; neither side conclusively proved its case. The committee had listened intently to all speakers. They had asked tough questions of both sides, and at least tried to appear objective in their approach. But the parents walked away with very mixed feelings. Their side had done well today: the science looked sound and most of the presentations were effective. But the meeting was confusing and the message muddled. No one expected the IOM committee to make any groundbreaking new pronouncements when it issued its report in May.

"I wish we were walking out of here feeling victorious, but I don't think we are," Lyn said to Sallie when they filed out of the auditorium. Even so, the women felt they had achieved something. The mercury-autism theory was still alive.

Laura Bono was steeped in mixed emotions. "I'm hopeful that something will come of this, you know what an optimist I am," she told her husband, Scott. But Laura also thought the committee had not given their side a fair hearing, that most of the panel members had already made up their minds. "I just can't believe that so many people could hear the evidence we presented and still not see the light," she said. "The meeting seemed like a bunch of blind people in a room full of deaf people."

Like most of the parents, Laura and Scott were impressed with Jeff Bradstreet. "He pulled all the research together into one congruent conclusion," Laura said. "And I was pinching myself that we had come so far. But it breaks my heart to think how many years it took to get here. How many children were affected as our public health officials went through their lives in denial? What if someone in power had listened to us earlier?"

"So many what-ifs . . . ," Scott said, "and we will probably never know."

When they got home, many of those present shared their thoughts with each other.

"As I flew home, I was thinking about the meeting, and it struck me as ridiculous," wrote Boyd Haley, the University of Kentucky researcher.[337] "Here was a Full Professor of Chemistry/Biochemistry testifying before one of the most highly regarded medical committees in the USA and perhaps the world, and I was trying to convince this committee that it was a bad idea to inject an extremely neural-toxic compound into a day-old infant. This does not reflect very well on our society or American medicine."

Liz Birt had done some thinking on her flight, too. "I kept thinking about what has happened to my life," she wrote to the other parents. The sight of so many thimerosal defenders at the IOM was sickening, she continued in an achingly emotional tone. "Their arrogance has led to the largest mass scale poisoning this country and world has ever seen. The day will come when they will have to answer for their negligence and disregard for the lives of the children that they were entrusted to treat with care. I will do everything possible to make sure justice is served."

And even though Liz would have done anything "to reverse the course of events that led to Matthew's illness in a heartbeat," she said, "I can't imagine going through this without your support. The next step is to 'FREE VSD,' and Jim Moody and I are working on it. Without good epidemiology we are going to have a tough time making our case and getting help for these children and their families."

Press coverage of the IOM meeting was considerable and, for the most part, balanced. Reporters noted that CDC researchers had found "no consistent link" between vaccines and autism, but almost invariably added that the contention was disputed by other scientists. It showed how much progress the "crazy" mercury people had made.

The *New York Times,* for instance, reported that medical experts had "squared off" at the meeting, and portrayed the proceedings as a showdown between epidemiologists and toxicologists.[338] Most of the epidemiologists doubted that thimerosal was responsible, the *Times* said. "But a few toxicologists said they had become more and more convinced of a potential link." Mercury levels were higher in children with autism, they said, suggesting that those kids "might have biochemical defects that prevented them from processing the metal as efficiently as do normal children."

Boyd Haley told the panel that "his studies had shown that testosterone might fuel the toxic effects of mercury," the *Times* continued, noting that "autism overwhelmingly affects boys." In addition, "two outsiders," Mark and David Geier, "examined the CDC data and came to the conclusion that thimerosal was causing autism." Such respectful, mainstream coverage of the mercury-autism theory, the parents knew, would have been unthinkable even a few short months before.

But then the *Wall Street Journal* weighed in, again.

On February 18, 2004, the paper lashed out against the flood of protest that had erupted after its last editorial attacking the parents and their avaricious attorneys.

"Everyone in our business learns to take a punch, but even we've been surprised by the furious response to an editorial a few weeks ago about vaccines," the column began. "Lost in the controversy has been a little thing called science."

The editors believed it was important to note "that nothing currently exists in the medical world to justify this furor."

To the editor's surprise, they had "wandered into a hornet's nest of moral intimidation." They claimed to have received letters and e-mails accusing them of "fraud," a "terrorist act." "We've been told we belong to a vast conspiracy—including researchers, pediatricians, corporations, health officials and politicians—devoted to poisoning their children. A few have harassed our secretaries and threatened an editorial writer. . . .

"We aren't about to shut up," the editors continued, noting that "these activists are using the same tactics in an attempt to silence others with crucial roles in public health and scientific research. Doctors who have spoken about the benefits of vaccination—Paul Offit and Samuel Katz (the co-creator of the measles vaccine)—have been targeted as baby killers and compared to Hitler.

Aided by trial lawyers, the intimidation has spread to Congress. Vaccine makers receive some liability protection from the federal Vaccine Injury Compensation Program—which pays out to the rare family whose child is injured by vaccines. But tort lawyers have exploited loopholes to file billion-dollar thimerosal suits that could bankrupt the few remaining vaccine makers. When Republican Majority Leader Bill Frist tried to modernize VICP—and require autism claims to go through the program like everyone else—the autism police went to work. They camped out in Washington and convinced three Republican Senators to kill any liability protection."[339]

MARK GEIER had been quoted in the *New York Times* coverage, but he wasn't getting any respect at the CDC. In mid-February 2004, the Geiers began receiving letters from HMOs that participate in the Vaccine Safety Datalink, suspending permission to peruse their patient files. Before long, all seven HMOs in the system had rejected the Geiers, even managed care companies they had never contacted for permission.

The HMOs told the Geiers that permission was suspended until they responded to "issues" raised by the CDC. They had no idea what the issues were, until one of the Kaiser-affiliated HMOs sent them a copy of the letter they had received from the CDC. The CDC letter said that the men had breached patient confidentiality and had run programs for an "illegal" vaccine analysis: they had proposed studying the effect of DTaP on autism and other disorders, but they had not specifically written in their proposal that they would be looking at thimerosal-free versus thimerosal-containing shots.

In the letter that the researchers were never meant to see, the CDC also accused the Geiers of trying to illegally take copies of the data out of the facility.

The Geiers brought the matter to Dave Weldon, who tried to intervene on their behalf. "There is no way we could have copied that and taken it out," David Geier told Weldon. "We are talking about many hundreds of megabytes. It would take a whole pile of CDs to hold all of that."

Now that they were frozen out of the data, they would not be able to publish what they had found. "The CDC claims it is contraband information, obtained illegally," David Geier told Weldon. "No one will publish it now. They must be in seventh heaven at CDC."

The Geiers were not the only ones under fire from the public health establishment. Andrew Wakefield, the English doctor who had associated regressive autistic symptoms with MMR, was embroiled in controversy yet again.

In late February, the editor of the *Lancet,* which had originally published his MMR study back in 1998, said the publication had found that Wakefield had a "fatal conflict of interest" after it emerged that the doctor had not disclosed he was also carrying out a study for a legal aid association on behalf of parents who believed the vaccine had harmed their children.[340] Had he known, the editor said, he would never have published the paper. The UK's health secretary, John Reid, asked the General Medical Council, a doctors' watchdog group, to investigate Wakefield "as a matter of urgency."

Wakefield refused to back down. In fact, he openly welcomed an inquiry.

News of the Wakefield scandal made headlines around the world. Most reports mentioned that fears over the MMR jab had sparked a drop in vaccination rates in Britain, and outbreaks of measles in various parts of the country.

LISA SYKES, the soft-spoken pastor from Richmond, Virginia, with an autistic son, the woman who had closed the IOM meeting with her impassioned testimonial, had been quietly pursuing a different approach. Lisa came from a "federal family," she liked to say. Both of her parents had been CIA employees, and her father had received the Intelligence Medal of Merit. Lisa was raised to respect the federal government: most of her immediate family worked for federal agencies or in law enforcement.

Lisa had been writing letters to government officials about mercury in vaccines since 2000, when her autistic son Wesley had excreted so much of the metal after his second round of chelation that the line of his lab results literally ran off the charts. She asked for a total recall of vaccines containing more than a trace of thimerosal.

At first, she directed her correspondence to the FDA, the CDC, the AMA, the AAP, and the White House. She truly believed that, when notified of the debilitating effects of mercury on her son, these agencies would surely respond quickly. For good measure, she sent a letter to Vice President Dick Cheney.

The responses came back expressing deep sympathy—and an utter lack of interest in doing anything about the matter. The reply from Cheney's office said that Lisa's "comments about the need to recall thimerosal containing vaccines have been carefully noted."[341] But, it added, "Your letter indicates that you have already been in contact with the FDA, as well as state and federal elected officials in your advocacy effort." It was a polite way of saying: "Go away."

"Thank you for taking the time to make the Vice President aware of this important issue," continued the letter, signed by Cheney's correspondence aide, Cecilia Boyer. "Vice President and Mrs. Cheney send their best wishes to you and your family and their hope for Wesley's full recovery."

Lisa had to laugh at one. Full recovery? Recovery from what, exactly?

Apparently Ms. Boyer wasn't aware of the fact that most federal researchers considered autism to be genetic—and incurable.

With this inaction, Lisa's trust in the federal government began to erode, but her resolve increased. Instead of focusing on the health agencies of the federal government, now she began to write to agencies with oversight and investigative powers. Early in 2004, she had written to the Office of Investigations for Health and Human Services. HHS dismissed her concerns as "moot," refusing even to forward them on to any other agency, and asserting that mercury was out of the vaccine supply, except for trace amounts.

Outraged, Lisa turned to a new level of action. She had considerable contacts within the federal government. Since the "appropriate channels" had failed her, she turned to well-placed friends and family, including one family member who worked in federal investigations, for advice.

"Have you tried the OSC?" the family member asked Lisa. Lisa had never heard of it. "The Office of Special Counsel," she was told, "it's an independent and politically insulated federal investigative and prosecutorial agency. You should write to them."

The primary mission of the OSC is to "safeguard the merit system by protecting federal employees and applicants from prohibited personnel practices, especially reprisal for whistleblowing," according to the agency's Web site.[342] "OSC receives, investigates, and prosecutes allegations of prohibited practices" and is authorized to "seek disciplinary action against individuals who commit [them]." The OSC is not to be confused with the Office of Independent Counsel (OIC), a position made famous by Kenneth Starr, who investigated President Bill Clinton in the Lewinsky matter.

Lisa needed help. To be successful, she learned that her letter to the OSC would have to be air-tight, and it would have to be copied to state and federal officials as well as media. The more expansive the list, the better the chances of success.

Lisa also wanted parental input on crafting a list of grievances for the Special Counsel. She turned to a small group of parents who were involved in the effort to convince state attorneys general to file class-action suits against the vaccine makers. It was a faction of some fifteen parents around the country. Lisa sent an e-mail to everyone, and Kelli Ann Davis, a mother of immense energy and organizational ability, from Fayetteville, North Carolina, was the first to respond. A stay-at-home mom, Kelli jumped at the chance to volunteer for the project, and she and Lisa became partners in steering it.

Other parents involved in the OSC campaign included Laura Bono and Lori McIlwain who contributed editorial advice, Jo Pike, who handled Internet postings and press releases, and Linda Weinmaster, a mother from Nebraska.

The group of fifteen took a few weeks to hash out a letter that was sound enough for the most seasoned and jaundiced federal investigators. It was Lent, and for Lisa the pastor, it was an endeavor of faith. Copies of the letter were mailed to all their press and research contacts, as well as the entire U.S. Congress, during Holy Week. Each letter was accompanied by copies of Lisa's "rejection letters" from the national health agencies and the vice president. In all, the group mailed out some nine hundred packets.

"We have resolved to bring this scandal to national prominence," their letter to the Special Counsel, Scott Bloch, said. "Seeking to enlist your oversight and resources in investigating this serious issue, we make the following charges:[343]

- The CDC is characterized by egregious conflicts of interest, which have compromised the safety of the vaccine supply, while putting our nation's children at risk. Placing pharmaceutical profits and patronage above our children's health, the CDC has failed to evaluate objectively the cumulative mercury exposure incurred through the standard immunization schedule. Furthermore, officials have refused to recall products containing this neurotoxin, despite the objections of clinical researchers and parents.

- The CDC, FDA and pharmaceutical companies met at the Simpsonwood Retreat Center on June 7 and 8, 2000. At this closed meeting, a CDC study authored by Dr. Thomas Verstraeten was discussed. The participants acknowledged the statistical correlation between mercury exposure through pediatric vaccines and neurological disorders in children. This version of the Verstraeten study was never released to the public. Evidence of their collusion is recorded in the Simpsonwood Transcripts.

- Dr. Verstraeten later denied a link before an IOM panel on July 16, 2001, and released a different version of the same study showing no correlation between Thimerosal and neurological disorders in the November 2003 *Pediatrics* journal.

- According to official communication from the CDC, various datasets compiled for the Verstraeten Study showing a relationship between Thimerosal and neurological disorders no longer exist. We fear loss or destruction of data, and therefore ask that steps be put in place IMMEDIATELY to safeguard the VSD Database.

• Independent researchers have been arbitrarily restricted from the VSD after previously being given access. This *taxpayer-funded* database must be open to all researchers regardless of CDC or government affiliation. We accuse the Internal Review Board (IRB) of denying access to the VSD—under the false pretext of privacy issues—to independent researchers Dr. Mark Geier and Mr. David Geier, who have published over 50 peer-reviewed articles. Additionally, we believe this action may have violated the Data Quality Act and Data Access Law, requiring further investigation from you.

• The methodology of government-sponsored studies of Thimerosal and its connection to neurological disorders in children has been exclusively statistical and epidemiological in nature. Such studies cannot assess the genetic vulnerability of subpopulations. Additionally, the ever-expanding clinical evidence amassed by clinical researchers is being ignored.

• Claims for Thimerosal-induced vaccine injuries from government-mandated vaccines are being hampered and delayed in the National Vaccine Injury Compensation Program (NVICP). Additionally, the statute of limitations for pursuing compensation excludes most families from gaining legal restitution from the American Government.

• Injecting mercury in excess of EPA standards without prior informed consent represents a significant and widespread violation of civil rights.

"Without immediate action from the federal government," the letter concluded, "confidence in the national immunization program will continue to erode. There is not a more pressing issue, nationally or internationally, than the epidemic of autism and the devastated lives left in its ruins. The cost of this negligence will be measured economically, intellectually and politically for years to come."

Out of nine hundred letters, only one response came in. It was from *Mothering Magazine,* which wanted to do a story for the July issue. The mainstream media were uninterested.

But within a week, Linda Weinmaster, the Nebraska mother, got a call from an old friend who knew Special Counsel Scott Bloch. Entirely coincidentally, Bloch had just been appointed, and he was to oversee the preliminary investigation into the thimerosal controversy. He asked Linda to send him copies of everything. A few days later, he sent her a message via their common acquaintance.

"Wow, I am blown away by this," Bloch reportedly told the contact. "This is really big stuff. You parents need to be careful. There are some big players involved here."

Bloch also relayed the message that he was going to suggest a formal inquiry. "But we need the parents to back off with the media for now," he said. "Don't do any more press follow-up until there is an authorization for a full investigation. We don't want the media calling around and scaring people away from cooperating."[344]

The parents agreed to suspend their PR campaign, and they asked *Mothering Magazine* to hold off on their reporting.

In mid-April, Bloch called Weinmaster directly. "We have given you a case number," he said. "That is the next big step to a formal investigation. But I want you to know: It is extremely difficult to be given a case number if the OSC doesn't feel there is a rational basis for looking into the allegations. Congratulations." Bloch told her that most people on the OSC staff were parents. Nearly everyone knew an autistic child. "We are devastated," he said, "that nothing has ever been done about this until now."

BY 2004, thimerosal (except in trace amounts) had been removed from every vaccine made for the childhood schedule. But it was still found in tetanus, diphtheria-tetanus, and meningitis vaccines, which are sometimes given to children.

The big remaining question was the flu shot. Most versions of the vaccine still contained 25 micrograms of ethylmercury. The CDC's Advisory Committee on Immunization Practices had voted to recommend the shot for pregnant women, and a pediatric version (two shots with 12.5 micrograms each) for children between six and twenty-three months of age. The panel refused to recommend thimerosal-free vaccines.

On April 1, the *Los Angeles Times* broke the news that the CDC would not recommend mercury-free flu shots. "Hundreds of thousands of infants and toddlers who get flu shots starting this fall could be exposed to a mercury-laced preservative that has been all but eliminated from other pediatric vaccines due to health concerns," it said.[345]

CDC officials "have confirmed that they won't advise parents and doctors to choose a mercury-free version of the flu vaccine," the story said. The decision was made "despite pleas from parent activist groups and some experts," and seemed "to be at odds with recent federal warnings about exposure to mercury, a potent neurotoxin, and with the government's successful effort to see mercury removed from other vaccines."

The mercury-free flu vaccine, made by Aventis Pasteur, would be more expensive, by about four dollars per shot, "because it is somewhat harder to make in large quantities than the alternative," the article said. "If the CDC were to warn parents, demand for thimerosal-free shots would rise, possibly squeezing supplies. Some experts said there was a greater risk in infants and toddlers failing to be vaccinated against the flu because of a shortage than in their being vaccinated with shots containing mercury."

The CDC, in a separate statement, asserted that "available scientific evidence has not shown thimerosal-containing vaccines to be harmful."

The agency came under "blistering attack" from parent groups, the article said. Barbara Loe Fisher, of the National Vaccine Information Center, said the government was "violating the precautionary principle which reminds doctors that, when in doubt, take an action which minimizes the risk of harm."

Dave Weldon was even harsher. The CDC's refusal to recommend mercury-free shots was "medical malpractice," he told the paper. As a physician, he said he would not permit his young son to have a mercury-containing shot.

And Boyd Haley said it was "'preposterous and ridiculous' for the government to warn about methyl mercury in fish but sanction ethyl mercury being injected into kids," the paper said. "The CDC decision is 'unconscionable,' he said. 'If it were my grandchild, there's no way in hell you'd give them a vaccine containing thimerosal.'" The CDC had ordered some two million doses of thimerosal-free flu vaccine for the coming fall, "'to be sure there is enough for health departments that request it,' said Roger Bernier, senior scientist with the CDC's immunization program," the paper said. But if the agency had stated a thimerosal-free preference, this would "drive the demand even more aggressively," he said. There was no need, given the "lack of proof of harm."

Still, it was unclear if demand for preservative-free vaccines would disrupt supplies. Len Lavenda, a spokesman for Aventis, said the company encouraged parents who were concerned to ask their doctors to order thimerosal-free vaccines. He didn't think that demand for the mercury-free product would be a problem. "We will be able to produce a sufficient amount," Lavenda told the paper, "providing we're notified early enough."

IF THE CDC would not agree to remove thimerosal from vaccines, Dave Weldon decided he would try to make them do so.

On April 2, Weldon and Rep. Carolyn Maloney, a liberal Democrat from Manhattan's Upper East Side, introduced a House bill to eliminate mercury from vaccines. "Given the increasing concerns about mercury exposures and our ability to eliminate this particular exposure," Weldon told the media, "this bill completes actions begun five years ago to ban mercury from vaccines."[346]

The government, he noted, "is poised to recommend the flu vaccine later this year without recommending that infants and pregnant women get the mercury-free version of the inoculation." The bill was therefore needed to "ensure that we don't roll back the clock when it comes to eliminating this mercury exposure to developing fetuses and infants. We can eliminate this exposure now and it is inexcusable not to."

"It's a simple concept: kids shouldn't be given anything that's toxic," Maloney added. "Who would argue against that? Vaccines can be made without mercury, so why not remove the mercury and remove any doubt?"

The bill would establish definite timelines for the elimination of mercury from vaccines, and provided a phase-in stage to allow for retooling of production facilities while ensuring firm deadlines for compliance. It would specifically eliminate exposure to mercury from the flu vaccine for the upcoming flu season by prohibiting mercury-containing flu vaccine from being administered to children after July 1, 2004.

By January 1, 2005, no childhood vaccine would be allowed to have more than 1 microgram of mercury; by January 1, 2006, mercury would be removed completely from all childhood and adolescent vaccines; and by January 1, 2007, all adult vaccines would contain no more than 1 microgram of mercury.

The bill was referred to the Subcommittee on Health. Meanwhile, Weldon was roundly criticized by some House colleagues, including Rep. Henry Waxman. Critics were upset that Weldon, by introducing the bill, was implying that proof of harm from thimerosal had been established. And, they said, it would disrupt distribution of flu shots.

Weldon reminded his critics that Aventis said it could meet demand for mercury-free flu vaccines if given enough notice in advance, but that claim did not pacify them.

Weldon was interviewed by Melissa Ross, a reporter for First Coast News, an ABC/NBC affiliate in Jacksonville, in his home state of Florida. "This is one of the most toxic substances on the planet, and I want to make sure no thimerosal-containing flu shots are given this year," he said. "Because anyone who would knowingly inject a little baby with mercury," he said again, "I would consider that malpractice."[347]

Ross went on to discuss the Geiers' findings, and the Simpsonwood transcripts.

"But the CDC tells First Coast News the concerns are overblown, and says the Geiers' research, along with other studies supporting their position, are not credible," she said. "Furthermore, the Geiers are no longer being allowed to access the CDC's vaccine database, because the CDC claims the Geiers did not follow proper privacy procedures."

Ross then interviewed Dr. Steve Cochi, the newest acting director of the CDC's National Immunization Program. "The studies showing a potential link have not been subjected to sufficient peer review," he said. "They have not been replicated."

As for Simpsonwood, Cochi said the transcripts "offer no proof thimerosal has the potential to harm. It is far more critical that we immunize everyone against influenza, which is a serious threat, than endanger the supply of vaccine over a theoretical risk."

The CDC had already begun stockpiling flu vaccines—with and without thimerosal—"to safeguard against possible shortages such as those the country saw last year," Ross reported. "And Cochi says if Weldon's legislation passes, a mandate of only mercury-free flu shots could squeeze an already tight supply."

Weldon's "malpractice" remark drew this response from the CDC official: "Any politician can champion a cause, whether it is based on fact, or whether it is not based on fact. And one must consider the consequences of unfounded fear."

"AND NOW for some possible good news," the Sacramento father Rick Rollens wrote to the Schafer Autism Report on April 18, 2004. "For the first time in over 20 years, a consecutive two quarterly (six month) reporting period has shown a DECREASE in the number of new cases compared to other reporting periods: a 6% decrease in 2004 over 2003. This may or may not be a trend. Time will tell."[348]

This was the news everyone was waiting for. If the drop in cases really did represent a trend, and if it continued, it would be damning evidence against thimerosal.

Rick had helped establish the MIND autism research institute in Davis, California, and had access to data on new caseload reports coming into the state's Department of Developmental Services, which tracks the numbers of "classic" full-blown autism only. The department had documented that it takes up to five years for a birth cohort year to fully flush all the full-syndrome cases of autism into the system.

Back in 2001, Rick, Mark Blaxill, and others had predicted that if thimerosal were a cause of the epidemic, then new cases of autism should begin to drop sometime around 2004 or four years after mercury removal began—which is precisely what happened, with steeper declines to follow.

"California's system does NOT include children under the age of three years old," Rick explained in the Schafer Report. "What this means is that those children born in 2000 and some in 2001 are just now entering the system. For those who are carefully watching the effect on autism rates and the reduction of the use of certain mercury containing childhood vaccines which began in 2000, these next few months to a year or so could be very interesting."

It was wonderful news for the parents. Whether autism was linked to thimerosal or not, at least the numbers were finally, for some reason, going down rather than up. And it jived with what the unnamed monitor at the CDC computer center had said, when she told Mark and David Geier that "we're watching the numbers drop."

WORD was getting out among parents about the new cutting-edge research into diagnostics and treatments coming to light through Defeat Autism Now!

By April of 2004, the rising stars in the mercury-autism world were investigators such as Richard Deth, the Northeastern University professor who described how minute doses of thimerosal and other toxins can interfere with critical processes of methylation; Marvin Boris and Allan Goldblatt, the Long Island M.D.s who were discovering that certain variations in the MTHFR gene were more common in autistic kids than controls; and Jill James, from the Arkansas Children's Hospital Research Institute, who was finding that autistic children have impairments in methylation and sulfation, and subsequent deficiency in proteins like cysteine and glutathione, two sulfur-based thiols, or mercaptans, the "capturers of mercury."

These new theories were gaining such a strong hold over the true believers that some parents were now testing their children for the telltale genetic variances in their MTHFR gene. Many more were beginning to experiment with a new vitamin B-12–based "cocktail" treatment that Jill James and some of the DAN! doctors were developing for affected kids. The idea was to repair the "critical metabolic pathways" that were supposedly blocked—victims of an unlucky confluence of the wrong genes and the wrong toxins at the wrong time.

James had studied 20 autistic children (compared with 33 controls) and found they had significantly lower levels of metabolites like methionine, cysteine, and glutathione. It was a metabolic profile, she said, consistent with impaired methylation and increased oxidative stress.

James had treated 8 of the 20 autistic children with a dietary intervention of folinic acid and betaine, which are needed for the methylation of homocysteine into methionine. That process completes the "methionine cycle" and provides methyl groups for the methylation of DNA, RNA, and neurotransmitters and the production of myelin, which in turn insulates nerve cells. After three months of treatment, nearly all the children had metabolites rise to the normal range. This indicated that methylation and transulfuration had improved considerably.[349]

But in 6 of the 8 kids, the treatment did not boost glutathione levels, nor did it reduce the ratio of glutathione to oxidized glutathione, indicating that oxidative stress was still occurring. For the last month of the four-month trial, James added twice weekly injections of vitamin B-12 into the betaine-folinic acid "cocktail" being given to the 8 children. B-12 is needed for the regeneration of homocysteine into methionine, by reacting with methionine synthase (already deficient in people with certain variants in MTHFR).

Adding the injectable methyl B-12, she found, reduced levels of oxidized glutathione and the glutathione ratio. It also significantly increased levels of cysteine and glutathione, as compared with folinic acid and betaine alone. Although folinic acid and betaine (intervention one) were effective in normalizing methionine cycle metabolites, the combined regimen (intervention two) was successful in bringing into the normal range all critical enzymes.

James's research had two big potential implications. The first was diagnostics. "If the observed decreases in methionine, cysteine, and glutathione levels in autistic children are confirmed in a larger study, low levels of these thiol metabolites could provide metabolic biomarkers for autism," she wrote in a draft paper.

The other big promise, of course, was new treatments. "Clinical improvement in speech, cognition, and seizure activity were noted by the attending physician," James wrote, although she noted that "these were not measured in a quantifiable manner and are therefore not reported here. The clinical aspects of targeted nutritional intervention in children with autism will be the topic of a follow-up study currently underway."

James presented her methyl B-12 findings at the semiannual DAN! conference, held April 15–19 at the Hilton Hotel in McLean, Virginia. The place was packed to overflowing. Lyn, Liz, and Sallie had never seen so many people at a DAN! conference. Much of the buzz centered around the new triple treatment cocktail, and the anecdotal evidence coming in that it was having some extraordinary effects on kids, especially when combined with behavioral therapy and detoxification.

Some of the children, especially the younger ones, had reportedly been brought back from the brink of darkness altogether.

During one morning session, a New York pediatrician named Sidney

Baker introduced three mothers whose sons were treated with the cocktail, or variations on it.

One of the mothers was Brenda Kerr, from Rhode Island. Kerr was the parent of a boy with PDD-NOS named Eric. Eric was born in August 1999, one month after the Joint Statement on Thimerosal was released. He was among the last group of kids in America to get the full load of mercury-containing vaccines. Eric was just beginning to speak when he regressed into autism at just one year, and then stopped talking.[350]

In 2002, the Kerrs had weaned Eric off dairy and grains, and immediately saw "phenomenal improvement," Brenda Kerr said at the conference. He started to speak again. Then, in the summer of 2003, under Dr. Baker's supervision, they started giving their son glutathion and a form of thiamine (vitamin B-1) called TTFD, which Baker said had been shown to enhance detoxification and increase cellular energy.

"It was a cream, and we put a pea-sized dab on his foot," Kerr said. "And I swear, in five minutes his eye contact and speech improved like I had never seen it before," she said, though there was no way to verify such a remarkable claim. "And then, he started stinking like a skunk for the next four days, because the toxins were just pouring out of him. We ran around the house opening windows," she said, "our eyes were watering."

In November 2003, the Kerrs began adding the twice weekly injections of B-12. "That was the kicker," Brenda Kerr said. "His social communication took off and his eye contact returned dramatically. Fine motor coordination improved considerably. His teachers at school asked me what had happened to him, because suddenly he was starting to talk like a normal kid."

The only problem with the injections was that Eric would be a little hyper on the first day, normal on the second, and then start to crash a little on the third. But as soon as he got his next injection, he improved again. Obviously, this treatment had a long way to go. And it didn't sound like a cure for autism. But it might be a way to convert the disease into a chronic but manageable illness, much like HIV.

There wasn't a parent in that room who did not want to rush home to try the strange and unproven cocktail on their own kid.

JILL JAMES and Richard Deth may have been the darlings of the April DAN! conference, but not everyone was singing their praises. In the same April issue of *Molecular Psychology* in which Deth published his report on methylation and thimerosal, Dr. Paul Offit and his colleague at the Children's Hospital of Philadelphia, Dr. J. Golden, took Deth to task for his methodology.[351]

The two Philadelphia pediatricians echoed previous criticism about Deth, that he had merely conducted an in vitro (test tube) study, rather than tests in living organisms. Deth's work assumed that ethylmercury readily crossed the blood-brain barrier and was as toxic to the central nervous system (CNS) as methylmercury.

But methylmercury "enters the CNS by an active transport mechanism, whereas ethylmercury does not," Offit wrote. "Also, because its half-life is much longer, methylmercury is more likely to accumulate than ethylmercury, causing higher levels of mercury in the blood. Exposing cells in vitro to ethylmercury assumes absolute availability in vivo, eliminates the most important difference between those two forms of mercury, and ignores the fact that ethylmercury is unlikely to enter the CNS at concentrations likely to be harmful."

Deth and colleagues had also used cells derived from a cancerous nervous system tumor, called neuroblastoma cells, "to make predictions about developing healthy cells of the CNS," Offit and Golden wrote. "If the authors were interested in making claims about the developing CNS they should use cells derived from the developing CNS. This failure is not trivial. At the very least, the authors should confirm their observations in other cell types, including several other cell lines."

Such limitations "should have been addressed prior to, not after, publication," they wrote. "People whose children suffer autism are desperate to find the cause or causes of the disease. Studies like this, although severely limited by their design, may be a focus of media and parental attention and offer the false hope that avoidance of thimerosal will lessen the risk of autism. However, by avoiding vaccines the risk of autism will not be lessened and the risk of vaccine-preventable diseases will be increased. The editors should be mindful that unreasonable extrapolations from in vitro studies to in vivo events may do more harm than good."

Deth's letter of rebuttal ran in the journal's July 2004 issue. "Clearly ours was an *in vitro* study," he wrote. "That said, the assertion that 'ethylmercury is unlikely to enter the brain at concentrations likely to be harmful' is wishful thinking and simply untrue." As for the neuroblastoma cells, Deth claimed they were "the most widely employed cultured human neuronal cell line" in this type of research. He also noted that thimerosal exposure in children occurs "during a period of exceptionally active" nerve growth and that "impaired methylation during this period could have profound and long-lasting consequences for cognitive function." As for parents being "misled by our *in vitro* findings," he said, "this is precisely the knowledge that parents are seeking and it is the appropriate role of scientific inquiry and scientific journals to provide such new information."

. . .

THOMAS VERSTRAETEN had returned home to Belgium to work for Glaxo-SmithKline in 2001. Since then, he had consistently refused requests from the media to discuss his VSD activities. His company also made it clear he was not authorized to comment. Verstraeten, having moved to Belgium, was protected from U.S. congressional subpoena power and he refused to return to the United States for a face-to-face interview under oath with Chairman Burton and his Government Reform Committee staff. Instead, the former CDC employee answered a few questions on a telephone call with staff members, who found his answers to be "entirely unsatisfactory," according to Beth Clay.

But in a letter printed in the April 2004 issue of *Pediatrics,* Verstraeten's voice was finally heard. He defended himself without sounding defensive.[352]

Verstraeten said that the first phase of the study had found a "positive" association between thimerosal and certain outcomes. But because the findings were not replicated in the second phase, "the perception of the study changed from a positive to a neutral study.

"Surprisingly, however, the study is being interpreted now as negative by many, including the anti-vaccine lobbyists," he said. "The article does not state that we found evidence against an association, as a negative study would. It does state, on the contrary, that additional study is recommended, which is the conclusion to which a neutral study must come."

This neutral take came as news to Safe Minds (who never considered themselves "anti-vaccine"). It seemed as if Verstraeten was backpedaling away from the CDC party line, which had not regarded his work as a "neutral study," but had cited it as evidence supporting the CDC's assertion of no link between thimerosal and autism.

Verstraeten said that the study, which was published in *Pediatrics,* "has been subject to heavy criticism from anti-vaccine lobbyists. Their criticism basically comes down to the following two claims: the CDC has watered down the original findings of a link between thimerosal-containing vaccines and autism, and GlaxoSmithKline (GSK) has hired me away from the CDC so as to convince me to manipulate the data further." Verstraeten listed his "personal opinions" on the allegations:

> Did the CDC water down the original results? It did not. This misconception comes from an erroneous perception of this screening study and other epidemiological studies. The perception is that an epidemiological study can have only 1 of 2 outcomes: either an association is found (or confirmed), or an association is refuted. Very often, however,

there is a third interpretation: an association can neither be found nor refuted. Let's call the first 2 outcomes "positive" and "negative" and the third outcome "neutral." The CDC screening study of thimerosal-containing vaccines was perceived at first as a positive study that found an association between thimerosal and some neurodevelopmental outcomes. The original plan was to conduct the second phase as a case-control study, [but] we soon realized this would be too time consuming. The validity of the first phase results needed urgent validation in view of the large potential public health impact.

Did the CDC purposefully select a second phase that would contradict the first phase? Certainly not. The push to urgently perform the second phase at [Harvard Pilgrim] came entirely from myself, because I felt that the first-phase results were too prone to potential biases to be the basis for important public health decisions. [It] was the only site known to myself and my coauthors that could rapidly provide sufficient data that would enable a check of the major findings of the first phase in a timely manner.

Continuing the debate on the validity of the screening study is a waste of scientific energy and not to the benefit of the safety of US children or of all children worldwide that have the privilege of being vaccinated. All discussion on how and why the results presented at different stages of the study may have changed slightly is futile for the same reason. The bottom line is and has always been the same: an association between thimerosal and neurological outcomes could neither be confirmed nor refuted, and more study is required.

Did GSK hire me away to manipulate the data before publication? Definitely not. This suggestion could be viewed as simply silly, were it not that it offends the ethical integrity of both the company and myself. Although I have been involved in some of the discussions concerning additional analyses that were undertaken after my departure from the CDC, I did not perform any of these additional analyses myself, nor did I instigate them. GSK was at no point involved in any discussions I had with former CDC colleagues on the study, nor were details of these discussions ever discussed between myself and GSK. The company and I had a very clear deal from the very start of my employment that I would finalize my involvement in the study on my own time and keep this involvement entirely separated from my work at GSK. I regard myself as a professional scientist who puts ethical value before any personal or material gains. I believe that I am currently employed by a company that has the same high ethical standards as myself. Therefore, any suggestion that GSK intended to have me manipulate this data is nothing short of an insult to both my and the company's integrity. Although I deeply regret such statements, I call on any party that truly has the safety of our children and the advancement of the health of the world's children at heart to move beyond such pitiable attitudes and focus on the future of the ongoing research.

BY THE END OF APRIL, Pastor Lisa Sykes had assumed the role of point person in the group of fifteen's discussions with Scott Bloch at the OSC.

"Okay, now comes the hard part," explained Tracy Biggs, one of the OSC's lead attorneys. She and Catherine McMullen, the disclosure officer for the OSC, explained to Lisa the legal requirements needed to give their office jurisdiction.[353] In order to launch a full investigation, the OSC first needed a whistle-blower, a current or former employee within a federal health agency, to come forward with a complaint of malfeasance.

"We need somebody to say that, 'Yes, federal officials were aware or concerned that improper things were going on,'" McMullen said. "Whatever wrongdoing they observed in the course of their professional duties." Anyone who came forward would be given federal whistle-blower protection status.

Lisa, Laura, and a few other parents set out on a scavenger hunt for canaries within the bureaucracy's coal mine. For good measure, they asked a few of the DAN! doctors to cold-call potential whistle-blowers as well, and try to appeal to them as fellow medical professionals. Surely, the moms thought, there must be at least one present or former employee at the FDA or CDC who would step forward, especially if given protection.

By the first week of May, they had found five people.

Each of the five candidates said they had significant inside information to disclose, but none of them met the requirements entirely. Some worried about retribution. Even with OSC whistle-blower status, their careers in public service would effectively be over. Whistle-blowers could not be fired, but they rarely got promoted, either. The moms gave each candidate a number at the OSC to call if they decided to talk.

Lisa and Laura spoke almost nightly about progress with their candidates. Fearful that their phone lines might be tapped (as Lyn suspected), they never mentioned the potential whistle-blowers by name, but only by number.

On May 5, Laura called Lyn to brief her on the progress. "We've got number one on board already," Laura said. "They are a strong witness, and they are just waiting until the others are entrenched before they call the OSC. Witness number two is going to be a wonderful asset, with knowledge of the activity of lots of people in different agencies. Then there's number three, I think number three is a godsend, they are being very helpful. The person is not yet sure if they are prepared to make the call. They are very upset. They think this is a big case to make. But it's a really big step for them."

Lyn could understand, but she wasn't sympathetic. "If these people are sitting on information that could shed light on the truth, they should come forward, finally, and fucking do it," she said. "What about number five?"

"They are mad for all the right reasons. They *do* want the truth to come out. Lisa is working on them now."

Lyn had big news of her own. CDC director Dr. Julie Gerberding had asked Dave Weldon to arrange a meeting with the parents.

"You're joking! Right?" Laura said. "What could be motivating this woman all of a sudden? Now she wants to fly from Atlanta up to Washington to meet with a lowly bunch of parents?"

"She wants to hear why we are angry at the CDC," Lyn said. Both women laughed.

News of the surprise meeting, scheduled for May 12, was kept to the few parents who would be attending—Lyn, Liz, Sallie, Scott and Laura Bono, and Mark Blaxill—and two researchers, Jill James and Mady Hornig, the Columbia University professor who had presented her rat and mice study findings to the IOM in February.

The group could not help but wonder what was driving Gerberding. Was it the parents' communication with the OSC? She must have known about that initiative. Was it all that media coverage over thimerosal in the flu shot, just as the CDC was about to order supplies for the following season? Was it the dropping numbers in California?

"I know what I want to say to her, if I get the chance," Laura told Lyn. "You have only been at CDC for a year. You didn't create this mess. You can either be a hero, and fix it; or you can choose to cover it up like everybody else. Either way, the truth will eventually come out. It always does."

LIZ BIRT now felt that Matthew, who had been sick all winter, was well enough to begin vitamin B-12 injections and folinic acid supplements. She started the experimental treatment shortly before the DAN! conference and, within weeks, saw dramatic changes.

Matthew's behavior improved at home. He was more obedient and attentive. Liz could get him ready and out the door in record time. Before the B-12 injections, each school morning was an ordeal. It took an hour or more to chase Matt around the house, get him to sit down and eat, and coax him into his clothes. Now, she could do it in fifteen minutes.

Matt was much less hyperactive. He could sit quietly for an hour without squirming, crying, or trying to get up and flee. He was sleeping better at night, and his sound sensitivity had diminished. Until recently, any loud noise would send him into fits of tears, and now that happened far less frequently.

His ability to go from receptive language to action picked up, too. He was much more responsive to questions, much quicker on the uptake, and more decisive than ever. When Liz asked him what cereal he wanted, for example, Matt would go directly to the cupboard, select the box he wanted, carry it to the table, and sit down to eat. Before the B-12 treatment, this process could last thirty minutes or more, as Matthew pointed to each box, pulled out each one, put some back, and threw others on the floor.

Of course, it was possible that Liz had fallen prey to some transferred placebo effect, that the improvements were all in her head, that she so desperately wanted the new treatments to work she began to see things that weren't there. But Liz didn't think so, and neither did the teachers at Matthew's school.

Matt was now ten, and in fourth grade. By early May 2004, his teachers were marveling to Liz about how compliant and attentive he had become in class. There were no more outbursts, no screaming, no biting, hair pulling, or shoe throwing.

They said that Matt's comprehension, accuracy, and computer skills were excellent. Matthew couldn't speak, but he could answer questions on a computer monitor with the click of a mouse. Suddenly he could read entire paragraphs with ease, and answer all the questions that followed. His comprehension had gone from 50 percent to 100 percent. He could also now correctly match images with written phrases on the screen, without making a mistake.

Liz's marriage was over and her life was not what she wanted it to be. She still struggled to spend time with Sarah and Andrew, and was warring with her estranged husband over custody, still proving her "fitness" as a mother.

But Matthew was getting better, and Liz could think of no better news than that. She was hearing miraculous tales of kids on the cocktail (combined, usually, with chelation and behavior therapy), who were speaking again after years of silence. Some of them, she was told, were no longer diagnosed with autism. Some were even having their special education services cut because their schools felt these services were no longer needed.

The last time Liz had heard her son say anything had been in 1995, during a family vacation to Seal Beach, Oregon. They had spotted a colony of harbor seals lazing on some smooth black rocks, and Matthew was tickled by his first glimpse of marine life.

"Seals, Mommy!" he squealed, running down the beach. "Seals, seals, seals!"

The kids had bought Liz a little gray stuffed seal on that trip, and she still kept it. She was waiting for the day that Matthew could tell her what it was.

EARLY ON THE MORNING of May 12, Lyn kissed Tommy, Will, and Drew good-bye and drove out to the airport for her flight to Washington and the big meeting with Dr. Gerberding. Her presentation was ready, and so were her nerves. Lyn would be calm, polite, and respectful, she thought, even though inside she was churning with anger. Lyn had an abundance of questions for the director, as did all the parents heading for Washington that morning. To wit: If thimerosal was not responsible for autism's surge in the 1990s, then what on earth was? And why wasn't the CDC in a hurry to find out?

The meeting was held in a small hearing room in the Rayburn Building, not far from Dave Weldon's office. Lyn, Sallie, Mark Blaxill, Scott and Laura Bono, Mady Hornig, and Jill James gathered beforehand, to gird themselves.

It gave Lyn time to share some vague but intriguing news she had heard. The IOM vaccine-autism report was ready. Lyn was hearing rumors that an IOM staffer had told a reporter that the document was "going to be an eye-opener." Lyn had also heard that vaccine companies were "scrambling" to respond to the bombshell pronouncement.

This came as somewhat of a surprise. After all, the February IOM meeting had seemed like a wash to the parents and researchers. They suspected that the panel would issue a muddled report, very similar to what the IOM had put out back in October 2001. An "eye-opener," the parents thought, could well mean good news for their side. And what else would drug companies be "scrambling" to do, except remove thimerosal from the 2004–2005 influenza vaccine, which was going into production for fall distribution?

Giddy with the prospects of a favorable IOM report, the group entered the conference room, where they found a woman seated alone at the end of the table. Her named was Lorine Spencer, and she had recently been appointed by Gerberding as the CDC's new "community outreach liaison" for autism. Spencer didn't bother to stand up to introduce herself, nor did she seem very enthusiastic about being there. Odd behavior for a "liaison," Laura mused.[354]

Weldon and Gerberding entered and sat down next to Spencer, with the parents and researchers seated on the other side of the long table. Gerberding seemed to be sizing up the group, and the group was certainly doing the same. They were trying to read her body language (did she look angry? dismissive? bored?). The doctor was cordial and respectful, if not overly warm.

Mark Blaxill began by offering a brief review of all the autism "time trend" population studies based on U.S. published surveys (California, Brick

Township, etc.) that showed a clear correspondence between thimerosal exposure and autism rates.

Mark also picked apart the Verstraeten VSD analysis, with a hard-hitting PowerPoint presentation that included slides such as: "CDC prevalence surveys have been poorly executed and interpreted with respect to trend assessment; CDC and local public health authorities have contributed to confusion and complacency in interpreting and suppressing trend evidence; CDC epidemiology studies have been manipulated to project a false sense of security; Limited toxicokinetic research has been misinterpreted as proving thimerosal safety while broader IOM research recommendations were ignored."

Gerberding betrayed no emotion while listening to this attack on the agency she had been nominated to run just one year earlier.

Mady Hornig followed Mark with the Columbia University mouse study that she had presented at the February IOM meeting. At the IOM, Hornig had discussed how mice with an autoimmune genetic predisposition developed autistic-like behaviors after injections with thimerosal-containing vaccines. She had shown videos, with graphic, sickening depictions of mice grooming themselves repeatedly to the point of injury.

Hornig played the videos for Gerberding, who suddenly appeared stunned. She brought her hands to her face in disbelief.

Dave Weldon had a similar reaction. He stopped Hornig in the middle of her ghastly presentation. "Wait a minute," he said. "Am I understanding you correctly? You injected these mice with the same amount of mercury, relatively speaking, that infants receive, in vaccines, and you saw these kinds of mutilatory behaviors? You saw this mouse eat through the cranium of his *cage mate?*"

Now Hornig was the one not displaying emotion. "Yes," she replied calmly.

Weldon said he was awestruck. He had never seen that video clip before.

Jill James then presented her findings on the altered biochemistry of autistic children, including low levels of methionine, cysteine, glutathione, and other key markers. She also discussed how thimerosal could be interfering with critical enzyme pathways in children with certain genetic mutations, leading to impaired methylation and sulfation. She talked about autistic children's blocked inability to process vitamin B-12, and how methyl B-12 injections were working miracles in some children.

Lyn then delivered a robust critique of what she said the CDC had done—and failed to do—to fund studies on autism and its possible connection to environmental insults, such as thimerosal. And she attacked the "revolving door" policy of the National Immunization Program, claiming that officials who make key decisions about vaccine policy drift back and forth between the public and private sectors at will.

Laura Bono went next, ratcheting down the argument to a deeply personal level, with a detailed description of her son Jackson's condition before and after regression. She discussed how she and Scott had started their boy on "therapeutic intervention," and about the progress he had been making.

Laura spoke eloquently of the suffering—emotional, physical, and financial—that her family had endured since Jackson became sick. It was enough to bring Jill James, who was fairly new to this autism business, to tears. But Dr. Gerberding sat and listened without expression. Lyn thought it was unseemly.

"She should have tears, too," Lyn would tell Laura and Sallie after the meeting. "We as parents lost our tears a long time ago. But for anyone to listen to that story for the first time—well, I can't imagine it wouldn't make them at least a little misty-eyed."

Sallie closed the meeting with a list of "recommendations." They included:

- Declare autism a public health emergency.
- Convene an in-depth science review in Atlanta for top CDC leadership.
- Remove vaccine safety oversight responsibilities from the National Immunization Program.
- State a preference for thimerosal-free influenza vaccine for infants and pregnant women for the upcoming flu season.
- With the NIH, support a broad and immediate environmental autism research initiative, not just "self-conducted epidemiology".
- Investigate and redress conflicts of interest in deliberations of the Advisory Committee on Immunization Practices.
- Review conduct of NIP leadership, including cover-up, dereliction of duty, and general incompetence.
- Expedite *all* Safe Minds Freedom of Information Act requests.
- Replace internal NIP staff with independent researchers on thimerosal studies and use non-VSD data sets as well.

Gerberding listened politely and waited for her turn to speak. She thanked the parents, quite sincerely, and said that their talk had been "sobering." She added that she was "committed to dealing with the issues raised here today," and insisted she wanted to "get to the bottom" of the thimerosal question. She reminded the group that many things had been done at the CDC before her time, but as director, she would see the issue through to its end. "I am not afraid of controversy," Dr. Gerberding declared, "and I am determined to follow the science."

To the parents' surprise, Gerberding commented that CDC officials had come to realize that autism was epidemic, and that epidemics are not genetic. She told them she was aware of the Bradstreet, Holmes, and other studies showing mercury retention in autistic children, and said that she was "open-minded" on this issue.

Gerberding also announced that she was going to transfer the VSD to another location at the National Center for Health Statistics, and vowed to expedite all FOIA requests by groups such as Safe Minds on unpublished VSD studies.

On the down side, Gerberding refused to have the CDC state a preference for thimerosal-free flu shots in the coming season for pregnant mothers and small children, something the parents felt very strongly about. And though she announced that she would immediately name a "Blue Ribbon Panel" on vaccine safety monitoring, she added, in a low voice, that only "reasonable representatives" from the autism world would be invited to participate. Safe Minds, apparently, did not fall within that category.

Gerberding thanked the parents and researchers again and promised that it would not be the last time she met with them. "I am committed to an open, scientific debate," she said. "You bring your science and we'll bring ours, and we'll talk about it."

The meeting lasted two and a half hours, thirty minutes longer than planned. The parents walked out feeling heartened, even a little excited. Gerberding seemed earnest, she seemed honest, perhaps even trustworthy. And she had listened to them. That counted for a lot. Sallie and Lyn wondered aloud if the IOM report was so favorable that the CDC director felt compelled to be receptive. Maybe good news really *was* awaiting them.

Laura Bono certainly felt upbeat. After returning home to Durham, she dispatched an e-mail to parents who were not present, but eager to hear about the meeting.

"The meeting went well. I believe she is sincere," Laura said of Gerberding. "I believe she knows the grave news and, just like any other administrator, is putting all of her ducks in a row and bracing for the inevitable—and still hoping for a reprieve. If I had finally realized, like I think she must be doing, that 'Oh my God, it is true!' what would I do if I were head of CDC and didn't want to hide it (or couldn't) anymore? I think that is exactly what is happening."[355]

Lyn also left Washington feeling optimistic. Not only was the meeting positive, she thought, but she was also excited by something that Stuart Burns, Weldon's deputy chief of staff, had told her as she was leaving. Weldon, who sat on the powerful House Appropriations Committee, had identified fifty thousand dollars in untapped CDC research dollars that would be returned to the general fund if not allocated by the new fiscal year on September 1. Weldon wanted to earmark the funds for Safe Minds, to fund research into a better understanding of the harm that thimerosal could be causing in children. Lyn knew exactly what they would do with the money: grant half to Jill James and half to Mady Hornig.

Lyn was walking on air when she got to the airport, and treated herself to a glass of her favorite libation: chilled white Zinfandel. But during the flight home, she had time to reflect a bit more on the Gerberding encounter. Now that she thought of it, the director did not really commit to very much of what Safe Minds had asked for: no science meeting, for instance, and no stating a preference for thimerosal-free flu vaccines, even though the first IOM report had recommended doing so. She did not agree to declare autism a public health emergency; she said nothing about internal conflicts of interest and nothing about allegations of manipulation and cover-up of the VSD autism results.

Lyn was likewise unable to pin down Gerberding as to when their next meeting would be. By the time her plane landed in Atlanta, Lyn had soured on the meeting considerably. She was also beginning to have her doubts that the IOM report would actually herald good news for Safe Minds.

In truth, Lyn wondered what Gerberding's real motives were. "I'm afraid she's just as much a politician as a bureaucrat," Lyn told Tommy that night.

LYN REDWOOD'S darker premonitions were correct. By the weekend, it had grown painfully clear to the parents that the IOM report would not be good news for their side. It would be a near slam dunk against the thimerosal-autism hypothesis. This was the "eye-opening" aspect they had heard about. And what the drug companies had been "scrambling" to do was to invite health and science reporters onto a teleconference call with Dr. Marie Mc-Cormick of the Immunization Safety Committee, to hear the big news.

On Sunday, May 16, Sallie sent an e-mail warning out to the regulars. "The IOM report on autism and vaccines (thimerosal and MMR) will be released on Tuesday, May 18th," she wrote. "We have no further information except that rumors are the CDC and manufacturers are ecstatic, so we are preparing for a bomb."

On the morning of the eighteenth, Lyn woke up feeling sick to her stomach, a result of stress over what was about to come. At around 8:00 A.M. Stuart Burns called from Washington, where he was huddled with Beth Clay, poring over the just-released document.

"It's bad," he told Lyn. "It's worse than we thought."

Stuart faxed the executive summary down to Lyn. She sat in her office with a strong cup of coffee and a highlighter pen, took a deep breath, and began to read.

"The committee concludes that the body of epidemiological evidence favors rejection of a causal relationship between the MMR vaccine and autism," it said. "The committee also concludes that the body of epidemiological evidence favors rejection of a causal relationship between thimerosal-containing vaccines and autism."

Lyn's heart sank. This *was* worse than they expected.

"The committee further finds that potential biological mechanisms for vaccine-induced autism that have been generated to date are theoretical only," the summary continued. This was a direct reference to all the evidence presented at the IOM meeting concerning the work of Hornig, Bradstreet, Holmes, Haley, Deth, James, and others.

"The committee does not recommend a policy review of the current schedule and recommendations for the administration of either the MMR vaccine or thimerosal-containing vaccines. The committee recommends a public health response that fully supports an array of vaccine safety activities," the summary said.

It ended with what seemed to the parents to be a kick in the gut: "In addition, the committee recommends that available funding for autism research be channeled to the most promising areas. The committee makes additional recommendations regarding surveillance and epidemiological research, clinical studies, and communication related to these vaccine safety concerns."[356]

The panel noted that this was the eighth and "final" report of the Immunization Safety Review Committee on "the hypothesis that vaccines, specifically the MMR vaccine and thimerosal-containing vaccines, are causally associated with autism."

Put another way: this was most likely the IOM's last word on the matter. But this time the committee had only addressed the alleged link to autism, and not any of the other neurological developmental disorders it had considered in past reports.

The committee based the bulk of its thimerosal conclusions on the five epidemiological studies that had been completed within the past year (the three that involved Denmark, the UK study, and Verstraeten et al.). Back in 2001, when the committee had determined the biological plausibility of an association, the new report said, that conclusion "was based on the fact that there were no published epidemiological studies" at the time. The only two unpublished epidemiological studies that were available (Verstraeten, 2001; Blaxill, 2001) "provided only weak and inconclusive evidence of an association."

The committee discounted most of the biological evidence presented at the February 2004 meeting (as opposed to the epidemiological studies), noting "several factors that limit acceptance at this time of the hypothesis that vaccines cause autism."

The biological evidence included "data from in-vitro experimental systems, analogies between rodent behavior and human behavior, and clinical observations that are at least as well explained as being co-morbid [coincidental] disease expressions than as causal factors," the report said. "That is, it is possible that some people with autism, perhaps even a subgroup that could eventually be identified by genetic markers, have abnormal immune reactions and abnormal mercury metabolism, but that vaccination of these individuals does not cause these abnormalities or autism itself."

The panel critiqued nearly all the data presented by proponents of the mercury-autism hypothesis at the February meeting. Particularly harsh criticism was reserved for the work of Mark and David Geier.

The pair had presented "an unpublished analysis" of the VSD, the report noted. "Only one slide depicted this information, and it demonstrated an increasing relationship between autism relative risk and amount of thimerosal." But, the panel added: "The basis of this calculation was not provided and additional data and methods were not described. Overall, the committee found the results of their analyses using VSD data uninterpretable, primarily due to the lack of a complete description of their methods.

"Given this lack of clarity, it is unclear how the incidence rate and the estimate of the relative risk could be calculated," the report continued. "The committee finds the results uninterpretable and, as such, non-contributory with respect to causality." The same critiques were made of the Geiers' analyses of the Vaccine Adverse Events Reporting System (VAERS).

The report also discounted the evidence presented by Dr. Mady Hornig of Columbia University, which showed that mice with genetic autoimmune disorders developed autistic-like behaviors following vaccination with thimerosal-containing shots. Noting that Hornig's work was also "as yet unpublished" (the study was published just three weeks later, in the peer-reviewed journal *Molecular Psychiatry*), the panel questioned the very premise of Hornig's protocol because it "assumes that autism is caused by an autoimmune reaction," and there was a "lack of evidence of autoimmune-mediated central nervous system damage in the brains of patients with autism."

The committee also questioned the "relevance" of rodent models, arguing that it was "difficult to assess" because the rodent "clinical" end points "may not reflect the human ones, because there is limited understanding of the etiology of autism, and because the methods used to cause changes in the animals may bear no relationship to pathogenesis of the human disease."

Somewhat interestingly, the committee added that it "accepts that under certain conditions infections and heavy metals, including thimerosal, can injure the nervous system." It also noted that "these rodent models are useful for understanding some of the processes by which these agents may exert their damage. . . .

"However," the panel concluded, "the connection between these models and autism is theoretical."

The committee was equally unimpressed with the work of Richard Deth, of Northeastern University, which was presented largely by Dr. Jeff Bradstreet at the February IOM meeting. Deth hypothesized that thimerosal and other toxins block the production of dopamine and insulin-like growth factor 1 (IGF-1), which are needed to stimulate DNA methylation and enhance memory and attention. Thimerosal can also block production of sulfur-based proteins (the thiols, or "mercury-capturing" mercaptans) that bind with heavy metals, Deth reported.

The panel conceded that dopamine is a "neurotransmitter associated with movement, attention, memory, and many other brain functions, and IGF-1 does have protective effects in many cells, including those responsible for producing myelin in the brain. But the authors [Deth et al.] hypothesize that disruption of this pathway by thimerosal leads to autism, ADHD, and other developmental disorders. However, the committee is aware of no evidence that autism is caused by alterations in this biochemical pathway."

And because Deth reported that other toxins besides thimerosal (e.g., ethanol, lead, aluminum) can disrupt the same pathway, this "weakens the argument that thimerosal might cause autism through this mechanism."

Interestingly, though, in a later passage, the committee did concede that the "experiments showing effects of thimerosal on biochemical pathways in cell culture systems and showing abnormalities in the immune system or metal metabolism in people with autism are provocative." The report suggested that autism researchers consider areas of research "with some of these new findings in mind," even though "these experiments do not provide evidence of a relationship between vaccines or thimerosal and autism."

The committee likewise dismissed the baby haircut study led by Dr. Amy Holmes, which showed that autistic children had much lower mercury levels in their infant hair than control children. Among the concerns cited by the panel was "the biased sampling" of study subjects.

"The clinical practice from which the case children were derived is specifically interested in the role of vaccines in autism," it said, "and the control children were solicited via the internet and newsletters related to autism." Other weaknesses were that types of fish consumed "were not elaborated," nor were "enough details of the hair samples given to indicate the period of the infant's life the hair sample represented. Further, infant exposures to other sources of mercury postnatally were not ascertained."

354 • EVIDENCE OF HARM

The authors (Holmes et al.) interpreted their findings "as suggesting that children with autism do not excrete mercury into the hair, i.e., that the mercury burden remains bioactive within the body," it added. "Direct evidence for this hypothesis was not presented."

The committee also questioned the integrity of the published chelation study submitted by Dr. Jeff Bradstreet, who reported that autistic children on average excreted six times more mercury than controls, following a chelation "challenge." But the controls, the report noted, "were healthy children whose parents sought chelation therapy in response to their worries about heavy metal toxicity."

And even though children with autism "excreted significantly more mercury" than controls, the panel said, "the range of mercury excreted was 0 to 59 (with a mean of 4.1 micrograms of mercury), and a standard deviation of 8.6, suggesting that the data might be skewed in the direction that many if not most of the children with autism are excreting little mercury."

The report made very brief mention of the work done by Jill James on defects in sulfation pathways; by Bill Walsh on metallothionein deficiency in autistic children; and by Dr. Vasken Aposhian on heavy metal efflux disorders in genetically predisposed people, but provided little to no comment on the merits of these studies. In the end, not a single argument for "biological mechanisms" put forth by the entire mercury-autism group was accepted by the committee as evidence of causality.

"In the absence of experimental or human evidence that vaccination affects metabolic, developmental, immune, or other physiological or molecular mechanisms that are causally related to the development of autism," the report said, "the committee concludes that the hypotheses generated to date are theoretical only."

The committee again reiterated its opinion that "a significant investment in studies of the theoretical vaccine-autism connection" would not "be useful at this time." It also warned that the vaccine-autism debate itself could have harmful consequences for the national immunization program, which the panel defended rigorously:

> The nature of the debate about vaccine safety now includes the theory by some that genetic susceptibility makes vaccinations risky for some people, which calls into question the appropriateness of a public health, or universal, vaccination strategy. However, the benefits of vaccination are proven and the hypothesis of susceptible populations is presently speculative. Using an unsubstantiated hypothesis to question the safety of vaccination and the ethical behavior of those governmental agencies and scientists who advocate for vaccination could

lead to widespread rejection of vaccines and inevitable increases in incidences of serious infectious diseases like measles, whooping cough, and HiB bacterial meningitis. The committee has yet to see any convincing evidence that supports the theory that vaccines are associated with an increase in the risk of autism, either to the population at large or to subsets of children with autism. Although this area of inquiry is interesting, it is only theoretical.

Lyn felt as if she had been transported directly back to square one in a matter of minutes. "We put so much time and effort into fighting over this," she told Tommy, "and this was a done deal before it even started."

Prior to the 1 P.M. teleconference call with Dr. Marie McCormick, Lyn sent an e-mail off to Lenny Schafer (of the Schafer Autism Report) and included the summary for him to post online, along with a note saying how devastated she was. "The investigation was paid for by CDC and they were also able to give the IOM their 'instructions,'" Lyn wrote. "They relied heavily on population-based epidemiology studies like Verstraeten and Hviid, and appear to have given much less weight to actual clinical science like Horning, Baskin, Bradstreet."[357]

But, Lyn added, "They have a history of being wrong. Remember their first investigation of Agent Orange, where they found no link with leukemia? That one was retracted in 2003. And most recently, their report that said there was no association with SSRI's [anti-depressants] and suicide in adolescents. Laura Bono found a quote in the *Washington Post* from Congressman Peter Deutsch of Florida, Ranking Member of the Subcommittee on Oversight and Investigations, in reference to the NIH Money-for-Science scandal, that IOM could 'explain away the unexplainable.' I think that is what we will be hearing today. I would not be surprised if they even found thimerosal 'neuro-protective.' Expect the worst. I fear we will be set back 5 years by this report. Lyn."

Lyn, Sallie, and Barbara Loe Fisher had been invited to sit in on the conference call between Marie McCormick and the medical media, just as in 2001. This time, Laura Bono also managed to get on the call. But before then, Lyn's phone would not stop ringing. Reporters were already working on their story about the report, and Lyn fielded interview requests from AP, Reuters, the *Los Angeles Times, Boston Globe, Detroit News, Orlando Sentinel,* and others. Mark Blaxill, meanwhile, was speaking with the *New York Times*.

The conference call went pretty much as Lyn expected. The "take home message," as some media people call it, was that the time had finally come to lay to rest any suspicions over vaccines and autism, and set out to find the "real" culprit.

"The overwhelming evidence from several well-designed studies indicates that childhood vaccines are not associated with autism," McCormick told the reporters.[358] "Don't misunderstand: the committee members are fully aware that this is a very horrible and devastating condition. It's important to get at the root of what's happening, [but] there seem to be lots of opportunities for research that would be more productive than vaccines. Resources would be used most effectively if they were directed toward those avenues of inquiry that offer the greatest promise for answers. Without supporting evidence, the vaccine hypothesis does not hold such promise."

Lyn's blood was boiling, but she kept quiet. She knew that Sallie and Barbara must have been ready to explode, too. Then, during the question-and-answer session, a reporter asked McCormick about the removal of thimerosal from childhood vaccines and the impact that should have on autism rates if the hypothesis were true.

"Wouldn't we see a decline?" the reporter asked.

"Yes," McCormick said. "And they looked at this very closely in Denmark. But when the Danes removed thimerosal from vaccines, autism rates skyrocketed."[359]

Lyn saw an opening and she took it.

"As a follow-up to your comment about Denmark," she said, "recent reports from California show that new autism cases have actually declined for the first time in decades, as we have just seen for the second consecutive quarter this April. Can you please comment on that?"

"Well, we all know that California is facing a severe budget crisis," McCormick replied. "It is very likely that services for disabled children are being cut back in that state. Therefore, fewer children would be allowed into the system, and the numbers would naturally come down."

SAFE MINDS had three different press releases ready to go, depending on how the IOM report came out: a positive release, a neutral release, and a negative one. At 1 P.M. that day, they sent out the negative release on the PR Newswire.

"Safe Minds Outraged That IOM Report Fails American Public," the headline said. "The IOM has not only compromised their integrity and independence, but also failed the American public, especially mercury-injured children with autism, by toeing the CDC, FDA, vaccine industry line. This committee clearly chose to ignore groundbreaking scientific research on the mercury-autism link, and instead the IOM has issued a flawed, incomplete report that continues to put America's children at risk.

"The problem with this report begins with its violation of nearly every tenet of medical science," continued the Safe Minds broadside. "Respected researchers everywhere do not support the IOM belief that proof can be solely found in epidemiology. Yet, the IOM wants the public to buy into the absurd belief that this report, bought and paid for by the CDC, is complete, independent and trustworthy. Since the committee is disbanding following this report they will not have to answer later for their failures today."[360]

In a separate statement, Safe Minds said it had investigated alleged conflicts of interest among many of the authors whose work was "relied upon for the flawed IOM report attempting to purport a lack of evidence to the mercury-vaccine-autism link. . . .

"Disclosure of potential conflicts of interest is an essential tenet to good science," Sallie said in the statement, "but here we have a situation where authors of 'studies' are probably quite literally writing to preserve their jobs." For example, she said, the IOM "gave unusual weight to several authors from the Statens Serum Institut (SSI) in Denmark. What the American public needs to know is that the SSI is not only the Danish version—and frequent collaborative partner—of the CDC, but also that country's largest vaccine manufacturer."

Indeed, the investigation conducted by Sallie and Mark Blaxill painted an intricately tangled web of relationships between the authors of the three Danish thimerosal studies. They allege that nearly all the investigators were either employees of or had financial ties to the SSI, which "relies heavily on its vaccine products for revenue, growth and profitability, including from the vaccine export business," they continued. "SSI has a direct financial interest in the assessment of past mercury-containing vaccine safety issues, and they cannot be considered an objective party. They should be excluded from further work in vaccine safety assessments."[361]

The Safe Minds parents weren't the only ones to react swiftly. Rep. Dave Weldon issued a scathing indictment of the report just hours after it was issued.

"Today's report is premature, perhaps perilously reliant on epidemiology, based on preliminary incomplete information, and may ultimately be repudiated," Weldon began. "This report will not deter me from my commitment to seeing that this is fully investigated, nor will it put to rest the concerns of parents who believe their children were harmed by mercury-containing vaccines or the MMR vaccine."[362]

The report, Weldon predicted, "will only drag the IOM under the cloud of controversy that has currently engulfed CDC. This concern is what led me earlier this year to request that Dr. Julie Gerberding delay this meeting and report."

Weldon also condemned the IOM for narrowing its scope of inquiry. "In 2001 the IOM considered thimerosal's relationship with neurodevelopmental disorders as a whole, but here they only consider autism," he said. "This raises suspicions that this IOM exercise might be more about drawing pre-designed conclusions aimed at restoring public confidence in vaccines rather than conducting a complete and thorough inquiry into whether or not thimerosal might cause neurodevelopmental disorders."

Moreover, Weldon charged, many of the authors of the epidemiology studies had conflicts of interest that included "funding from vaccine manu-facturers, employment by manufacturers, or conflicts in that they imple-mented vaccine policies that are now being investigated."

The IOM, he warned, is not immune from error "and has been forced to reverse itself before, most recently reversing a long-standing finding that chronic lymphocytic leukemia was not due to Agent Orange. A similar rever-sal is a very real possibility here."

Weldon concluded by saying he was "troubled by the lack of liability or accountability by these decision-makers should they be proved wrong. I want more than just a 'sorry' from them should their conclusions be found erro-neous a few years down the road. Too many lives are at stake."

Other supporters of the thimerosal-autism hypothesis also weighed in, largely in the form of long, critical e-mails. Richard Deth, for example, wrote:[363]

> The report aims to close the door on concerns that mercury-containing vaccines might have contributed to the increased fre-quency of autism. Unfortunately it is obvious that the need to close the door was given a higher priority than reaching reliable scientifically-based conclusions. This is particularly evident when the report shock-ingly takes a hard-line against further research into this important question and goes on to endorse the inclusion of thimerosal in vaccine formulations for national and international distribution, dismissing any concerns about their ethylmercury-related toxicity. Having at-tended the IOM hearing in February, the report does not really come as a surprise. From the very outset, Dr. Marie McCormick displayed a pugnacious and adversarial attitude toward the presentation of in-formation suggesting a thimerosal/autism link, as opposed to that of a neutral investigator. She was curt and hostile, rather than welcom-ing new input. The report reflects a similar adversarial tone, with a welcoming, uncritical presentation of those epidemiological studies which failed to find a link contrasted to a hypercritical, dismissive ap-proach toward data supportive of a link.
>
> The IOM clearly valued the epidemiologic approach and de-valued results derived from autistic individuals. The report was a biased effort

at damage control. It did not have the interest of the American public as its central concern, but rather was an instrument to attempt to cover-up a very important public health problem.

Jill James, meanwhile, made these observations:

> They conclude that the available biological hypotheses for a causal relationship between autism and mercury "lack supporting evidence and are theoretical only." ALL scientific hypotheses are "theoretical" by definition—that is why we propose to test them! I am most disappointed that the committee chose to recommend that available funding for autism research be channeled to more promising areas—basically discouraging further research into a possible association—despite a huge body of evidence in the literature that mercury is both immunotoxic and neurotoxic. This recommendation was way out of line in terms of their original charge and is a gross misuse of their power.[364]

And Boyd Haley wrote:

> The observation of mercury level differences in birth hair of autistics versus normals that Amy, Mark and I published was replicated using a different approach by MIT researchers. It was also confirmed retrospectively by Dr. Bill Walsh. Why did the IOM totally ignore this in their report and call the thimerosal hypothesis "theoretical only"? It appears very solid that autistic children do not biochemically handle mercury as do normal children! This is not theoretical, this is biochemical fact—the IOM members just chose to ignore it as it does not fit into what they wanted to report. This data clearly shows that a small subset of the population is being affected by mercury that would be somewhat difficult to detect with a less than elegantly designed epidemiological study, and easy to miss or cover up. This biochemical data does not totally prove thimerosal is causal for autism, but it certainly should have prevented the IOM from saying they 'conclusively' proved thimerosal was not involved. If you do not believe in a hypothesis you replace it with another. That is how science is done.[365]

IT WASN'T until the next day, when the dust had settled and the reporters' phone calls slowed down, that Lyn had time to read the whole report. Buried deep in the body of the 160-page document, she came across several passages of caveats about the reliance on epidemiological evidence at the expense of biological data.

On MMR vaccine, the panel had this to say: "The committee's conclusion did not exclude the possibility that MMR could contribute to autism in small numbers of children, given that the epidemiological studies lacked sufficient precision to assess rare occurrences. Thus it was possible that *epidemiological studies would not detect a relationship between autism and MMR vaccination in a subset of the population with a genetic predisposition to autism* [italics added]. The biological models for an association between MMR and autism were not established, but nevertheless were not disproved."

And the panel conceded this: "Determining causality with population-based methods such as epidemiological analyses requires either a well-defined at-risk population or a large effect in the general population. Absent biomarkers, well-defined risk factors or large effect sizes *the committee cannot rule out, based on epidemiological evidence, the possibility that vaccines contribute to autism in some small subset* or very unusual circumstances [italics added]. However, there is currently no evidence to support this hypothesis." And later it also added this: "This hypothesis cannot be excluded by epidemiological data from the large population groups that do not show an association between a vaccine and an adverse outcome. Depending upon the frequency of the genetic defect, a rare event caused by genetic susceptibility could be missed even in large study samples."

13. Paying the Piper

TWO DAYS after the IOM's "eye-opener" of a report was issued, the Office of Special Counsel Scott J. Bloch dropped a bomb of its own. On May 20, 2004, the OSC sent a letter to Congress, specifically to Senator Judd Gregg (R-NH), chairman of the Senate Health Committee, and Rep. Joe Barton (R-TX), chairman of the House Committee on Energy and Commerce, requesting that they look into allegations of malfeasance among federal employees, as well as the toxic nature of thimerosal.[366]

Special Counsel Bloch sent the letter to Congress "notwithstanding a new Institute of Medicine study released yesterday that concludes there is no link between thimerosal and autism," said an accompanying press release. It said that Bloch "shares many of the concerns about the allegations, many of them from parents of children with autism or other neurological disorders." But it added that his office lacked jurisdiction over disclosures from private citizens.

And then the special counsel issued the equivalent of an open call for whistle-blowers. "In the event, however, that a federal employee comes forward with information on this issue," the press release said, "OSC would then have jurisdiction to determine whether there is a substantial likelihood that the information discloses a violation of any law, rule or regulation, or a substantial and specific danger to public health and safety."

When it came to thimerosal and damage to children, Bloch said: "It appears the science is inconclusive, not definitive. Based on my limited review of the literature, there appear to be equally qualified experts on both sides of the emotional, scientific and medical debate. This strikes me as a far-reaching public health issue that warrants further study and awareness, particularly because it affects the most vulnerable among us."

It is important, he said, that government agencies "be as certain as possible that these vaccines containing mercury, a known potent neurotoxin, have undergone sufficient, reliable scientific review definitively answering the legitimate medical questions, such as, whether there is any medically necessary reason for including mercury in vaccines given to children. Furthermore, parents and others should also know that they can request a mercury-free vaccine."

Bloch wrote that he had "recently received hundreds of disclosures from private citizens alleging a widespread danger to the public health, specifically to infants and toddlers, caused by childhood vaccines which include thimerosal." And though he lacked a whistle-blower, Bloch wrote, "based on the publicly available information, it appears there may be sufficient evidence to find a substantial likelihood of a substantial and specific danger to public health caused by the use of thimerosal/mercury in vaccines because of its inherent toxicity. . . .

"Due to the gravity of the allegations, I am forwarding a copy of the information disclosed to you in your capacity as Chairmen of the Senate Committee and House Committee with oversight authority for HHS. I hope that you will review these important issues and press HHS for a response to this very serious public health danger," Bloch wrote. He also said that some of the disclosures alleged that thimerosal "is still present in childhood vaccines, contrary to statements made by HHS agencies," and that, according to the information provided, "vaccines containing 25 mcg of mercury and carrying expiration dates of 2005, continue to be produced and administered. . . .

"In addition," the letter continued, "the disclosures allege, among other things, that some datasets showing a relationship between thimerosal/mercury and neurological disorders no longer exist, that independent researchers have been arbitrarily denied access to CDC databases, and that government-sponsored studies have not assessed the genetic vulnerabilities of subpopulations. Due to their heightened concern that additional datasets may be destroyed, these citizens urge the immediate safeguarding of the Vaccine Safety Datalink database, and other relevant CDC information, so that critical data are not lost."

The disclosures also alleged that the CDC and the FDA "colluded with pharmaceutical companies at a conference in Norcross, Georgia [Simpsonwood], in June 2000, to prevent the release of a study which showed a statistical correlation between thimerosal/mercury exposure through pediatric vaccines and neurological disorders, including autism, Attention-Deficit/Hyperactivity Disorder, stuttering, tics and speech and language delays. Instead of releasing the data presented at the conference, the author of the study, Dr. Thomas Verstraeten, later published a different version of the study in the November 2003 issue of *Pediatrics,* which did not show a statistical correlation. No explanation has been provided for this discrepancy."

There was "an increasing body of clinical evidence" of thimerosal's connection to neurological disorders, "which is being ignored by government public health agencies," he said, expressing "serious continuing concerns about the administration of the nation's vaccine program and the government's possibly inadequate response to the growing body of scientific research on the public health danger of mercury in vaccines."

Lisa Sykes was bowled over. She e-mailed a copy of the letter to her large and growing universe of activist parents. And though it was also posted on the Schafer Autism Report the next day, the news received zero attention in the mainstream media.

ONE YEAR EARLIER, the nation's leading autism organizations had been quarreling over how to reform the federal Vaccine Court—with more "mainstream" organizations like Cure Autism Now divided against more "radical" groups like Safe Minds. But when it came to the IOM report, every autism group was on the same page, united in opposition to the committee's conclusions: Autism One, Defeat Autism Now!, Cure Autism Now, the Autism Society of America, Unlocking Autism, Moms Against Mercury, the National Autism Association, NoMercury.org, the National Alliance for Autism Research, and Safe Minds all expressed vigorous objections to the report.[367]

On Saturday, May 29, 2004, Dave Weldon summarized this unanimous discontent in an unusually harsh speech to the annual Autism One Conference in Chicago—where Dan Burton had released his "Mercury in Medicine" report one year before.

"Just what is so wrong with the IOM report? What has caused all of the autism groups to unite against the IOM?" Weldon began. "In my ten years of service in the U.S. Congress, I have never seen a report so badly miss the mark. I have heard some weak arguments around Washington and I can tell you that those in the IOM's recent report are very weak. Examine this report in detail. It is plagued with serious flaws."

Then Weldon attacked the CDC. "A public relations campaign, rather than sound science, seems to be the M.O. of the officials at the CDC's National Immunization Program office," he said. "Let's look, not only at the timing of the IOM meeting in February, the content of the IOM report, but also at studies the IOM used as a basis for their decisions. The IOM bases their decision almost entirely on five epidemiology studies, all of which were conducted by researchers with an interest in not finding an association, all of which have short-comings, and all of which the IOM declares would miss an association if it were in a genetically susceptible subset of children."

Then the congressman made a very serious accusation. In the absence of epidemiological evidence to support causality, he charged the IOM had been "instructed" by the CDC to "give biological evidence little consideration, and was *prohibited* from allowing biological evidence to lend credence toward causality. Is it any wonder that the CDC has spent the past two years dedicating significant funding to epidemiology while starving funding for clinical and biological research?"

Weldon also accused the CDC of instructing the IOM to "narrow" its scope to look only at autism and not other neurological developmental disorders (NDDs). "Anyone familiar with the Verstraeten study knows exactly why the IOM's scope was narrowed," he said. "Because the 2003 Verstraeten study found associations between thimerosal and NDDs and some children with autism may have been misdiagnosed as having speech or language delay. By narrowing the scope—which largely went unnoticed by the media—the CDC has avoided acknowledging that thimerosal very well may have caused NDDs in some children.

"Does that sound like an agency interested in understanding whether or not thimerosal might be harmful, to some children?" he asked. "Or, does this response lead one to conclude that they are more interested in designing something to reassure an increasingly skeptical public? This latest IOM report is simply part of a P.R. campaign in my view. The IOM notes in their report that the epidemiology studies they examined were not designed to pick up a genetically susceptible population. Yet, they attempt to use these five flawed and conflicted statistical studies to quash further research into the possible association between vaccines and autism. This report is extreme in its findings and recommendations. The IOM process became little more than an attempt to validate the CDC's claims that vaccines have caused no harm," Weldon continued.

"This report will not deter me nor the autism community from our commitment to seeing that thimerosal and MMR research is properly done. This report will do nothing to put to rest the concerns of parents who believe their children were harmed by mercury-containing vaccines or the MMR vaccine. While this report will lead many clinicians to believe that thimerosal is safe and there is no problem with the MMR, it may contribute further to an erosion in the doctor-patient relationship."[368]

Weldon's fiery remarks received little play in the media. But all of his recent comments on the IOM did seem to catch the attention of CDC director Julie Gerberding. One morning in late May, Gerberding happened to be on Capitol Hill on CDC business, when she popped in unexpectedly to the Florida Republican's office. "Okay," she said to him, "what do we need to do to get to the bottom of this issue?"

"We need more research on mercury and autism, not just epidemiology," Weldon told her. "We need funding directly related to fully understanding the biological mechanisms that may be causing the neurological problems in these children."

"Fine," Gerberding said. "Can your office put together something? Can you get me a wish list of all the kinds of research protocols that *you* would like to see funded?"

When Gerberding left, Weldon's deputy chief of staff, Stuart Burns, called Lyn Redwood at home. "Hey, Lyn," he said excitedly, "do you think Safe Minds could put together a list of research projects on autism and vaccines you would like to see the federal government pursue?"

ON JUNE 8, 2004, just three weeks after the IOM issued its report, Dr. Mady Hornig's mouse study was published online in *Molecular Psychiatry*. A press release issued by the peer-reviewed journal said that the animal model was "the first to show that the administration of low-dose ethylmercury can lead to behavioral and neurological changes in the developing brain."[369] The work also reinforced previous studies "showing that a genetic predisposition affects risk in combination with certain environmental triggers."

Identifying a potential connection between genetic susceptibility and environmental triggers (i.e., thimerosal) was important, according to Hornig, because "it may promote discovery of effective interventions for and limit exposure in a specific population."

Safe Minds, which helped fund the Columbia University study, jumped at the chance to upbraid the IOM. They released a statement titled "New Columbia University Study Confirms IOM Vaccine-Autism Report Is Wrong."[370] The Hornig study, Lyn said, "is a perfect example of the scientific findings that the IOM ignored when creating their recent report. The IOM was well aware that studies such as these were due for release, but chose to ignore them—which is why Safe Minds called the IOM's report premature."

The findings, Lyn said, "make clear that the IOM was more interested in regurgitating CDC spin than incorporating hard science. Until the CDC and FDA stop hindering crucial medical research, and stop playing Enron-esque accounting games under the label of 'science' to protect their position, it will be up to independent organizations, like Safe Minds, to assure that every possible research avenue is funded."

The Columbia mouse study got ample play in the mainstream media, and served to counterbalance the seemingly incontrovertible conclusions of the IOM.

In particular, the *Los Angeles Times* and CBS News—the only two national outlets to follow the thimerosal controversy with the most aggressive reporting—covered the mouse story well. The *Los Angeles Times* interviewed independent researchers not involved with the study, who raved about its methodology. "The exciting thing is that this gives us a way forward in understanding why we have not seen more conclusive findings on either side of the fence, and how we need to design studies to pick up gene-environment interactions," said Ellen Silbergeld of the Johns Hopkins School of Public Health.[371]

"I believe this has enormous implications for public health," Dr. Julio Licinio of the University of California, Los Angeles, and editor of *Molecular Psychiatry,* told the *Times.* "Showing that genetic background impacts on the outcome of thimerosal exposure is a major breakthrough." He said that Hornig's study showed a clear link between vaccines and autism "for some groups and not for others."

Members of the IOM panel, perhaps not surprisingly, played down the study's significance. Dr. Steven Goodman, of the Johns Hopkins School of Medicine and a member of the IOM panel, told the *Los Angeles Times* that "it's a tantalizing little piece of evidence that requires a lot more work" in order to overturn the "tremendous amount of human work that doesn't find a clue of a connection."

At CBS News, health reporter Sharyl Attkisson on June 18, 2004, delivered a five-minute special report on Hornig's work—including an interview with the researcher in her lab—during the "Evening News with Dan Rather." And WebMD.com published a lengthy article titled "Mercury Linked to Autism-Like Damage in Mice." In it, medical writer Laurie Barclay wrote that "many thought the battle was finally over, laid to rest by a report released by the IOM," but that Hornig begged to differ. "We believe that these conclusions were rendered prematurely," she told Barclay.[372]

Dr. Steven Goodman was quoted in this article, too. To the parents, he seemed to be doing a bit of backpedaling on the definitive tone of the IOM report.

"It was clear from the report that we were not giving thimerosal a clean bill of health," Goodman said. "We didn't say that thimerosal is something that we should want in vaccines; we said that the safest vaccines are indeed thimerosal-free vaccines. We only said that the evidence favored that there was not a connection between autism and thimerosal exposure."

And, he went on, "We didn't say that investigations shouldn't continue in the lab on the effects of mercury, on the effects of thimerosal, and on the causes and profiles of autism. Where the committee thought that research dollars probably shouldn't go, at least for the moment, are these large-scale [public health] studies linking autism and thimerosal exposure."

Dr. Hornig, however, countered that the IOM report would most likely shut off federal funding for her work. "The pronouncement that research funds are better applied elsewhere effectively forecloses any possibility of federal funding for an entire field of research," she said. "The timing is particularly unfortunate given that we are only just beginning to define the mechanisms by which environmental factors such as thimerosal interact with immune response genes during early development." Indeed, Hornig told Lyn Redwood and others that she thought she might never again get NIH funding to continue her work with mice.

THE SEARCH for an OSC whistle-blower continued. The five original candidates that Laura, Lisa, Lyn, and others had identified were either unwilling to step forward or did not meet the criteria set down by the special counsel's office. Lisa was getting desperate. In early June, Lyn went through her entire address book, virtually everyone she had ever spoken with about thimerosal. She provided Lisa with the name of every person who could even remotely be a whistle-blower or know where to find one. One of the people on Lyn's list was an organic chemist from New Jersey named Paul G. King, an independent product safety compliance consultant to a number of drug companies, with experience with the FDA's vaccine program. In 2003 he was working on a research paper when he contacted Lyn about Safe Minds' mercury studies. King seemed astounded by what Lyn told him about the controversy, and said that if he could assist the parents they should let him know. Looking back on that conversation, Lyn realized that Dr. King, who had spent decades working with the public health bureaucracy, could become an outstanding ally in the whistle-blower manhunt. Lyn gave his name to Lisa.

It was a fortuitous union. King had a number of potential informants in mind. One individual in particular, an employee at the FDA's Center for Biologics Evaluation and Research (CBER), seemed like a prime candidate. He most likely met the OSC criteria for status as a federally protected whistle-blower.

Lisa contacted the man. He seemed interested, and said that he certainly did have incriminating evidence to reveal. After all, he been with the agency going all the way back to the 1970s. It was during this time, according to allegations in the legal papers filed by Andy Waters in the Counter case in

Texas, that Eli Lilly "lied to the FDA in a bid to avoid regulation." In 1972, Lilly had received an article alerting the company that thimerosal had caused six deaths from mercury poisoning in infants. The babies died after a thimerosal-containing solution was applied to their omphaloceles (a serious birth defect in which a portion of the intestines is exposed).

"Shortly thereafter, the FDA required Lilly to provide all the information at its disposal concerning the potential toxicity of thimerosal," the Waters lawsuit contends. "Lilly reported to the FDA, in a February 14, 1973 letter, that 'as with other chemicals of its generation, information relating to safety and efficacy of thimerosal in animal models is sparse.'" But Waters said Lilly went further, advising the FDA that the product was non-toxic. "It cited the fraudulent Jamieson and Powell study of 1930 [on dying meningitis patients] as its supporting scientific evidence. Despite knowledge to the contrary, Lilly continued to use the [study] to support its conclusions that the product was safe and 'non-toxic.'" Lilly's failure to inform the FDA of this and all the other evidence collected by the company was a criminal act, according to the potential mole.

But the man—and his sponsor, Paul King—was demanding the backing of a reputable and experienced law firm, in addition to any protections that the feds could offer. Lisa scrambled to find someone who had represented other federal whistle-blowers, but could not locate even one. Then Laura Bono told her about a nonprofit group in Washington, D.C., the Government Accountability Project (GAP), which specializes in such cases.

The OSC was getting closer to landing their whistle-blower, and Lisa kept Scott Bloch's office apprised of her progress.

Paul King was proving to be a terrific new recruit to the cause, a tactical wizard with several regulatory tricks up his sleeve. In mid-June 2004, King suggested a second prong of attack to Lisa, quite apart from any federal investigations. The two had been communicating by e-mail, and one day King told Lisa that the parents should file something called a "citizen petition" with the FDA.

Lisa had no idea what King was talking about. But when he explained it to her carefully, she jumped at the idea.

"There is a mechanism by which private citizens can call on the FDA to take action against products or policies that are believed to be harmful," King explained. "Not everyone knows about it. You could file one to formally ask the FDA to remove mercury from all vaccines given to children. You could demand a recall."

A citizen petition is a federally established avenue of recourse for the public to pursue a review of any aspect of the FDA's oversight of foods, drugs, medical devices, and cosmetics. By rule, the FDA has 180 days to respond to the petitioners' requests. If the agency fails to do so, or if the petitioner is un-satisfied with the response, the case may then be brought to a court of law for resolution.

Lisa put out word to the parents who had worked on the attorney gen-eral and OSC efforts, asking for volunteers. Lisa recruited Kelli Ann Davis, from North Carolina, as well as Mark and David Geier, who would work closely with King to lay out their legal and scientific case. Soon, a few more parents of autistic children were invited to join the little FDA working group, such as Brian Hooker, a Ph.D. from Washington State who was look-ing into conflicts of interest at both the CDC and the IOM, and issuing a flurry of FOIA requests on the matter; Leslie Weed, a mother from Ponte Ve-dra Beach, Florida, who had been collecting thousands of documents attest-ing to thimerosal's toxicity; and Bobbie Manning, the mother from Kansas City (who had now moved to Buffalo) who had experience working with the media and close ties to powerful people in the Democratic Party.

The group gave itself a name: the Coalition for Mercury-free Drugs (CoMeD) and, of course, launched a Web site. The site became an electronic depository for any parent, doctor, or researcher wishing to file supporting documents for the FDA petition, including personal testimonials, medical records, and research data on thimerosal's toxicity.

MANY of the same parents working on the FDA petition had also been busy trying to get their respective states' attorneys general to pursue lawsuits against the drug companies. Despite energetic efforts to make this happen, none of the attorneys general was ready to make the plunge into tobacco-style litigation, and none wanted to go first.

The most promising prospect was in Minnesota. A union of parents led by Nancy Hokkanen and backed up by Mark and David Geier had met three times with Attorney General Mike Hatch, an ambitious Democrat who was mulling over litigation on behalf of autistic Minnesotan children. In June of 2004, Hatch began interviewing law firms to represent the state for possible action against Eli Lilly and the vaccine manufacturers.[373] But by late August, he still seemed highly reluctant to make a move, according to Dallas attorney Andy Waters, who participated in a conference call with Hatch in late July. Waters said Hatch was under pressure from Republican Governor Tim Paw-lenty not to proceed (though the two rivals were barely on speaking terms). And, he said, the IOM report had made it much more problematic to take any kind of legal action. (Hokkanen, who was on the call, said she did not remember Hatch saying this. A spokeswoman for the attorney general said she could neither confirm nor deny any of the accounts.)

In North Carolina, Kelli Ann Davis was trying to meet with her own state's attorney general, Roy A. Cooper III, with little success. But Kelli had enlisted the help of a strategic ally: Senator John Edwards (D-NC), who was widely rumored to be John Kerry's pick for vice president on the Democratic ticket. Kelli had met several times with Edwards's staff since late 2003, and had conferred with the senator himself at a Washington, D.C., "Tarheel" gathering during the spring. There, she extracted a promise from the rising political star to meet with her personally on the issue.

Kelli is indefatigable and will rarely if ever take no for an answer. In November 2003 she convinced John Edwards's staff to have him send a letter to the North Carolina attorney general, in which he asked Cooper to meet with Kelli and Mark Geier "regarding mercury-based immunizations, in light of a recent report (Verstraeten et al in *Pediatrics,* November, 2003) on the link between thimerosal vaccinations and autism in children. Mrs. Davis has asked Dr. Geier to visit North Carolina to present his own findings on this link," Edwards wrote.[374]

"While previous research has found that children are 2.48 times as likely to become autistic if they receive an immunization with mercury, the recent report shows no link," the senator continued. "Given the seriousness of this issue and the effect that it can have on children across the state of North Carolina, it is important that we make educated decisions based on all credible and available information." In February 2004, Cooper agreed to meet with Kelli, the Bonos, Lori McIlwain, and the Geiers. But so far, he had declined to act.

By June of 2004, Kelli was seeking the sit-down meeting that John Edwards had promised her. His staff was helpful and sympathetic, but it was a frenetic time for the senator, who was being vetted by Kerry campaign officials for the VP spot. When Kerry announced his choice on July 6, Kelli knew that it would be even harder to get her meeting. She was disappointed, but sympathetic. A lifelong Republican, Kelli was not about to vote for George W. Bush and Bill Frist's GOP in November. And she did not give up. Kelli kept in touch with Edwards's staff, sending them late-breaking information on all the potential federal investigations bubbling up around Washington. Edwards's staff agreed to send a letter to the investigator general of HHS, Dara Corrigan, to let her know how extremely interested he was in the progress and outcome of the investigation.

John Edwards had also met personally with Mark and David Geier in Washington, on the day of the February 2004 IOM meeting. Edwards reviewed the internal VSD documents and was impressed by their incriminatory nature. "I think that these parents," the accomplished trial lawyer told the Geiers, "have a really good case." When the meeting ended, Edwards told the Geiers: "As long as I am in public life, I will work to make sure that every American has a fair day in court." And, he added: "Bill Frist may want to cut these people off so they can't sue. But we won't let that happen."[375]

BY LATE JUNE, the California bill to ban mercury in childhood vaccines (other than trace amounts) had gained extraordinary momentum. The bill, sponsored by Assemblywoman Fran Pavley (D-Agoura Hills), was approved by the State Assembly, 49–22. On June 23, the State Senate Health and Human Services Committee voted to approve the measure by a 9–1 margin.[376]

Up until that point, the state chapters of the American Academy of Pediatrics and the American Academy of Family Physicians had opposed the bill, warning that it might lead to shortages of some vaccines. But shortly before the Senate committee vote, the AAP suddenly switched to a "neutral stance" after Pavley agreed to a six-month delay in the ban, to July 2006, and a provision for temporary waivers in public health emergencies.

Myron Levin, a *Los Angeles Times* reporter who had begun to cover the thimerosal controversy more thoroughly than any other national correspondent, reported on June 24 that the state measure was being "closely watched by federal health officials and the vaccine industry," and it was "advancing at a time of mounting concern over environmental exposures to mercury, a potent neurotoxin. It also comes amid scientific debate and legal battles over whether thimerosal in children's shots has contributed to a sharp rise in reported cases of autism and other neurological disorders."[377]

Meanwhile, Aventis Pasteur, the only U.S. pediatric flu vaccine maker, did not oppose the bill, nor did it say it "won't be able to produce enough thimerosal-free vaccine by 2006," Levin wrote. An Aventis spokesman said his company had not taken a position on the bill, but said that "in general, we oppose any legislation that would interfere with the public availability of FDA-approved vaccines and unnecessarily undermines public confidence in national vaccine policy."

The Pavley bill was expected to pass the full legislature in late August 2004. It would then be sent to Governor Arnold Schwarzenegger at the end of the month, just as he was preparing to speak at the Republican National Convention in New York City.

DR. JULIE GERBERDING had asked Dave Weldon to prepare a research "wish list" on autism, and Lyn had no trouble finding things to put on it. In June, she finished the list and sent it back to Weldon, who passed it on to Gerberding. He also promised to send a letter to the NIH to request funding for at least some of studies. The list was broken down into three categories: epidemiology, toxicology, and clinical studies. Among the research projects that Safe Minds proposed were:

EPIDEMIOLOGY
1. An investigation into the rates of neurodevelopmental disorders including autism in vaccinated and unvaccinated populations (e.g., Amish, Christian Scientists).
2. An investigation into the rates of autism in vaccinated and unvaccinated control siblings, following the diagnosis of autism in a family member.
3. A study of the rate of RH-negative blood type in mothers of children with autism.
4. A study of cumulative effects from pre- and postnatal exposure to methylmercury and ethylmercury through environmental, dietary, and medicinal sources.
5. Epidemiological studies comparing the incidence and prevalence of autism before and after removal of thimerosal from infant vaccines in a defined population (i.e., Brick Township, New Jersey, or from the California data).
6. Open the VSD (without identifiers) to independent investigators.

TOXICOLOGY (cell and animal models)
1. Determine toxic end points in cultured blood cells from children with autism versus controls, to see if there is increased genetic sensitivity to thimerosal among the autistics.
2. Compare thimerosal neurotoxicity and mercury excretion rates between mice with genetic or nutritional depletion of glutathione and those with adequate glutathione. Restore glutathione levels in depleted mice and evaluate protective effect.
3. Evaluate neurotoxicity, immunotoxicity, and GI toxicity in primates given standard infant vaccination protocol (including MMR), and effects on blood-brain barrier integrity.
4. Further examine already existent primate brains exposed to both ethyl- and methylmercury to identify the exact location where mercury localizes in the brain.

CLINICAL STUDIES

1. Compare genetic mutations in metabolic pathways that lead to glutathione synthesis and oxidative stress between children with autism and controls, to see if there is a genetic basis for vulnerability to oxidative stress induced by thimerosal.
2. Study methylation pathways in children with autism.
3. Investigate metabolic profiles of children with autism in regards to their ability to effectively detoxify environmental toxins, including mercury.
4. Monitor a large cohort of children with autism versus controls for levels of mercury excretion during chelation, including metabolic markers and cognitive function.
5. Conduct placebo-controlled studies of nutritional interventions that have been reported to improve GI function, cognitive ability, and speech in autistic children.[378]

Safe Minds did not hear back from the director about their wish list. And they were still waiting to hear if Dave Weldon could secure that fifty thousand dollars in unused CDC research funds, to help keep the work of James and Hornig alive.

But Lyn, Liz, Sallie, and Mark Blaxill were also pursuing another financial avenue at the time. In early June, Safe Minds submitted two applications for several hundred thousand dollars in government research funds, under the aegis of Dave Weldon's office. The group said it would use the money to fund "research to determine whether low exposures to mercury from common, everyday sources result in adverse developmental outcomes in subpopulations of children." It would also seek to "detemine the biological pathways impacted" and help scientists to identify "subgroups who may be genetically most vulnerable. . . ."

"These findings may lead to biomarkers for identification of these subgroups, leading to preventive measures, and may also lead to treatments for those already exposed," Sallie wrote in the proposal. "It is expected that the studies will be reported in peer-reviewed journals, for the benefit of the scientific and medical communities."

IN THE MIDDLE of July 2004, the new California case numbers came in. They had dropped again—for the third time.

On July 14, Rick Rollens, the parent and Sacramento insider who helped found the MIND Institute at UC Davis, sent an e-mail to Safe Minds and other allies with the news. "According to information released today by the

FIGURE 14. Number of new autism cases (DMS=IV) added per quarter to the California State Department of Developmental Services statistics, January 2000–March 2004.

	No. of New Cases	Increase over Previous Three-Quarter Period	April Through June Increase from Previous Year
Jan.—March 2000	1,331	—	—
Jan.—March 2001	1,930	599	176
Jan.—March 2002	2,314	384	182
Jan.—March 2003	2,391	77	–15
Jan.—March 2004	2,194	–197	–108

Source: Rick Rollens, e-mail to Lyn Redwood, subject: "New Autism Cases Declining," July 14, 2004.

Department of Developmental Services (DDS), California's developmental services system has just experienced the first-ever nine-month sustained reduction in the numbers of professionally diagnosed new cases of full syndrome autism being added to California's developmental services system," Rick wrote. The data compared new intakes from the most current three consecutive quarterly periods (October 2003 through June 2004):[379]

"Not only did the most recent three consecutive quarter period produce the first sustained reduction in the 35 year history of California's developmental services system (197 fewer new cases than the previous October-through-June period)," Rick wrote, "but the most current quarter, April 2004 through June 2004, produced the all time largest reduction of any quarter (108 less cases)."

It's important to remember that the California system only reports diagnosed cases of full-syndrome DSM-IV autism, and does not include PDD-NOS, Asperger's syndrome, or any other autism spectrum disorder that might corrupt the data. California, with the "world's best record keeping system," Rick said, is the "de-facto canary in the coal mine in tracking new cases of autism. . . .

"What makes this historic development of this very recent reduction in new cases of autism so important is that those children from the birth cohorts of 1999 and 2000 are now entering the system," Rick continued. "First with the year 1999, and much more so with year 2000, these are the widely recognized first two years of the beginning of the serious effort to substantially reduce the amount of thimerosal in childhood vaccines. Could this be the beginning of the decline of the autism epidemic? Have we discovered a 'smoking gun' environmental factor that has contributed to the epidemic?"

The news was tantalizing, but by no means proof. Any number of factors apart from the removal of thimerosal could have accounted for the decline. On

FIGURE 15. Quarterly Trends in Number of Persons with Autism Added to the System (1994–2004).

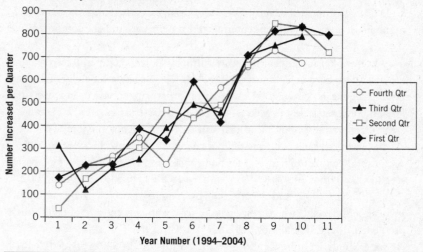

Source: Dr. Ron Huff, California Department of Developmental Services.

July 17, Rick briefed Lyn, Sallie, Mark Blaxill, the Bonos, and others on what the numbers might actually mean. There were several concerns: Though the rates of reported new cases were falling, they were still quite high. Then again, the switchover to thimerosal-free vaccines had been gradual, beginning in 1999–2000. Some children were still receiving mercury in their shots well into 2001, 2002, and possibly beyond. If thimerosal removal was causing the drop in cases, it would take another two or three years for the full effect to appear.

Everyone was cautious about whether the drop could be attributed to thimerosal or not. There were other possible causes. An obvious one, of course, was the severe budget crisis in California and a reduction in services (including autism programs) that might lead to fewer cases entering the system—something that was suggested by Marie McCormick in her teleconference with reporters.

Rick doubted that the fiscal crisis was to blame. He explained that the budget for direct services within the DDS program—which makes up 85 percent of the total—was cut by a mere seven million dollars in the current year, out of a total of three billion. "This would be easily absorbed by the twenty-one regional intake centers," Rick said. The DDS budget for construction and other operations was cut by forty-eight million dollars, but that would not affect new intakes.[380]

In fact, he noted, there had been no substantial cuts in the budget of this program for several years, "and historically, even in years where the budget was cut, it did not impact intake into the program. This was the case in 1990 to 1993, when the state faced even more dramatic cuts than today, and the numbers of cases of children entering the system with autism continued to skyrocket."

Another plausible explanation was shifting population figures. If fewer children had been born in California in 1999 and 2000, then fewer children might be entering the system in 2004. Alternatively, there might have been a drop in foreign immigration in the wake of tightened visa restrictions after 9/11, or increased emigration *from* California because of its struggling economy.

But birth rates in California did not change significantly in 1999 or 2000. As for total population figures, they had consistently risen for each of the past several years, from 34,431,000 on January 1, 2001, to 35,049,000 in 2002, 35,612,000 in 2003, and 36,144,000 by January 1, 2004.[381] If anything, there should have been a corresponding *increase* in new cases of autistic children entering the system, not a decline.

Safe Minds, in a press release issued on July 19, 2004, expressed "cautious optimism" over the third consecutive report from California to show a decline in new requests for autism services. But, they said, "even with this encouraging news, vigilance and continued research should be the course of continued action. . . .

"It has long been the scientifically supported belief of Safe Minds that such a trend would be witnessed following the decreased use of thimerosal, and this trend seems to support our research," Lyn wrote. "In 2002, CDC said they were waiting to see how the prevalence of autism may have been impacted based on the removal of thimerosal from vaccines. I guess now they have their answer."[382]

BY JULY OF 2004, Liz, Sallie, the Redwoods, the Bonos, and the Blaxills were ready to take another summer respite from the thimerosal wars—at least temporarily—to enjoy more time with their families, and each other. Tommy Redwood and Scott Bono went whitewater rafting in North Carolina, while Liz and Sallie started an "Extreme Sports Camp" for autistic kids in Aspen, near the Bernards' home.

But no one stopped working entirely. At this point, Safe Minds was concentrating its efforts on research and new treatments more than on lawsuits and investigations. The public policy fight was critical, to be sure, but the Safe Minds parents felt tantalizingly close to a medical breakthrough, to a new era of metal detoxification and methyl B-12 therapy as the standard of care for regressive autism.

For Safe Minds, the action right now was at the NIH.

At any rate, there was no shortage of parents of affected kids willing to step in to carry the banner on the political and investigative side. The reinforcements included: Lisa Sykes, the minister from Richmond, and Kelli Ann Davis from Fayetteville, North Carolina. There were Bobbie Manning and Kelly Kerns from Kansas, Teri Small of Wilmington, Delaware, Robert Krakow of Long Island, New York, Brian Hooker of Kennewick, Washington, Alan and Lujene Clark of Carthage, Missouri, and Nancy Hokkanen of Minneapolis.

Lisa Sykes had prompted the OSC investigation and, with the help of Kelli Ann Davis, Laura Bono, Lyn Redwood, and others, was still hot on the pursuit of a whistle-blower—needed for the special counsel to open a formal investigation.

When Lisa and the group first wrote to the OSC, they also sent copies to federal investigative bodies all over Washington. One of these was a little-known interagency task force called the President's Council on Integrity and Efficiency. The PCIE consists of leading investigators from nearly every department in the federal government. Each department has an inspector general (IG), and each agency, such as the FDA and CDC, that falls under the Department of Health and Human Services, has an Office of Investigation (OI). Most of these officials sit on the PCIE.

The PCIE is headed by White House deputy director of the Office of Management and Budget. The group is charged with "coordinating and enhancing governmental efforts to promote integrity and efficiency and to detect and prevent fraud, waste, and abuse in Federal programs," according to its Web site.[383] The PCIE also develops "plans for coordinated government-wide activities that attack fraud and waste and promote economy and efficiency in government programs and operations. These typically include audit and investigation of fraud and waste that exceed the capability or jurisdiction of an individual agency."

On July 12, Lisa received a letter from an official at the PCIE saying that the group was going to review the request for an investigation. In fact, the PCIE considered the matter to be of such gravity that it had cleared time in the next meeting's agenda to discuss the allegations.

"Here we go," Lisa thought, smiling, as she finished reading the letter. "This whole house of cards is about to start crumbling."

EVEN AS LISA, Kelli, and other parents worked on the Office of Special Counsel, the President's Council on Efficiency and Integrity, and the citizens' petition to the FDA, another group was pursuing its own avenues of governmental investigation. This group, headed by Teri Small, the mother of an autistic boy from Wilmington, Delaware, and aided by Mark and David Geier, took a slightly different approach to the feds.

In April 2004, Teri and other parents and activists had written to Dara Corrigan, acting principal deputy inspector general, HHS, and to Special Counsel Scott Bloch outlining a number of complaints against the CDC and FDA, including conflicts of interest with drug firms among employees and consultants; negligence and malfeasance among FDA officials who failed to monitor cumulative mercury exposures in vaccines; manipulation and cover-up of VSD data; illegal denial of public access to the VSD; illegal destruction of VSD data sets; and other misdeeds.[384]

At first their allegations seemed to fall on disinterested bureaucratic ears within the vast Department of Health and Human Services. Most officials preferred to shuffle the matter off onto other officials. But the group refused to back down. They sent letter after letter, document after document, demanding that the HHS inspector general look into the charges. By late spring/early summer, HHS investigators *were* taking notice. Three or four separate HHS investigations were under way, or at least under consideration:

> *HHS Office of the Inspector General and CDC Office of Investigation*—A special agent in charge was assigned to look into allegations that National Immunization Program officials deliberately manipulated taxpayer-funded data (from the VSD) to eliminate an association between thimerosal and NDDs.
>
> *HHS Office of the Inspector General and CDC Office of Investigation*—A second special agent in charge was assigned to investigate allegations that immunization officials were blocking access to VSD data by qualified researchers; and that they either lost, destroyed, or did not properly maintain previously analyzed data sets (Verstraeten), in violation of the federal government's Data Access Law (protecting the public's right to government research findings) and the Data Quality Act (which requires full and honest reporting by government officials of taxpayer-funded research).
>
> *FDA Office of Criminal Investigations*—Parents such as Teri Small and Kelly Kerns met with inspectors from the FDA at the Geier home in Silver Spring, Maryland, on three separate occasions. The agents were investigating the alleged withholding and/or misrepresentations made to the FDA by Eli Lilly and the vaccine manufacturers concerning safety data on thimerosal. If found to be applicable, the special agent in charge would present his report to the Department of Justice.

FDA Division of Internal Affairs—Yet another special agent was assigned to look into whether FDA personnel knew that pharmaceutical products (i.e., vaccines) were being marketed without an accurate package insert, and not taking appropriate steps to correct the situation. And also to investigate alleged "grievous injury being wrought upon children due to negligence and/or conflicts of interest on the part of FDA personnel due to a product that had never been adequately tested for safety."[385]

FEDERAL INSPECTORS were now crawling all over Washington, Rockville, and Atlanta—hunting for evidence in what seemed to be evolving into a bona fide thimerosal scandal.

On July 19, 2004, Lisa Sykes received a letter from the Office of the Inspector General of HHS, and it made her heart sing.

Michael E. Little, deputy inspector general for investigations at Health and Human Services, was writing in response to a communication he'd received from the investigations committee of the President's Council on Integrity and Efficiency concerning Lisa's "allegations that thimerosal is being used in order to increase the manufacturers' profit margins." Little had been asked by the PCIE to "provide a second review and take whatever action we deem appropriate. . . .

"Upon review of the correspondence you provided to the PCIE, in conjunction with further research into the matter, we have determined that your above allegations represent a potential conflict-of-interest issue which may be criminal in nature, and therefore falls within the Department's office of investigations authority to investigate. We are forwarding a copy of your info to Patrick Doyle, special agent in charge of our Philadelphia regional office, for his review and appropriate action."[386]

Patrick Doyle was the same special agent who had been asked to look into some of the allegations against the FDA that Teri Small and her band of parents had raised. The two inquiries would be dovetailed into one, it appeared.

Lisa ran to her computer, copied the letter into her system, and e-mailed it to all the parents working on the federal investigations. "Sweet taste of vindication!" she wrote. "Congrats, OSC Families! We did this together!!! Blessings, Lisa."

FOR THE THIMEROSAL ACTIVISTS, extraordinary news seemed to be breaking out all over. Now the tidings were about to get even better. On July 21,

2004, David Geier was sorting through some old documents at home when he came across a set of data charts that he had glanced at once a few years earlier and then tucked away in a closet.

The documents had come to Lyn from the CDC's Atlanta headquarters in 2001 as part of a FOIA request. In the fall of 2002, when Lyn began working with the Geiers, she made them copies of all her FOIA documents, and this one was among them. Lyn had also briefly glanced at the charts at the time, but an expert statistician told Safe Minds that the data were "raw and uninterpretable." She didn't know what they were, and the data seemed to be a bit shaky, with very large margins of error (or "95% confidence intervals") for many of the results listed.

The data were potentially explosive.[387] David immediately e-mailed copies of the CDC charts to parents and their researcher allies. "We have recently come across some really exciting VSD data linking thimerosal with neurodevelopmental disorders," he wrote.[388] "These data show some VERY large, statistically significantly increased relative risks the CDC found in their assessment of the VSD for thimerosal and neurodevelopmental disorders. Of specific interest are some of the following (this is by no means an exhaustive list)." All the results he listed were considered statistically significant because the low end of the margin of error (95% CI) did not go below 1.00.

"It should be noted that the CDC has never publicly acknowledged a statistically significant correlation between thimerosal exposure and autism," David wrote, "but the results show that the CDC found [the correlation] in three separate analyses."

- *Autism*
   (Study A) Relative Risk = 7.62 (95% CI: 1.84–31.5) [this is an example of a statistically significant result], comparing children receiving more than 25 mcg of mercury from thimerosal-containing vaccines to children receiving 0 mcg by age 1 month
   (Study B) Relative Risk = 11.35 (95% CI: 2.70–47.76), comparing children receiving more than 25 mcg to children receiving 0 mcg by age 1 month[389]
   (Study C) Relative Risk = 2.15 (95% CI: 1.04–4.43), comparing children receiving increases of 7.5–10 mcg over 1 month, to children receiving less than 5 mcg over 1 month

- *Specific Disorders of Sleep of Nonorganic Origin*
   (Study A) Relative Risk = 4.98 (95% CI: 1.55–15.94), comparing children receiving more than 25 mcg to children receiving 0 mcg by age 1 month

(Study B) Relative Risk=4.64 (95% CI: 1.12–19.25), comparing children receiving more than 25 mcg to children receiving 0 mcg by age 1 month

- *Somnambulism or Night Terrors*
(Study A) Relative Risk=5.76 (95% CI: 1.38–24.05), comparing children receiving more than 25 mcg to children receiving 0 mcg by age 1 month

- *Attention Deficit Disorder*
(Study A) Relative Risk=2.88 (95% CI: 1.05–7.88), comparing children receiving more than 75 mcg to children receiving less than 12.5 mcg by age 3 months
(Study B) Relative Risk=2.84 (95% CI: 1.03–7.85), comparing children receiving more than 75 mcg to children receiving less than 12.5 mcg by age 3 months

- *Attention Deficit Disorder without Mention of Hyperactivity*
(Study A) Relative Risk=6.38 (95% CI: 1.56–26.09), comparing children receiving more than 25 mcg to children receiving 0 mcg by age 1 month

- *Attention Deficit Disorder with Mention of Hyperactivity*
(Study A) Relative Risk=8.29 (95% CI: 2.03–33.89), comparing children receiving more than 25 mcg to children receiving 0 mcg by age 1 month

- *Developmental Speech or Language Delay Disorder*
(Study A) Relative Risk=2.09 (95% CI: 1.08–4.03), comparing children receiving more than 25 mcg to children receiving 0 mcg by age 1 month

- *Other Developmental Speech or Language Disorder*
(Study A) Relative Risk=2.32 (95% CI: 1.20–4.48), comparing children receiving more than 25 mcg to children receiving 0 mcg by age 1 month

- *Unspecified Delay in Development*
(Study A) Relative Risk=2.08 (95% CI: 1.03–4.19), comparing children receiving more than 25 mcg to children receiving 0 mcg by age 1 month

In contrast, "some other disorders that are not necessarily biologically plausibly linked to mercury did not show a statistically significant correlation with thimerosal-containing vaccines (i.e. illustrating that above effect is a specific effect of thimerosal, and not the methods of analysis)," David wrote.

The striking tables represented some of the earliest VSD thimerosal data ever circulated among CDC officials, David surmised. These were most likely the first figures that Verstraeten came up with when he began running the numbers in late 1999. Meticulous and conscientious, the statistician had initially taken patients from the original four West Coast HMOs and compared them by various exposure categories. In many cases, the difference in the number outcomes among kids who received higher doses of mercury compared with those who received little to none was striking.

"Everyone is aware of the CDC's Phase I VSD Thimerosal study report of 2/29/00 (with the 2.48 increased autism RR), but these data actually pre-date the 2/29/00 report, and were produced by Tom Verstraeten on December 17, 1999," David wrote.

How did David come to that conclusion? The now notorious, somewhat cryptic e-mail that Verstraeten sent to Robert Davis and Frank DeStefano on December 17, 1999, with the subject line: "It just won't go away." That e-mail had contained the exact same exposure category codes as the tables that David had rediscovered. "This is an email that many may have seen previously, but have been really unable to place in context," he said. "This email also makes the comment, 'As you'll see, some of the RRs increase over the categories and I haven't yet found an alternative explanation. Please let me know if you can think of one.' This email contains an explicit declaration by Verstraeten stating that thimerosal is causing harm in children."

The e-mail, David continued to speculate, "reveals the basis for the panic" expressed by Verstraeten in a previous communication, on November 29, 1999. At that time, Verstraeten wrote that "after running, re-thinking, re-running, re-thinking . . . for about two weeks now, I should touch base with you, I think, to see whether you can agree with what I came up with so far. I'll attach the SAS programs hoping you or one of your statisticians can detect major flaws before I jump to conclusions."

The "worst nightmare" of the CDC had come true, David offered. The theoretical discussions held in June 1999, when the AAP, CDC, and FDA issued the Joint Statement on Thimerosal, "now had been shown to cause broad-based harm in children. Verstraeten was in total panic mode considering the broad-based effects of thimerosal on childhood neurodevelopmental disorders, as revealed in the Tables I sent to everyone," David wrote.

"Now for the first time, we see a much larger and more significant plot of potential alteration and manipulation that the CDC has employed in order to remove the initial effects of thimerosal that they found—i.e. it was not a very limited 'weak' statistical correlation between thimerosal and childhood neurodevelopmental disorders, but was really a broad-based 'strong' [i.e., relative risks in many cases greater than 2, and in some cases relative risks over 50] statistical correlation."

David and Mark had found statistically significant relationships between thimerosal and NDDs in their own analyses, he noted, "but we have never found such a large broad-based statistically significant relationship. It is apparent that our studies have in many cases significantly underestimated the effects of thimerosal on neurodevelopmental disorders in children. This is very powerful additional internal CDC data showing a direct linkage between thimerosal and specific neurodevelopmental disorders," David concluded. "It was not released to the public and needs to be released immediately to everyone, including our media contacts."

ONCE AGAIN, Dave Weldon had come through for Safe Minds. Lyn Redwood was on vacation when she got the call. It was July 30 and Lyn was staying with her family at a tidy little beach house in Destin, Florida, when her cell phone rang. She walked out on the sunny terrace, where the reception was better. It was an official from the CDC calling to say that the fifty thousand dollars in research funds had been allotted for Safe Minds, provided that the group could submit a detailed proposal and could meet a long list of qualifications.

All the paperwork, pages and pages of documentation and certification, was due by August 17. "So much for the beach," Lyn thought. But she was happy to do it.

Also in late July, Lisa Sykes, Paul King, and the CoMeD parents had finished writing their citizens' petition to the FDA. It was a sixty-five-page document backed up by more than a thousand pages of supporting studies, transcripts, data sheets, analyses, and reports. The group decided to deliver the papers in person to the FDA's Rockville, Maryland, headquarters, on Wednesday, August 4.

The petition demanded that HHS Secretary Tommy Thompson and/or acting FDA Deputy Commissioner Lester Crawford immediately issue an order "barring the administration of any thimerosal-containing vaccine, or other such mercury-containing pharmaceutical products, that contained more than 'trace' levels of mercury to pregnant women and children under the age of 36 months."[390] It also called on the FDA to suspend the approval or licensing of any FDA-regulated product that contained more than 0.5 micrograms of mercury per dose, and demanded a Class I recall of all batches of multidose vaccines that contained more than "trace" levels of thimerosal.

"Recent studies, cited in this petition, clearly prove the causal link between mercury exposure and neurodevelopmental disorders (NDDs)," the petition said. "These studies also establish that, *though susceptibility to NDDs is genetically linked and mitigated by other factors,* mercury is the causative agent. These NDDs are currently at epidemic levels. The quicker the agency grants each CoMeD request, the sooner the FDA will begin reducing the risk of irreversible neurological harm to susceptible individuals of all ages."

On August 3, the day before they were to deliver the documents to the FDA, Kelli Ann Davis met once again with the staff of Sen. (and now Vice Presidential candidate) John Edwards at his Capitol Hill office. She invited Lisa, Bobbie Manning, Leslie Weed, and the CoMeD group to join her. She briefed Edwards's staff on the FDA petition and the various nascent inquiries and secured a promise that Edwards would write a letter to the inspector general at HHS in support of the internal investigations.

The next morning, Kelli met Lisa Sykes, Paul King, Bobbie Manning, and Leslie Weed outside the FDA, and they all walked in together, carrying reams of papers to deliver at the agency's dockets department. They were accompanied by a reporter and photographer from *Mothering Magazine* and a television crew from CBS News.

After the FDA, the parents dropped off copies of the petition at the office of HHS Secretary Tommy Thompson, and then went to the Hill to visit the staff of Sen. Judd Gregg (R-NH) asking why there had been no response to the letter from the Office of Special Counsel and stating that a whistle-blower was about to step forward in the case.

"You guys can't sit on this anymore," Kelli told the staff, "because we're not going away. Our numbers are getting bigger and our voices are getting louder."

Another stop that the CoMeD parents made while in Washington was at the headquarters of the Democratic National Committee, where Bobbie Manning worked her various contacts. She had arranged a meeting with Becky Ogle, who handled health and disability issues for the party. This time, David Geier came along as well. The group laid out the entire thimerosal controversy to Ogle, who looked flabbergasted.

"I am going to walk this over to the top strategy people at the Kerry-Edwards campaign and put it right on the table for all of them to see," Ogle told the group when they finished. "This deserves to be on the front burner." As they got up to leave, extremely pleased with their meeting, Ogle stopped to say: "Can I ask you a question? Why aren't you running through the streets, blocking traffic, screaming at the top of your lungs and burning down government buildings?"[391]

THE COMED PARENTS returned from Washington feeling pretty good about what they had achieved, and excited at the prospects of potentially forcing the FDA to finally ban thimerosal from childhood vaccines. Near the end of their third day in Washington, on Friday, August 6, Mark Geier got an unexpected call from the Institute of Medicine. The IOM, Mark learned, had just scheduled a special meeting in Washington for August 23 "to discuss the VSD database, among other things," a staffer told him, adding that the IOM would post more information about the meeting on its Web site by the end of the day.

Mark did not know what to make of the call. A meeting about the VSD? Was the IOM actually going to address the many roadblocks to access that the Geiers had endured? Would they finally open the books on the secretive database and its five generations of analyses—in which no evidence of harm was eventually found? And what committee of the IOM would hold this meeting? After all, Marie McCormick's Immunization Safety Committee had finished its work and disbanded.

Word got out quickly about the IOM announcement. Lyn, Sallie, and Laura Bono were initially optimistic. Something was up, they thought: all these investigations must be making some powerful people very nervous. "IOM is backtracking now," Laura said. "They want to cover their rears because they know this is about to blow wide open."

Paul King, the biochemist who crafted most of the FDA petition, also thought the announcement portended good news.

"Coupled with the filed 'Citizen Petition,' the buttonholing of certain Congressional staffers, and the news coverage by CBS and *Mothering Magazine*, it would seem, based on an apparent scheduling of an IOM meeting on 23 August 2004, that HHS, CDC and the drug industry have 'noticed' that: A) We have just begun; and B) The FDA has been put on notice."[392]

A few hours later, a bulletin for the meeting was posted on the IOM Web site. Most of the parents stopped smiling when they read it.

The review was to be conducted by the IOM's Committee on Health Promotion and Disease Prevention. The committee would be charged with reviewing the "design and implementation of the new VSD Data Sharing Program to assess compliance with the current standards of practice for data sharing in the scientific community," the Web site said, and to make recommendations to the NIP "for any needed modifications that would facilitate use, ensure appropriate utilization, and protect confidentiality."[393]

This last line could have been interpreted either way. "Facilitate use" would imply opening up the database, while the words "protect confidentiality" would indicate a desire to crack down on access. The panel would also "review the iterative [repetitive] approaches to conducting analyses that are characteristic of studies using the complex, automated VSD system," the announcement said. "Examples of recent studies to be examined are a completed screening study on thimerosal and vaccines [Verstraeten]."

Based on the above review, the committee was to then consider "whether, when, and how preliminary data about potential vaccine-related risks obtained from the VSD system should be shared with other scientists, communicated to the public, and used to make policy or recommendations to CDC." It would also make recommendations to the CDC "on the release of such preliminary data in the future."

The word *whether* set off alarms among many parents and researchers. This would imply that preliminary data should, perhaps, *never* be released to the public, under any circumstances. When Lyn read it, she recalled how Jim Moody and other attorneys had said that CDC information officers were neither authorized nor obligated to include preliminary research documents in FOIA requests. Such "preliminary data" would include the Verstraeten analysis that found a relative risk for autism of 2.48 and, presumably, the very early (and potentially damning) charts that David Geier had recently rediscovered and sent out via e-mail to dozens of people.

Whoever had stuck those documents into Safe Minds' FOIA box back in 2001 had acted either out of ignorance or subversion, the parents surmised.

The tentative agenda also looked somewhat ominous, for the parents at least. Following a background discussion on the VSD Data Sharing Program by an as yet unnamed official, the "charge to the committee" would be delivered by Roger Bernier, a leading vaccine official at the CDC.

Later, Mark and David Geier were scheduled to testify about their "experience with the VSD Data Sharing Program," followed by an HMO rep who would present the "perspective of a managed care organization involved in the VSD," and then comments by "a consumer group on access to VSD data."

It was bound to be an explosive meeting.

Mark Geier called Stuart Burns from Weldon's office. "Why are they in such a hurry to set something up?" he said. "Why have an emergency meeting? What are the vaccine boys *up* to?" Geier worried that the IOM, under pressure from the CDC, was going to determine that "it's inappropriate to look into intermediate data sets on studies like Verstraeten," he said. "And they are going to say that congressmen like Weldon shouldn't interfere with the workings of the CDC and that no one should have access. I am confident the CDC is trying to get IOM to clear them, just like they did before!"

Outrage spread quickly through the autism world. Teresa Binstock, the developmental researcher who helped Safe Minds write its original mercury paper, denounced the meeting in a well-circulated e-mail. "The purpose of the 'hearing' is to create a paper trail giving the illusion of public input," she wrote. "The hearing's conclusions are stated in the agenda: (i) keep VAERS and VSD data as secret as possible, (ii) control which researchers have access to the data, and (iii) control what gets written and publicly shared by researchers who've had access to the data."[394]

The IOM and CDC, Teresa charged, "know full well that extensive neurologic damage has occurred across the nation, and that evidence for such damage exists." She called the hearing a "formalizing of what shall remain/become an ongoing cover-up of the damage," and "blatantly intended to enforce hiding the data and thereby keeping from the American public the ramifications of the data showing widespread neurologic damage from thimerosal, etc. Thus an issue that needs major attention is the IOM's deliberate attempt, via the forthcoming hearing, to HIDE THE EVIDENCE OF HARM."

IT WASN'T the only startling news of the day for many parents. That morning, Myron Levin reported in the *Los Angeles Times* that Aventis Pasteur, the only manufacturer of pediatric flu vaccine, "is trying to rally opposition to state legislation that would bar use of a mercury-based preservative in vaccines administered to infants and pregnant women in California."[395]

Aventis, Levin wrote, "is raising the specter of shortages that could leave the state vulnerable to a mass outbreak of flu." But, he noted, "Earlier this year, an Aventis spokesman said the company should be able to produce enough thimerosal-free vaccine to fill all orders, given sufficient notice. Aventis representatives did not return calls seeking clarification." Rick Rollens was quoted as saying that Aventis's stand was indefensible and "a bully tactic by a large pharmaceutical company."

Aventis, "in a late charge against the bill," had recruited an "important ally"—the California Conference of Local Health Officers, which represents chief medical officers of all fifty-eight California counties. "The group's president, Dr. Scott Morrow, acknowledged this week that the group decided to oppose the ban after being contacted by Aventis," Levin wrote. But then Morrow contradicted himself: "In response to inquiries by *The Times* Morrow said he discovered that Aventis sought the group's help on the bill—something he said he didn't know at the time he signed the letter," Levin wrote. " 'I'm very disappointed,' he said. 'It feels to me very disingenuous.' Nonetheless, he added that the group has taken the correct position, 'regardless of how it came to us.' "

The next day, Levin published an in-depth front page story on the entire thimerosal controversy. It was one of the most comprehensive, insightful articles ever printed on the subject in a major daily newspaper. In it, Levin called it a "dispute overflowing with bitterness and rancor." Parents, he wrote, "are pushing a disturbing theory: that their children were casualties of the war on disease, suffering brain damage from thimerosal by itself or in combination with measles virus in the measles-mumps-rubella vaccine. They blame mercury from vaccines and other sources for an epidemic rise in autism and related neurological disorders."

Lyn had been working closely with Levin for a number of months, and he wrote about the struggles of the Redwood family. Lyn, he said, recalled that Will "started to walk, talk and generally do things on time, before suddenly regressing and slipping away. 'He stopped looking at us. He stopped playing. It was like *Invasion of the Body Snatchers*,' she said. 'Somebody had taken away my baby's soul and just left a shell of him in there.' "

Levin, with his contacts in the pharmaceutical industry, wrote that drug companies and the government were bracing for a fight. "Big vaccine makers such as Merck, Wyeth and Aventis-Pasteur, along with Glaxo, are watching with trepidation," he wrote. "Though safe from liability in the vaccine court, they are anxious because claims have begun to leak into the civil courts."

But vaccine makers "insist that their defense is rock-solid," Levin said. "The evidence 'is so overwhelmingly one-sided that we are confident that juries will overcome their natural sympathy for plaintiffs and decide these cases as science dictates,' said Daniel J. Thomasch, lead outside counsel for Wyeth. 'There's simply no reliable scientific evidence' that thimerosal causes autism, said Loren Cooper, assistant general counsel for GlaxoSmithKline."

Privately, however, Levin said that "some industry figures conceded that when it comes to sick children and brokenhearted parents, science doesn't always win the day. The companies 'are terrified' of huge jury awards because 'the injuries are so grave,' said Kevin Conway, a lawyer for parents."

Meanwhile, Dr. Stephen Cochi, head of the CDC's National Immunization Program, told the *Times* that only "junk scientists and charlatans" supported the thimerosal-autism link. He blamed the uproar on those eager "to capitalize on the tragedy of parents with children who have autism, because they see a huge pot of gold at the end of the rainbow," Levin reported. " 'That's the other side of this story,' Cochi said, 'that it has the potential to be a gigantic scam on the American taxpayer.' Of all the resentments of the parents, the idea that they are out for a buck seems to gall them the most."

But the *Los Angeles Times* seemed to disagree with Cochi. The same day, in an editorial titled "Safer Vaccines for Children," the paper endorsed the Pavley bill to ban mercury in vaccines for infants and pregnant women.

"There is a sharp and unresolved scientific debate over whether thimerosal in vaccines has contributed to a steep rise in reported autism cases," it said. But "common sense and prudence argue for the bill's passage."

LYN RETURNED HOME from vacation with a lot of work left to do. It was now August 8, and the CDC research proposal was due in just over one week. The trip to Florida had been idyllic. Will seemed to be getting much better, Lyn thought. She marveled at how engaged her son was on vacation: playing in the water like a normal kid, hugging his dad after a long walk down the powder-white beach.

Back in Tyrone, Lyn sat at her computer and looked up at the Mercury Monkey, still tacked to her wall after all these years. It seemed as if she had been in that office for centuries. And yet here she was, still working, still fighting, still trying to convince powerful people of her belief that mercury in medicine had poisoned her son and so many other children. She was still trying to prove that effective treatments were at hand.

Lyn prayed that the endless war over thimerosal would reach a conclusion. But the prospects were dubious. The IOM had issued its report, and more epidemiological studies showing no link to thimerosal, including the UK investigation presented by Dr. Elizabeth Miller at the IOM meeting, were about to be published in *Pediatrics*.

Lyn took a break from her work and switched on CNN, to try to catch news from the campaign trail, where John Kerry and George Bush were duking it out in a dead-heat election. CNN was showing images of the war in Iraq. Thick black smoke billowed from the rooftops of the ancient city of Najaf, where rebel Shiite forces were holed up in a holy mosque, fighting to the death. Meanwhile, Pvt. Lyndie England, accused of being a major player in the Abu Ghraib prison scandal, was just beginning her trial at Fort Lejeune, North Carolina. The Pentagon had announced back in January that it had opened an investigation into abuses at the prison. But no one in the media had bothered to look into the story until those ghastly photos surfaced. The scandal was a catastrophe for the United States. It was a giant misdeed that had already happened, and the press had been silent about it. It wasn't until the photos came to light, until there was irrefutable evidence of abuse in living color, that the media snapped out of its collective myopia.

What the mercury-autism story lacked was a photo finish. There was no clean or damning verification. Nearly five years after the Joint Statement on Thimerosal was released, there was evidence of harm, but still no proof.

When Lyn thought of war, she often thought about Will. When soldiers return from war, she thought, they are acknowledged for their bravery. Some even receive medals and hero status. And our kids? she thought. They receive strange looks and pity, or ridicule for their injuries, with no public acknowledgment of the sacrifices they made to protect our country. Our children are heroes and they deserve that same recognition from our country. Our children deserve to have their injuries and disabilities acknowledged and compensated by our government and those responsible. The nation's mandatory vaccine program acknowledges that there will be some casualties, but harming our kids is acceptable for the "greater good."

And yet Lyn was encouraged by her own situation. Will had done so well already on oral B-12 and folinic acid. Will was getting better. To be sure, he still had a distance to go before he became a completely "typical" kid, but he was doing a lot of typical things for a ten-year-old. He had gone on his first overnight trip with kids from school. Will had never been away from home on his own. Even a year ago it would have been unthinkable. But he had begged his parents to go, and he had a blast.

Will was now speaking in complete sentences instead of the two or three words he used to blurt out. Sometimes his enhanced communication skills were a mixed blessing: Will was so good at talking that he was starting to sass back—but just a little. Overall, Lyn thought, her son was one of the sweetest, most loving, and guileless human beings she had ever met.

And yet she couldn't deny the signs of a developing, typical, at times cocky teenager. A few nights earlier, Lyn had driven Will to Blockbuster Video, where he had a game pass. That meant he could check out a video game, play it, and then exchange it for another game in a few days. But when they arrived at Blockbuster, Will discovered he had grabbed the wrong video to return. The young man behind the counter said they would have to return the right game in order to get a new one. Lyn drove her son home and then back to Blockbuster. Will walked into the store and plunked the game down on the counter.

"There," he said to the clerk. "I hope you're happy." Lyn was mad at Will, and she made him apologize to the young man. But inside, she was giddy. Will was reacting to the world around him, just as any growing boy would.

Will was also starting to notice girls. It was something that every parent of an autistic child wonders about: What will happen when they are adults? How will they ever find intimacy, romance, love? Most autistic kids in America were still too young to face that issue. But now, Will Redwood was smitten with a girl at school. He came home one day walking on air. Lyn had never seen such delight in his eyes. Will even called the girl one evening, holding his own in conversation. When Tommy heard about Will's new courtship, he was beside himself. "That's pretty damn good for a child we thought would never be talking again!" he told Lyn, all smiles.

Lyn prayed that the world would eventually come to realize what had transpired. Slowly, squarely, the puzzle was coming together. The work of so many dedicated people. Richard Deth, Jill James, Mady Hornig, Jeff Bradstreet, Boyd Haley, Mark and David Geier, Amy Holmes, David Baskin, the Safe Minds parents, and many others, each had contributed a key piece to the scientific riddle. Lyn thought they were getting close.

So much was happening that it was hard to keep track of it all. There was the decline in numbers in California, for instance. There was the OSC investigation and the newly unearthed whistle-blower. There were the FDA criminal investigation and at least three other internal HHS inquiries looking into wrongdoing at the FDA and CDC. There was movement among the state attorneys general, who were mulling over class-action suits. There was growing controversy over the flu shot, and the bill by Weldon and Carolyn Maloney to ban mercury in vaccines. Meanwhile, a handful of thimerosal suits were proceeding in civil courts.

Then, on August 8, 2004, Lyn logged onto her computer once again to check out what was happening in the world of autism. There was astonishing news out of England: the UK Department of Health had just announced that it was immediately and unconditionally, without comment or fanfare, removing thimerosal from the DTP vaccine routinely administered to children.

Several outlets, including the BBC, reported that it was Mady Hornig's Columbia University study that had tipped the scales.[396] But Dr. David Salisbury, head of immunizations at the UK Department of Health, said the decision was in no way connected with worries over a link between the preservative and autism.[397]

To Lyn, it didn't matter. Research that Safe Minds had helped to fund and bring to the media—the Hornig mouse study—was clearly having an impact. It was essential to keep Hornig's work alive. Lyn put the finishing touches on her CDC proposal for a fifty-thousand-dollar grant to support her work at Columbia and that of Jill James in Arkansas. When Lyn finished, she gathered the documents into a binder, got in the car, and began the thirty-minute trip into Atlanta, to the CDC.

On the drive, Lyn began thinking about all that she wanted after these years of great effort. She wanted more research, to solve the mysteries of mercury and its effect on infant minds and bodies, and to develop effective, proven therapies to treat, if not cure their children.

Lyn wanted mercury removed from all medical products immediately, not only in the United States, but worldwide. She thought of the millions of kids who are vaccinated every year in developing countries with mercury-laced shots provided by the American government and U.S. relief organizations. The intentions were wonderful, but the results could be disastrous.

What an abysmal legacy it would be if America were one day found to be responsible for autism epidemics around the world.

Lyn wanted justice and compensation: for Will and for tens of thousands of other kids and their families. Their lives had been mangled and their futures left uncertain. Who would pay for all that tending and treatment? Who would take care of these people when their parents were gone?

Lyn wanted something else. She wanted recognition. She wanted someone in a position of authority to tell the American people—and the world—that a generation of children had been placed at unnecessary risk, at times with devastating consequences. Lyn wanted someone to take responsibility, something that seemed to be in dwindling supply in American civil society. She wanted those responsible to be held accountable. She wanted someone to admit that a terrible blunder had been made.

And there was one more thing, Lyn thought, as she wove her way through the heavy traffic, the postmodern skyline of Atlanta rising into the warm, humid haze. She wanted an apology.

Epilogue

November 5, 2004

THIS SPRAWLING, interwoven story is far from over. Evidence to both support *and* refute the thimerosal-autism theory continues to trickle in from research under way around the world. Until the question is definitely resolved, the controversy will bubble and simmer. Meanwhile, determined parents will not relent in their search for new and promising treatments that could, perhaps, bring their ailing children one small step closer to "normalcy." There is now tantalizing evidence—but still no definitive scientific proof—that this is possible.

What follows is a summation of many of the unresolved issues in this controversy. It's impossible to know which, if any, will be settled by the time this book is published.

The Legal Front

Civil Litigation

Though most lawsuits filed in civil court currently remain in jurisdictional purgatory, pending movement within the federal Vaccine Court (including those filed by families such as the Bonos and Redwoods), a small number of cases have quietly moved forward. In Texas, a suit filed by the coalition led by Andy Waters, of Waters & Kraus, has been allowed to proceed, and the trial date has been set for March 23, 2005.[398] In another case filed by Waters & Kraus in Federal Appeals Court in New Orleans, the court ruled in August 2004 that claims against Eli Lilly are not preempted by the Vaccine Injury Compensation Program, because thimerosal is not a vaccine and Lilly is not a manufacturer under the law.

Thimerosal, the court ruled, "is not the finished product itself, and on its face the statute governs only lawsuits filed against manufacturers of completed vaccines."[399] In other words, Lilly and the makers of thimerosal, at least, are not covered by the VICP and thus not immune from lawsuits. This was the very issue addressed by the notorious "Lilly rider" that was inserted into the 2002 Homeland Security Act.

The court, however, went one step further in upholding the right of parents to sue Lilly in private lawsuits outside the VICP. "Congress could not have been much more plain in its desire *not* to preempt tort claims filed by persons who are ineligible to recover in Vaccine Court," the ruling said. "There is nothing in the Vaccine Act [that] prevents this suit from going forward."

In late October 2004, Andy Waters finally secured the ability to depose Thomas Verstraeten, and he flew from Dallas to Belgium to complete the long-awaited task. Waters said he could not discuss the content of the former CDC researcher's remarks.

Meanwhile, none of the dozen or so state attorneys general who met with parents and the Geiers have yet decided to move forward with tobacco-style litigation against Lilly and the vaccine makers. It is believed that the IOM report of May 2004 discouraged some of them from proceeding further. By the fall of 2004, parents such as Nancy Hokkanen, who had placed great hope in Minnesota Attorney General Mike Hatch, conceded that he probably would not be moving forward with legal action anytime soon. Other parents, including Robert Krakow of New York, are hopeful that Elliot Spitzer, New York's ambitious and successful Democratic attorney general, might one day take up the fight.

Vaccine Court

In July 2004, Special Master Hastings rejected the petitioners' request for discovery of industry documents related to Merck's MMR vaccine.[400] Hastings referred to the February 2004 IOM meeting to justify his decision. It did not bode well for the pending thimerosal cases, even though Hastings said his decision would not affect his ruling on causality, nor was it clear what impact, if any, this would have on the demand for discovery materials in the thimerosal cases. Hastings also set a hearing for September 23, 2004, on the petitioners' request for all raw data from the Vaccine Safety Datalink (VSD). Attorneys for the families said they would present the recently rediscovered "Generation Zero" analysis to the court as proof that full release of the VSD data was warranted.

Federal Investigations

As of this writing, the potential federal whistle-blower inside the FDA's Center for Biologics Evaluation and Research was still in the process of formalizing his protection status in order to bring charges to the Office of Special Counsel. Special Counsel Scott Bloch's office did not return calls seeking comment. Likewise, there was no response from the Office of the Inspector General at the Department of Health and Human Services, which is looking into allegations of fraud, malfeasance, and conflicts of interest among employees of the FDA and CDC. And Special Agent Richard S. Bacherman of the Special Prosecution Staff at the FDA's Office of Criminal Investigation, said he could neither confirm nor deny that his office was investigating fraud charges against Eli Lilly and other companies (that allegedly violated federal law by withholding from the FDA data showing evidence of harm). Meanwhile, the FDA still has a few weeks before it must respond to the citizens' petition filed by Lisa Sykes, Kelli Ann Davis, and the parents of the CoMeD coalition.

If any crimes are charged, they may take years to go through the courts. Still, Rep. Dave Weldon said he was "very suspicious of malfeasance" among CDC officials. "There is conflict of interest on the part of those people, clearly, they bounce from the vaccine manufacturers to the CDC, back and forth all the time," the conservative Republican from Florida said in an interview. "Verstraeten listed himself as a CDC member when in fact he had been employed for two years by a manufacturer under litigation."[401]

But without a whistle-blower, there is no case. Weldon expressed near contempt for the CDC monitor who told the Geiers that the agency was scrutinizing the VSD database each week and "watching the autism numbers come down. . . .

"If you publish that, she's toast. And frankly, if she's hiding information I don't care. The whole thing stinks, in my opinion. The whole thing is shabby." The woman, reached at her home, refused to be interviewed.

Weldon expressed confidence that CDC director Dr. Julie Gerberding would look into the charges. "I talk to her all the time, and she clearly recognizes that there's a problem here, a problem with perceptions," he said. Still,

Gerberding never "intimated" that thimerosal was causing autism. "The problem with her on this issue is, when she became the CDC director she kind of took ownership of this. And the big thing everybody's afraid of is, if anything came out like this, it would erode public confidence in vaccines," Weldon said. "People wouldn't vaccinate their kids, and their kids would end up dying. But that's been the problem since the beginning of vaccines."

A thorough airing of the nation's immunization laundry, no matter how dirty, Weldon believes, could only serve to help, not hurt confidence in the vaccine program. "People are not stupid," he said. "Some people on the fringe may not vaccinate their kids, but the vast majority of people understand how dangerous those diseases were. I almost wonder if [vaccine officials] are trying to protect their careers more than they're concerned about increased immunization uptake. Actually, when they engage in that kind of cover-up behavior, I think that precipitates people refusing to vaccinate their kids."

Access to VSD Data

In July 2004, Kaiser Permanente Northern California reapproved access for Mark and David Geier to examine data from their HMO.[402] But that didn't mean the father-son team could return to the CDC computer center without delay.

On August 23, 2004, the Institute of Medicine held its hastily called meeting on the sharing of VSD information and "preliminary" data with researchers outside the government. Mark and David Geier testified, and several groups, including Safe Minds, the National Autism Association, CoMeD, and others, issued a joint statement to protest any discussion that could "potentially further limit or permanently restrict access for independent research and review of taxpayer funded VSD."[403] Among the many concerns was the "urgency of this meeting," given the request for a mid-September interim report, just prior to the September 23 VICP hearing on releasing VSD data for legal discovery.

But even if full VSD access were granted, the data sets (the actual groupings of children) assembled by Thomas Verstraeten and colleagues seemed to have been lost or destroyed. One contractor testified at the August IOM hearing that he was ordered to destroy data sets to "protect privacy." It would be virtually impossible for anyone to reconstruct the exact same groupings of patients on their own. The CDC had asserted to Dave Weldon that the data sets were provided to the Geiers, but the Geiers insisted that the sets contained no data and were "totally unusable." The same assertion was confirmed to the Geiers by their CDC monitor at the computer center in Hyattsville.

The CDC also claimed that it no longer monitored the VSD for adverse thimerosal effects after the year 2000. Dave Weldon, who had been told by the Geiers that the CDC was quietly mining the data every week for signs of bioterrorism, wrote to the agency to inquire when it would provide an update. "If CDC is not going to update the VSD, why was this decision made?" he asked.

And given that thimerosal had been removed beginning in 1999, Weldon wanted to know, "how will the failure to update the VSD adversely impact the ability to track changes in outcomes, if thimerosal has been a contributing factor?"[404]

"This is outrageous," Weldon told Gerberding, point-blank, in his Capitol Hill office in May 2004. "You took the mercury out of the vaccines, and you're stopping the collection of data immediately *afterward?* Wouldn't you want to collect that data and know whether there's a trend downward?" Gerberding conceded he had a "good point," and said she would get back to him. "And I'm reminded just now that she never got back to me," he said in an August 2004 interview. "The whole thing stinks to high heaven."[405]

Ominously, many parents allege that the CDC secretly instructed the IOM vaccine safety committee not to find any associations between thimerosal in vaccines and neurological disorders, a claim the IOM vehemently denies. Brian S. Hooker, the parent from Washington State, charged as much in a letter to Dr. Julie Gerberding on August 21, 2004. He also filed a FOIA request for all communications on the matter between the CDC and IOM. In August, Hooker received a letter from the CDC saying that his request would be fulfilled, but with one glaring exception. "We are withholding a one-page predecisional internal communication," the letter said, "the release of which would interfere with the agency's deliberative process."[406]

Finally, concern was raised by parents such as Lujene and Alan Clark of Missouri, among others, that the CDC had established a private, offshore organization called the Brighton Collaboration, in which all vaccine safety data would be deposited, free from the prying eyes of U.S. subpoenas and FOIA requests.

The Political Front

Legislation

On August 26, 2004, the California state assembly, by a margin of 48 to 21, approved the final measure to remove thimerosal from vaccines given to infants and pregnant women. Earlier in the week, the state senate passed the bill by 22 to 13, despite opposition from Aventis Pasteur.[407] On September

28, following intense pressure from both sides, Governor Schwarzenegger quietly signed the measure, making California the second state after Iowa to pass this measure.

Meanwhile, Rep. Dave Weldon's federal bill to remove mercury from childhood vaccines seemed to be stalled, at least until the new Congress convened in January 2005. "It's frustrating," he said. "I talk to my colleagues in Congress. They turn around and they talk to the CDC, or they talk to their pediatricians. And they come back to me and say, 'Oh, there's nothing to it. Those people are off the deep end.' "[408]

Some opposition to his bill comes from liberals. "It's strange for me, because I'm a conservative," Weldon said. "It's usually the liberals doing this: the whistle-blowers, the histrionics, the Wellstone types. And I've got liberals like Waxman accusing me of being *fringe*. Why are these guys going berserk over mercury emissions from smokestacks, but go mum on injecting mercury into babies?"

Attempts to reform the Vaccine Court would surely be held over for the new Congress as well. Parents like Laura and Scott Bono were still pushing hard for their own version of a reform bill that would allow children allegedly injured by any vaccine or thimerosal—going as far back as 1986, when the court was established—to enter the program before reaching the age of eighteen, with the right to "opt out" preserved. Some attorneys, including Andy Waters, feared that Senator Frist and others would allow these families into the program but then, once they were in, move to prevent them from leaving the VICP to sue in civil court.

The 2004 Election

As of this writing, President George W. Bush had just won reelection and an increased majority in the House and Senate. This could have considerable bearing on the outcome of this story, particularly where the legal rights of affected families are concerned. Most observers agree, it could strike a grave blow against parental attempts to sue drug companies in civil court.

President Bush made tort reform a pillar of his reelection campaign and promises to make it a leading agenda item in his second term. Bush routinely belittles "frivolous" medical lawsuits when rallying against gluttonous trial lawyers. Bill Frist, who will return to the majority leadership as the Bush administration's point man on tort reform, will surely resume his drive to cap punitive damages in malpractice awards at $250,000. And some version of his vaccine compensation bill is almost certain to resurface in 2005.

Could a Republican reelection victory have a stifling effect on the various investigations of malfeasance among government employees? In theory, it should not. Then again, "the Administration and the Justice Department are the ones who would have to do the prosecuting, and I'm not sure they're of the mind to do that," said Dan Burton in an interview. "Of course, if we could find a flagrantly visible violation, then we might be able to get something done."[409]

Meanwhile, the Bush administration has quietly been going to court to obstruct lawsuits involving government-approved drugs and medical devices. "The administration contends that consumers cannot recover damages for such injuries if the products have been approved by the Food and Drug Administration," reported Robert Pear in a July 25, 2004, *New York Times* article.[410] The Justice Department admitted in court papers to a "change in governmental policy" on this issue.

"Allowing consumers to sue manufacturers would 'undermine public health' and interfere with federal regulation of drugs and devices, by encouraging 'lay judges and juries to second-guess' experts at the FDA, the government said in siding with the maker of a heart pump sued by the widow of a Pennsylvania man," Pear wrote. "Moreover, it said, if such lawsuits succeeded, some good products may be removed from the market, depriving patients of beneficial treatments."

Drug Money Influence

During the 2004 election cycle, pharmaceutical dollars continued to flow into political coffers, but with two substantial changes over 2000. First, the ban on "soft money" had slashed total contributions from corporations for political races. Lilly, for example, shelled out $1.6 million in 2000, but only $575,500 in 2004. Interestingly, most drug companies chose to cut the lion's share of their contributions from the Republican column, meaning that the percentage of money contributed to Democrats rose considerably.[411] Could this be why the Democratic ticket remained silent on this issue? Many parents think so. (Calls to the Democratic National Committee were not returned.)

"It's all very bipartisan," said Jim Moody, the libertarian Washington lawyer who advises Safe Minds. "Drug companies aren't doing anything that any other large corporation isn't doing. They're just buying favors from politicians from both parties who are for sale."[412]

What the vaccine makers get for their millions, Moody contended, is "fast-track drug approvals, less regulatory scrutiny, litigation protection—and mandatory use of their products." Returns on their political investments are

FIGURE 16. Percentage of political contributions to Republicans and Democrats made by five major drug companies, 2000 and 2004 election cycles.

Company	% of money to Dems 2000	% of money to Dems 2004
Pfizer	15	33
Bristol Myers	13	30
Glaxo	16	34
Lilly	19	27
Aventis	22	31

Source: Center for Responsive Politics, www.opensecrets.org.

considerable, he added. "They're buying quite a little package. I can't think of any other industry that gets both mandated product use *and* immunity. Usually, you get one or the other. To get both, to get this deal—'you have to use it and we can't get sued for it'—well, that's sweet. Get me some of *that*."

Moody is convinced that the immunity afforded to companies under the 1986 Vaccine Injury Compensation Act "encourages them to be less safe than they could be." With the belief that they could no longer be sued for mercury-related injuries, he said, "any incentives were removed to behave as safely as they can," he said. "And if they're let off the hook for good, which Bill Frist wants to do, then it would destroy any remaining incentive. The connection between political money and regulatory oversight can lead to failures that can hurt kids. We can't trust this system. We *have* to be skeptical."

The Scientific Front

Search for a Cause

Incontrovertible proof that mercury causes autism remains elusive. Tantalizing data suggesting a link continue to be published, but consensus among most public health officials that there is no evidence of harm seems to have solidified, if anything.

Experts from the FDA, the CDC, the American Academy of Pediatrics, Eli Lilly, Merck, and other vaccine makers have all expressed confidence that thimerosal in vaccines cannot and does not cause autism, ADHD, speech delays, or other disorders. They have denied the existence of any conflicts of interest or undue influence by the drug companies over federal health policy. They have insisted that, because thimerosal is safe, there is no need to force its removal from the pediatric flu vaccine, or any other shot for that matter. Some have said that thimerosal-based lawsuits are baseless and frivolous.

One of the harshest critics to emerge from the debate recently is Dr. Steve Cochi, acting director of the CDC's National Immunization Program. Cochi has called evidence to support a thimerosal link "junk science and disinformation," concocted by "charlatans" seeking to stir up "unfounded fears" among the public. These junk scientists, presumably, include researchers from Columbia University, Harvard, Northeastern University, UC Davis, the University of Kentucky, and Baylor College of Medicine.

Perhaps it should come as little surprise that no employee at the FDA, CDC, or AAP or in the drug industry would agree to be interviewed for this book, despite numerous requests. At the FDA, spokespersons repeatedly referred queries to the agency's Web site, while the AAP wrote to say that "limited resources" prevented the academy from "assisting authors with extensive research requests or critiquing of information."[413]

On June 19, 2003, CDC public affairs officials abruptly canceled an interview scheduled with the author in Atlanta with Robert Chen, Roger Bernier, Frank DeStefano, and Walter Orenstein, twenty minutes before its slated time. The interview had been arranged weeks in advance, but HHS lawyers nixed it at the last minute, citing "pending litigation," even though the CDC, it should be noted, faced no lawsuits in relation to thimerosal. And though officials did offer to look at questions in writing, requests for interviews with Dr. Julie Gerberding and Dr. Steve Cochi were flatly ignored.

The CDC has, however, set up a "Blue Ribbon Panel" on vaccine safety issues to discuss improvements and Mark Blaxill from Safe Minds has been invited to sit on the panel. The agency is also conducting two separate follow-up studies on the Verstraeten VSD report, which will include physical and neurological evaluations of some of the children enrolled in the HMOs. Results of these studies are expected in 2005 or 2006. And in August 2004, the CDC announced that it would seek public comment on its vaccine safety program at a series of hearings to be held around the country.[414]

Without access to CDC officials to interview, the best alternative is the agency's Web site, which includes a Q&A on the VSD. Here are some excerpts.[415]

On the Verstraeten Study—"The final results of this study found no consistent statistically significant associations between exposure to vaccines that contained thimerosal and a wide range of neurodevelopmental problems, including autism, attention deficit disorder (ADD), language delays, sleep disorders, emotional disorders, and tics. None of the results found any associations with autism or ADD."

On the Early Findings—"In the first phase of the research, there were some statistically significant associations between exposure to thimerosal-containing vaccines and two categories of neurodevelopmental problems, 'tics' and language delay. However, these results were not consistent—that is, the relationships were only found with one of the health maintenance organization (HMO) databases, rather than in all three that were used in the study. Such a pattern suggests that an association does not exist, but that further research should be done."

On Thimerosal and Autism—"In one of the first analyses there was a weak result that found a possible increased risk for autism, but this result was not statistically significant and was later found to have been based on incorrect data." These results, however, "cannot be considered definitive since the study was not specifically designed to assess a complex condition such as autism but to guide the development of follow-up studies at CDC. These studies will investigate more rigorously possible associations between thimerosal in vaccines and a number of neurodevelopmental disorders."

On Simpsonwood and the Four Study Generations—"Thanks to suggestions from other scientists, researchers, and organizations, improvements were made in the databases, research methods, and statistical procedures used to analyze the data. It is accepted and sound scientific practice, especially with complex and important research issues, to seek and use the advice and recommendations from both internal and external reviewers to strengthen a study as much as possible before publishing a final paper. In this case, four major improvements were made after the initial findings were presented in 1999. The methods used to analyze the data were refined and improved based on expert input from inside CDC and from outside CDC. Errors in the data were corrected (e.g., mistakes in medical records, errors regarding the thimerosal content of certain vaccines) to make the results more accurate. More children with diagnoses of interest were identified as the study progressed and the children at the HMOs became older."

On Verstraeten's Alleged Conflict—"One of four CDC scientists involved in the study left CDC to work for GlaxoSmithKline (GSK). Dr. Thomas Verstraeten worked at CDC during the critical time when the study was designed and the data were analyzed. As a result, the journal *Pediatrics* listed Dr. Verstraeten's affiliation as the CDC." To avoid any "perceived" conflict of interest, "CDC should have assured that Dr. Verstraeten's current employment status, as well as his status when the work was carried out, were both disclosed in the journal article."

On VSD Access—"External researchers can submit research proposals to conduct new studies of vaccine safety or reanalyze study-specific datasets from published VSD studies. [They] have the opportunity to submit research proposals for new vaccine safety hypotheses that include any or all of the data variables available in the VSD." (This statement is contradicted by the fact that the original Verstraeten data sets appear to have been lost or destroyed.)

What Opponents Say

Some people who contest the thimerosal-autism theory were willing to speak on the record. Mostly they cited the May 18, 2004, IOM report and a trio of studies published in September 2004 refuting any connection between thimerosal and autism. Two of them, large population studies conducted in the UK, showed no "significant link between thimerosal-containing vaccines and abnormal neurological development," according to WebMD.[416] Both studies (one of which was presented by Dr. Elizabeth Miller at the February 2004 meeting) were published in the September issue of *Pediatrics*. Remarkably, these two studies showed a "protective" effect against neurological disorders compared with children who received mercury-free shots. Many critics said the surprising findings were the result of overeagerness to eliminate any signal in the data. The third study, a "careful review of all research published thus far," WebMD said, also found a preponderance of evidence to refute the mercury-autism theory. (Safe Minds and other groups had not finalized their response to the articles at the time of this writing.)

As for the IOM report, "What I think the IOM is saying is, it's been a lot of work to evaluate this, obviously, and the best work in multiple countries is not showing that there was a link," said Dr. Walter Orenstein, who was director of the CDC's National Immunization Program and is now an associate director at the Emory Vaccine Center at Emory University.[417]

"As the IOM says, you can never really rule out anything," he added. "And for the people very heavily invested in this, I don't think any study will ever persuade them, other than to find an alternative cause. I think the issue, though, is the vast, vast preponderance of the information that supports the fact that vaccines are not playing a role in autism. I think the vast, vast majority of people, myself included, think the data strongly does not support a relationship."

Dr. Orenstein went on to defend both the methodology and the integrity of his former colleagues at the CDC. "Nobody wants to harm people or to conceal that harm," he said. "I can't see anyone consciously trying to do that [purposefully manipulate data to eliminate a thimerosal "signal," as alleged by some]. These things always come to light. You're always, in my opinion, a lot better off getting it out, even if you have to take your lumps." And, he added, "To me, regardless of everything, if indeed thimerosal causes autism, then I think those people are entitled to compensation. That's why we have a Vaccine Injury Compensation Program."

Orenstein claimed that he and his colleagues had been roundly criticized by some health officials for releasing preliminary data, for example, at the June 2000 meeting of the Advisory Committee on Immunization Practices in Atlanta, because it was still in a very preliminary fashion. But, he continued, "We believed we were better off getting the information out than, God forbid, something bad is found, and it was later found out that we were sitting on that information. I don't feel we did. We felt people needed to know, and we needed to know whether policy positions needed to be altered."

Dr. Marie McCormick, chairwoman of the now-defunct Immunization Safety Committee of the IOM, also agreed to be interviewed. "The average consumer should be reassured that we could find no evidence of either immunologic or much beyond a theoretical biologic model that would associate vaccines with autism," she said.[418] At any rate, she added, the debate "trades off a theoretical risk for a very real risk of disease. It isn't remote, it's only one plane ride away, because these conditions are still quite present in the rest of the world."

Dr. McCormick also dismissed allegations that her committee was "doing the bidding" of the CDC, as many parents charged. She also denied that committee members had any conflicts of interest, despite allegations made by Dallas attorney Andy Waters in a Texas case, outlining specific conflicts of several members. "What's being said is that, because CDC and NIH paid for [the report], it's not independent. The fact of the matter is it's quite independent," McCormick said. "We're buffered by a number of mechanisms that allow us to work quite independently of our sponsors."

Moreover, she said, "the committee was selected to have had no prior pharmaceutical experience, no experience on a vaccine advisory committee, made no known statements about vaccines or vaccine policy, and taken no recent funding from the CDC [or] the pharmaceutical industry." That, she added, "was very controversial, because it was seen as setting a strict precedent for the staffing of other vaccine advisory committees. But this was quite literally to have this committee as squeaky-clean as possible, and I don't think anyone has ever challenged the fact that the committee had any conflicts in that regard."

McCormick conceded that more weight was given to epidemiological data than to the biological studies presented to the committee. The IOM, she said, has a "ten-year tradition in terms of looking at the issues of vaccine safety" with more emphasis on population studies than on lab or clinical work. "There are a lot of things you can do in the lab that will never show up in the real world," she said. "And so the issue of looking at epidemiological evidence, can you see it in the real world? Because you can do a lot of manipulation in the laboratory, and hold things constant and put things in very constrained circumstances as proof of the principle that a reaction occurs."

But isn't epidemiological data also easily manipulated? "Of course, any data can be manipulated," she said. "But you have confidence that the person who is working the data is working it through in a systematic and logical fashion. I'm telling you, we took very seriously the concerns that had been raised about [data manipulation], particularly through the Simpsonwood process. But it doesn't change very much the results."

Another willing interviewee was Dr. Paul Offit, chief of infectious diseases at the Children's Hospital of Philadelphia, and a vocal vaccine defender. Offit believes that thimerosal is patently safe. "It's a very gentle bacteriostatic agent," he said, one that was often confused with its "more toxic" cousin, methylmercury.[419]

"That carbon atom makes a difference in terms of how quickly the molecule gets excreted from the body," he said. "That's why ethylmercury was chosen, back in the 1930s, as a preservative. A good example of that is ethyl alcohol; it's what you drink in wine or beer. It's nice and relaxing. If you drank methyl alcohol when you went home at night, you'd go blind. That one carbon atom makes a tremendous difference."

Offit provided another analogy: "If I sat here and drank ten gallons of water quickly, I would feel sick. But it doesn't make water unsafe. It just means I shouldn't take ten gallons at once. I feel the same way about these substances, which are in the environment already. I think the way they're presented in vaccines, they are at levels which are helpful, not harmful."

The thimerosal debate itself was dangerous, Offit warned. The controversy had threatened confidence in the national vaccine program and needlessly, dangerously driven some parents away from immunizing their children. Offit did not mention the fact, however, that U.S. child vaccination rates were reported to be at record highs (79 percent of all kids) in July 2004. "We gave thimerosal a scarlet letter," he said. "We precipitously pulled it out of vaccines, and the consequence was immunization programs were disrupted. We disrupted the hepatitis-B [shot] and so people got hepatitis-B. I think we took a real risk and substituted it with a theoretical risk, which is never a good idea."

Offit said he knew of six cases of pediatric hepatitis-B in the Philadelphia area after the birth dose vaccine was delayed. "And there was the death of a three-month-old in Michigan. You could argue that's one more child than was hurt by thimerosal. . . .

"Frankly, until thimerosal is out of all vaccines, nobody's going to be comfortable, which is sad," he continued. "I think we scared people unnecessarily. And you did more harm than good in sort of, quote/unquote, allowing the parent to be fully informed. There's no politically correct way to say this, but being fully informed is not always the best thing. You can take that out of context and make me look like a jerk, but you know what I'm saying. You need to be appropriately informed. You need to have information in a context. That is what I think gets lost in this."

What Proponents Say

Rhetoric on the other side is equally volatile. "You tell Dr. Offit that Boyd Haley said he is full of crap," the chairman of the Chemistry Department at the University of Kentucky, known for his colorful southern sound bites, said in an interview. "If ethylmercury is so damn safe, let's have him take a couple of milligrams" (a few thousand micrograms).[420]

"The difference in the toxicity of ethylmercury and methylmercury is oink and oink, oink," Haley said. "I have no doubt methylmercury is more toxic than ethyl. But if we were to take rats and start injecting them with methanol and ethanol, the methanol would probably kill them quicker, but both would kill them. And you want to argue that ethylmercury can't be toxic enough to cause autism, to cause neural damage? That's preposterous. It's like when you can't get drunk on wine, but you can get drunk on whiskey because it's got higher alcohol. That's not an argument."

Haley said that if thimerosal were not a major cause of autism, the CDC seemed to be in no rush to find out what was. "Why isn't the CDC putting their money into a reasonable hypothesis, or asking for grants to come up with a reasonable hypothesis for what's causing the epidemic? That's what bothers me. It makes me feel like, well, maybe I'm right. There doesn't seem to be any money for a search for an alternative cause, [only] more money for doing studies that will deny that thimerosal is the cause."

The CDC, Haley alleged, "has people just to evaluate this data and come up with the answer they want. But to me the evidence is beginning to be overwhelming, because I can't imagine another rationale. With the testosterone enhancement, the estrogen protection, mercury in birth hair, the level of thimerosal that you *know* is needed to cause neurons to quit growing is even lower than what we're talking about for killing them. It's getting overwhelming. But it's hard to convince everybody, especially people who don't want to be convinced because they will be held accountable."

Haley holds accountable both bureaucrats and pediatricians. "These are M.D.s, the people who consider themselves the smartest in the world," he said. "And yet they sat there and injected into babies a compound that was listed in the PDR [*Physicians Desk Reference*] as an extremely toxic compound. It's listed in there as a percentage of weight. It's freshman chemistry to convert that to micrograms of mercury. And no one ever did. And so now they all look like a bunch of damn dummies, and they're very sensitive to this. I think it's ego and face-saving. I wish I had the answer. To me, it's trying to avoid severe embarrassment."

As for bureaucracies, he said, "they don't have a heart, they don't have a brain, but they do have one helluva strong survival instinct."

Meanwhile, the work of science continues. Richard Deth is further examining the role of dopamine and growth factors in autism and ADD, and how the interaction of thimerosal with certain variations in the MTHFR gene can block the methionine synthase enzyme and thus interfere with methylation and proper nerve growth.

"A single mutation in the MTHFR in and of itself probably isn't enough to cause thimerosal sensitivity," Deth said in an interview.[421] Such "polymorphisms" are hardly rare, he said. At least one MTHFR "polymorphism" occurs in 15 to 20 percent of the population. "It's probably one of several polymorphisms in combination that provide a background of risk that is otherwise generally latent—unless it's brought out by the additional insult that thimerosal provides." Risk factors for thimerosal sensitivity, Deth added, probably result from a number of different genes and their respective proteins. Deth also believes that heavy metal exposure may one day be linked to other epidemic and near-epidemic disorders, including asthma, diabetes, multiple sclerosis, and amyotrophic lateral sclerosis (ALS).

Jill James continues with her studies of low sulfation and methylation levels in autistic children, and the potential promise of treating kids with interventions like the injectable methyl B-12 vitamin. Mady Hornig, at Columbia University, will attempt to continue her work with genetically susceptible lab mice, even if the NIH refuses to grant her a dime.

Then there is that highly provocative early VSD data that David Geier unearthed out of his closet showing elevated, statistically significant relative risks for a variety of outcomes. The data had been culled by Verstraeten in November and December of 1999, when he first grouped together all the children in the four original HMOs. It is not clear what impact the release of these papers will have on the debate.

In August 2004, Mark Blaxill prepared an analysis on the original findings, which he called "Generation Zero" (because up until now, everyone thought that the secret February 2000 report by Verstraeten, showing a 2.48 relative risk for autism, was the first analysis of all; it wasn't).

"These 'Generation Zero' analyses followed a straightforward methodol-

FIGURE 17. One-Month Exposure (Linear Scale).

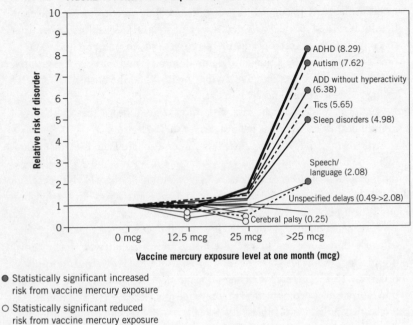

Source: Mark Blaxill, Safe Minds.

ogy that was relatively unaffected by biases applied later, and [were] considerably more sensitive with respect to detecting mercury exposure effects than the later reports," Mark wrote.[422] "Most notably, these initial analyses compared disease risk in the *highest exposure* population groups to disease risk in *zero exposure* population groups."

Moreover, these groupings of children (data sets) had not yet been subjected to "numerous exclusions and adjustments" that were applied later. The cumulative effect "was to reduce the reported impact of mercury exposure on children's health outcomes," Mark wrote. He also prepared some slides to illustrate his point. One slide in particular dramatically shows the increased risks among children who got more than 25 micrograms or more by one month of age.

Another slide shows just how drastically the CDC team managed to reduce the risks between Generation Zero and Generation One. Keep in mind that the data wasn't published until Generation *Four*, when virtually all risks for outcomes had disappeared.

"The results of the Generation Zero analyses are striking and more supportive of a causal relationship between vaccine mercury exposure and child-

FIGURE 18. Selected Diagnoses Comparing Generation Zero to Generation One Results from February 2000.

	Generation Zero 1999 analyses (relative risk)	Generation One 2/29/2000 report (relative risk)	Percent reduction
Autism (399.0)			
• 1 month	7.62/11.35	1.58	79–86
• 3 months	2.00/2.19	2.48	12–19
Attention deficit disorder (314.0)			
• 1 month	3.76/3.96	2.14	43–46
• 3 months	2.88/2.84	2.45	14–15
Developmental speech delay (315.39)			
• 1 month	2.32	0.80	66
• 3 months	0.99	1.30	(31)
Sleep disorders (307.4)			
• 1 month	4.98/4.64	1.74	62–65
• 3 months	2.75/2.74	n.a.	n.a.
Low/high exposure level			
• 1 month	0 to > 25 mcg	0 to > 12.5 mcg	
• 3 months	0 to > = 75 mcg	<37.6 to > 62.5 mcg	

Source: Safe Minds, Generation Zero: Thomas Verstraeten's First Analyses of the Link Between Vaccine Mercury Exposure and the Risk of Diagnosis of Selected Neuro-Developmental Disorders Based on Data from the Vaccine Safety Datalink: November–December 1999, September 2004.

hood developmental disorders (especially autism) than any of the results reported later," Mark continued. He noted that investigators "have wide discretion in the results they choose to report, depending on whether they are interested in reporting a positive or negative finding. In their words and actions, Verstraeten and his supervisors demonstrated clear biases against reporting positive results and made numerous deliberate choices that took positive findings in a single direction, towards insignificance."

Mark said the pattern of behavior "constitutes malfeasance" and "should not be permitted to stand. It is time to remove the parties involved from their role in vaccine safety assessment and to subject the VSD data base to open and independent review."

Methodological errors, meanwhile, continue to plague some of the research put forth as evidence against a thimerosal-autism hypothesis. The most notable recent example is the correction posted on the Web site of the Institute of Medicine, in reference to the NIH study that compared the distribution and durability of methylmercury versus ethylmercury in exposed primates.

The correction was not insignificant. At the February IOM hearing in Washington, Dr. Sager had reported that ethylmercury was "washed out" from primate brains in eighteen days, while methylmercury took fifty-nine days to clear. But in the corrected data, it was revealed that ethylmercury did not wash out of the brains for twenty-eight days. That is probably long enough, proponents of the thimerosal-autism theory argue, for mercury ions to come in contact with, and damage, healthy neuronal cells.

Finally, considerable doubt has been cast on the significance of the declining autism cases reported in the past year in California. On October 15, 2004, Sacramento parent Rick Rollens sent an e-mail to the autism online community detailing case numbers from the just-completed quarter. It painted a murky picture, one that was not particularly favorable to the thimerosal-autism hypothesis (though neither was it catastrophic).

According to information released by the California Department of Developmental Services (DDS), "the number of new professionally diagnosed full syndrome cases of DSM IV autism for the quarter ending October 2004 dropped slightly compared to the October 2003 quarterly report: 749 new cases in October 2004 vs. 786 new cases in October 2003," Rick wrote.

Even so, those 749 new cases represented an *increase* of 26 new cases compared to the previous April 2004 to July 2004 report and represented the second largest number of new cases ever reported for an October reporting period in the history of California's thirty-five-year-old developmental services system.

Complicating matters further, Rick reported that in July 2003 California adopted a new additional "substantial disability" criterion for eligibility into its developmental services system. Now people with mental retardation, epilepsy, cerebral palsy, and autism were required not only to be professionally diagnosed, but they must also demonstrate "significant functional limitations in three or more of the following areas of major life activity: Self-care; receptive and expressive language; learning; mobility; self-direction; capacity for independent living; and economic self-sufficiency."

Since the new law took effect, Rick continued, "there has been a decrease in the number of new intakes in all four categories of disabilities in California's system. In some categories the decrease in the number of new intakes has been substantial." He said that new intakes between July 2002 to July 2003 (prior to the new requirements) and July 2003 to July 2004 (the first full year since the implementation of the new requirements) showed a decline in cerebral palsy of 60 percent, while epilepsy intakes declined by 59 percent, mental retardation by 29 percent, and autism by 1 percent.

"As expected, children with full syndrome autism generally fail in at least 3 and as many as 6 of the areas of 'major life activities' as defined above, therefore one would expect that autism would be the least impacted of all the categories by the new, additional requirements for eligibility," Rick wrote. "The 1% reduction in autism, compared to 60%, 59% and 29% reductions respectively in Cerebral Palsy, Epilepsy, and Mental Retardation, bears that out."

So where does the removal of thimerosal fit into this confusing picture? "The question will be answered here in California in the near future," Rick predicted. "We now know how sensitive California's system is to reporting changes in the number of new intakes when a new factor has been introduced. We also know that California's system does not include children under the age of three years old. Therefore, if one believes that the real decline in the mercury exposure began in 2001 and further declines in mercury containing vaccines over subsequent years, then the first impacted birth cohort (birth year 2001) should start showing up in our system in 2005. We will watch and report the upcoming California quarterly reports with great interest."[423]

Search for a Cure

Is autism treatable? Some people clearly think so, including Bernard Rimland, founder of the Autism Research Institute and Defeat Autism Now! In fact, the Autism Research Institute is preparing a major media campaign called "Autism Is Treatable." Rimland explained in an interview that his organization had "kept track of treatment modalities that we have heard about. We now have fact sheets on seventy-seven different treatments."[424] By far, he said, chelation therapy was consistently shown to have the most dramatic impact on improving the clinical condition of children with autism spectrum disorders. The use of injectable methyl B-12, he added, was too new to have been studied thoroughly.

Rimland said he had collected testimonials from the parents of more than a thousand children "who are now reported to have been taken off the autism spectrum, or who are improving dramatically and becoming normal."

And what, exactly, constitutes "normal"? "We wouldn't call a kid recovered unless they were speaking fully," Rimland said. "And we have lots of kids who have recovered. In fact, we had about a dozen or so attending the last conference," at the end of September in Los Angeles.

Now a newer form of chelation therapy has emerged on the scene, and some doctors and parents insist that it is tantalizingly close to the much-coveted autism "cure," if not the remedy outright. The chelating agent in question is called DMPS, a sulfur-based substance and cousin of DMSA, the oral chelation treatment that most parents use on their autistic children.

The use of DMPS in treating autism was pioneered by Rashid A. Buttar, D.O., vice chairman of the American Board of Clinical Metal Toxicology and visiting scientist at North Carolina State University. His son, Abid Azam Ali Buttar, was born in January 1999 and began speaking at fifteen months. But by eighteen months he descended into silence, and at thirty-six months he was firmly within the autistic spectrum.

At first, Dr. Buttar tried chelating his son with oral DMSA, but little to no mercury came out of the boy. Then he tried administering the more "aggressive" agent, DMPS, delivered in skin patch form on a measured basis into his son's system. By the third "challenge" with transdermal DMPS, Buttar said, Abid was found to have mercury levels in his urine that were 400 percent over levels considered to be safe.

Five months after starting the transdermal DMPS, Buttar's son began speaking again "with such rapid progression that his speech therapist commented how she had never seen such rapid progress in speech in a child before," Dr. Buttar said.[425] "Today at the age of five, Abid is far ahead of his peers, learning prayers in a second language, doing large mathematical calculations in his head, playing chess and already reading simple three- and four-letter words. His attention span and focus was sufficiently advanced to the point of being accepted as the youngest child into martial arts academy when he was only four. His vocabulary is as extensive as any ten-year-old, and his sense of humor, power to reason, and ability to understand detailed and complex concepts constantly amazes me."

This, Buttar added, "led me to the conclusion that a more aggressive method of treatment was necessary compared to the DMSA and various other treatments I had to date employed." In early 2004, Buttar embarked on a study of thirty-one patients with ASD. All thirty-one patients were tested for metal toxicity as measured in urine, hair, blood, and feces, at baseline, two months, four months, six months, eight months, ten months, twelve months, and then every four months thereafter. All thirty-one patients showed little or no levels of mercury on the initial baseline test results.

"Compared to the baseline results, all thirty-one patients showed significantly higher levels of mercury as treatment continued," he said, noting that one child excreted 350 percent more mercury after two months of treatment, over baseline.

More notably, patient improvement "correlated with increased yield in measured mercury levels upon subsequent testing," he said. "As more mercury was eliminated, the more noticeable the clinical improvements and the more dramatic the change in the patient." Evidence for clinical improvements included many observations but was "specifically quantifiable with some patients who had no prior history of speech starting to speak at the age of six or seven, sometimes in full sentences. Patients also exhibited substantially improved behavior, reduction and eventual cessation of all stemming behavior, return of full eye contact, and rapid potty training, sometimes in children that were five or six but had never been successfully potty trained," he added.

Some parents reported additional benefits, including increased growth rates, better adherence to instructions, increased affection and socialization with siblings or other children, appropriate response behavior, and rapid acceleration of verbal skills. "The results in many of these children have been documented on video," Buttar said. "Other physicians involved with this protocol have been successfully able to reproduce the same results."

Buttar believes that DMPS is the wave of the future in the treatment of autism. Oral DMSA, he said, cannot achieve the same remarkable results as the more powerful DMSP. Not only is it a superior chelating agent to DMSA, according to Buttar, but the transdermal delivery system bypasses the GI tract and moves directly toward affected tissue. Meanwhile, he claims, "the constant and continuous 'pull' of mercury, by being able to dose it every other day," is key to the treatment's success.

But chelation therapy for autism remains controversial, and DMPS is most controversial of all. The treatment is not FDA approved for this type of use in the United States, and doctors who prescribe it conceivably run the risk of disciplinary action from medical boards.

In addition, one company that makes DMPS, Heyltex Corporation, issued a letter to pharmacies in August 2004 warning of adverse reactions in autistic children who received transdermal DMPS as a chelating agent. The reactions occurred at the patch site, the letter said, and ranged from mild skin rash to severe reactions involving bleeding and scarring. It was not clear if the DMPS caused the problems or if the delivery agent in the transdermal patch was to blame. Either way, Heyltex recommended against the use of DMPS in transdermal form and urged caution among its pharmacy clients, urging them to "consult with the prescribing physician if you receive a prescription order for a compounded transdermal DMPS product."[426]

It will be some time before DMPS pans out as a proven treatment, and clinical trials are urgently needed, researchers and parents say, to find out. Meanwhile, many parents are not willing to wait. Some of them report extraordinary results.

J. B. Handley is a manager of a San Francisco investment firm who has a young son with autism. Handley began transdermal DMPS in 2004, shortly after his son's diagnosis, and now claims that the boy is beginning to talk and behaving like any normal twenty-six-month-old would. Handley, who has spoken to dozens of parents with the same remarkable success stories to share, is as good as convinced.

"Transdermal is a significantly better way to deliver the agent because it bypasses the gut, which presented major issues for kids with chronically bad guts," Handley claims. "It's better than an IV drip—how do you give that to a kid?—and it is gentle enough to use every other day.

"I believe that Dr. Buttar will go down as the defining figure in the battle to cure autism," he enthusiastically put forth. "Many DAN! doctors are switching 100 percent of their patient populations to TD-DMPS, seeing amazing results, and watching mercury pour out of kids they thought had been fully chelated. His presentations have sparked a treatment revolution. Within a year, you will quite literally see hundreds of fully recovered kids who used Buttar's protocol to get there. He has taught us that autism is nothing more than mercury poisoning: It can be cured; there is a protocol to cure it, and he has the data to prove it is working."[427]

Skeptics, of course, are waiting for publication of Buttar's data in a respected and peer-reviewed journal before they pass their own judgment.

Then there is injected methyl B-12. It seems far-fetched to think that a *vitamin* might hold a clue to the medical management of autism. Researchers like Richard Deth, however, insist it is anything but far-fetched. "We have found that children with autism have an absolute requirement for methyl B-12," he said. "We've figured thimerosal is basically blocking the body's ability to synthesize the methyl 12 itself, because it also impairs methionine synthase."[428]

In the test tube, at least, thimerosal caused methionine synthase activity to "go down to zero," Deth said. "It was rather striking. Usually things will change a little bit down, but it won't be zero. And it turns out that it's zero because the cofactor, methyl B-12, is an absolute requirement for methionine synthase. And when we treated cells with thimerosal, it went away completely."

Conversely, Deth said, his team was able to reactivate the methionine synthase enzyme fully by giving it back the methyl B-12, "in which case it was perfectly happy again." But if they treated the enzyme with a nonmethyl form of B-12, "it had no activity at all." Thus, he said, thimerosal interferes with the formation of methyl B-12, which in turn "explains in a rather dramatic way why methyl 12 injections treat autism," he said. "Because they bypass the very steps that thimerosal inhibits."

Most of the parents in this book—including Lyn, Liz, Sallie, Mark Blaxill, and the Bonos—have tried some form of B-12 therapy on their children, and all of them report at least some improvement in cognition and behavior, especially when combined with chelation. Furthermore, all the kids who have been tested showed at least one "polymorphism," or genetic variance, in the MTHFR gene.

Dr. Jim Neubrander, a physician in Edison, New Jersey, said he had treated more than five hundred children with ASD, and administered thirty to forty thousand methyl B-12 shots. For several years, Dr. Neubrander treated patients with injections of nonmethyl forms of vitamin B-12, as was being done by many DAN! doctors.[429]

"B-12 is a family," Neubrander explained. "There are five different kinds." At first he used whatever form he could find. "Occasionally the patient might give me a little eye contact and focus, but not much else." Then, after the methyl form of the injectable vitamin was made available in the United States, he began to use that version.

"I had no idea that the methyl form would be better," Neubrander said, "it was just the new one available." In May of 2002 he administered his first injection of methyl B-12. "Seven days later, the parents literally ran down the hall with their five-year-old, shouting with joy," he said. "The child previously had no spontaneous speech, only cryptic four-word sentences. And now he would not shut up. He was speaking in complete sentences, with adjectives and pronouns and everything else. They were freaked out, and so was I." Neubrander began trying the new vitamin form on other patients and "out of sixteen kids, twelve responded very positively. That was my initial study, I guess."

By early 2003, Neubrander had treated scores of patients, and more than eighty-five parents wrote to him with the results. Sixty-three of them (74 percent) reported positive outcomes, including improvement in executive function, awareness, cognition, speech and language, socialization and emotion, he claimed. "Half reported moderate to significant improvements and the other half were moderate to mild. But if I can keep them on the regimen for a year to a year and a half, it will make even more of a difference."

Methyl B-12 is hardly a cure, however. It is no magic bullet. Many kids regress within days or weeks without another injection, Neubrander said.

The doctor has dozens of case studies that he likes to cite to support methyl B-12 intervention. One mother, in June 2003, brought a girl into his office who was "one of the worst cases of autism I'd seen," he said. At the time, the child could only make out a syllable or two, and that was on a good day. Exactly two weeks after starting methyl B-12 treatment, after thirty minutes of doing "block therapy" with her mother and special ed teacher, she suddenly looked at both of them—directly in the eyes—and firmly announced: "Okay, I'm finished with the blocks now!" Now, Neubrander said, the girl is "totally off the autism spectrum" and is even advanced in many areas.

"It's not infrequent for a child to be taken off the spectrum a year or so after starting methyl B-12 therapy," Neubrander said. "Doctors will often tell the parents, 'Gee, I'm sorry, I misdiagnosed your child. He doesn't have autism. There's no way he ever could have.' One doctor, during a follow-up visit, told a mother: 'Your son must have been having an awful day a year ago when I diagnosed him with autism. Now, the most I can give him is mild ADD, with some hyperactive overtones.'"

THIMEROSAL'S LEGACY?—A FINAL NOTE

Thimerosal is a known neurotoxin that is not 100 percent effective against bacterial contamination. So why are we still relying on it?

On October 6, 2004, the nation was stunned and frightened to learn that half of the flu vaccine supply produced for the upcoming season, more than 45 million doses, had been abruptly pulled from the market after bacterial contamination was found in the mix. The vaccine, Fluvirin, produced by the California-based company Chiron, was made in a factory in Liverpool, England, that had been cited on numerous occasions for a wide range of sterility problems in the production line.[430]

Health officials in the United Kingdom announced they had detected the potentially dangerous *serratia* bacteria in the final vaccine product— presumably in all the lots that were made. According to the vaccine's label, Chiron used preservative thimerosal as a sterilizing agent in making Fluvirin, to prevent exactly this type of contamination.[431] The company also uses thimerosal as a preservative in the multidose vials. By definition, no thimerosal-containing solution should have live bacteria present in its final formula period.

Making flu vaccine is risky business. Because chicken eggs are used, microorganisms can grow in the brew used to produce the flu shot. The potentially contaminated solution is treated with thimerosal, as a sterilizing agent, to kill the bugs.

It's possible that sterility control at the plant remained substandard because technicians knew they would be treating the solution with thimerosal, assuming it would kill any potential contamination that had occurred in production. But it didn't turn out that way. Their apparent reliance on mercury to make up for less-than-sterile production codes might have been a big mistake.

If the factory were truly a sterile environment, there would be no need to use thimerosal in the production line. Many vaccines today are made without thimerosal, but they are produced in 100 percent sterile environments, with the utmost in quality control, consistent monitoring, and meticulous documentation, all at great expense.

The question, then, becomes: With all that thimerosal in the mix, how was the bacteria able to survive?

Organic mercury can kill certain specific strains of bacteria, but there are differences between strains in their vulnerability. Some are highly sensitive to mercury, while others have high survival rates. Many studies have found that serratia has a particularly high degree of mercury resistance, and thimerosal might not have made much difference in removing this contaminant from the vaccine.[432] Meanwhile, contact lens solutions that contain thimerosal explicitly state on their label that the preservative does not protect against serratia contamination.

Serratia can be deadly if it gets into the bloodstream.[433] It can cause infection of the inner layer of the heart, acute and chronic bone infections, blood poisoning, pneumonia, and meningitis. It is a notorious hospital pathogen and naturally resistant to a number of antibiotics.

It's a good thing the British government caught the contamination in time. As a nation, we may have really dodged a bullet. Still, millions will go unvaccinated this year, and people could die because thimerosal failed to perform its job. Government and industry must work to develop a safe and effective way of making flu vaccine. This is especially true given emerging infectious threats such as the avian flu virus.

Finally, while it's true that mercury has been phased out from most pediatric vaccines given in the United States, this is hardly the case with countries overseas.

In late 1999, shortly after the release of the Joint Statement on Thimerosal, the administration of President Bill Clinton agreed to purchase some fifty million dollars' worth of thimerosal-containing hepatitis-B vaccine from the drug companies and donate it for use in Third World countries.[434] Since then, American-made vaccines have been exported to nations throughout the developing world.

Most of these vaccines contain thimerosal. When dealing with mass immunization programs in poor countries—unquestionably a lofty goal— reliance on multidose vaccine vials is paramount. Single-dose (preservative-free) formulations are simply not viable in terms of production, distribution, storage, and refrigeration. Multidose vials require a preservative, and thimerosal is the cheapest, most abundant vaccine preservative there is. Moreover, thimerosal is needed in the production of most vaccines to maintain sterility. By removing the thimerosal at the end of production, manufacturers lose up to 30 percent of the vaccine solution. This would make vaccines prohibitively expensive for poor nations.

Autism has rarely been reported outside of industrialized countries, at least until recent years. A good example is China, where companies such as Merck and GlaxoSmithKline have begun an aggressive pediatric marketing campaign, selling millions of dollars in vaccines to the Communist government, including pediatric hepatitis-B, DTP, Hib, MMR, and others.[435] On August 11, 2004, the official Chinese news agency, Xinhua, reported that the number of children suffering with autism in that country had suddenly and unexpectedly skyrocketed. In a few short years, the number of reported cases had jumped from nearly nothing to some 1.8 million children in 2004.[436] One researcher "estimated that the number of Chinese children with autism was growing at an annual rate of 20 percent, even higher than the world average of 14 percent," the news agency reported.

Other increases in autism cases are currently being reported in such far-flung countries as Indonesia, Argentina, India, and Nigeria, though improved medical attention may be part of the reason.

If thimerosal is one day proven to be a contributing factor to autism, and if U.S.-made vaccines containing the preservative are now being supplied to infants the world over, the scope of this potential tragedy becomes almost unthinkable.

The United States, at the dawn of the twenty-first century, is not exactly the most beloved nation on earth. What if the profitable export of our much vaunted medical technology has led to the poisoning of hundreds of thousands of children? What then?

NOTES

INTRODUCTION

1. Institute of Medicine, Committee on Immunization Safety, *Immunization Safety Review: Vaccines and Autism,* "Executive Summary" (Washington, DC: National Academies Press, 2004).
2. "Prevention and Control of Influenza: Recommendations of the Advisory Committee on Immunization Practices," *Morbidity and Mortality Weekly Report* 52 (RR08), April 25, 2003, 1–36.
3. Ibid.
4. U.S. Food and Drug Administration, Center for Evaluation and Research, "Mercury in Drug and Biologic Products," August 5, 2003; updated March 30, 2004.
5. Sources for 1 in 5,000 figure: Only two autism prevalence studies were conducted in the United States in the 1980s: one showed a rate of 1 case per 10,000 children, and the other showed a rate of 3.3 per 10,000 (or 1 in 3,030). This typically has been averaged out to 2 per 10,000 (or 1 in 5,000). Source for 1 in 500 figure: Marie Bristol et al., "State of the Science in Autism: Report to the National Institutes of Health," *Journal of Autism and Developmental Disorders* 26, no. 2 (1996): 121–57. Source for 1 in 250: In 2002, the CDC conducted a prevalence study in Brick Township, New Jersey, showing a rate of 4 per 10,000 (or 1 in 250). CDC, National Vaccine Program Office, "Vaccine Fact Sheet on Autism." Source for 1 in 166 figure: CDC, Medical Home Initiatives and First Signs, "Autism A.L.A.R.M."
6. Centers for Disease Control and Prevention, Medical Home Initiatives and First Signs, "Autism A.L.A.R.M."
7. C. Gillberg and M. Coleman, *The Biology of the Autistic Syndromes,* 2d ed. (London: MacKeith Press, 1992, 90.
8. Denmark source: K. M. Madsen et al., "A Population-Based Study of Measles, Mumps, and Rubella Vaccinations and Autism," *New England Journal of Medicine* 347, no. 19

(November 7, 2002): 1481. UK source: Medical Research Council, UK, "MRC Review of Autism Research—Epidemiology and Causes," December 2001.

PROLOGUE

9. Sheryl Gay Stolberg, "A Capitol Hill Mystery: Who Aided Drug Maker?" *New York Times,* November 29, 2002.
10. Jonathan Weisman, "A Homeland Security Whodunit; In Massive Bill, Someone Buried a Clause to Benefit Drug Maker Eli Lilly," *Washington Post,* November 28, 2002.
11. Sheryl Gay Stolberg, "A Capitol Hill Mystery: Who Aided Drug Maker?" *New York Times,* November 29, 2002.
12. See Thomas Frank, "Special Interest Items Part of Homeland Security Bill," *Newsday,* November 16, 2002.
13. See www.frist.senate.gov.
14. Bob Herbert, "Whose Hands Are Dirty?" *New York Times,* November 25, 2002.

1: MOTHERS ON A MISSION

15. Cure Autism Now Web site, www.cureautismnow.com.
16. Ibid.
17. Liz Birt's husband did not wish to be identified by name in this book.
18. These remarks, while almost identical to those made at the Chicago conference, were taken from testimony by Dr. Singh at a hearing called "Autism—Present Challenges, Future Needs—Why the Increased Rates?" on April 6, 2000, held by the U.S. House Committee on Government Reform and Oversight. Source: *Congressional Record.*
19. A. J. Wakefield et al., "Illeal-Lymphoid-Nodular Hyperplasia, Non-specific Colitis, and Pervasive Developmental Disorder in Children," *Lancet* 351, no. 9103 (February 28, 1998).

2: INJECTING FEAR

20. "Wakefield Stands By MMR Claims," *Panorama,* BBC News, London, January 27, 2002, 22: 15 GMT.
21. R. T. Chen and F. DeStefano, "Vaccine Adverse Events: Causal or Coincidental?" *Lancet* 351, no. 9103 (May 2, 1998), 611–12.
22. H. Peltola et al., "No Evidence for Measles, Mumps, and Rubella Vaccine Associated with Inflammatory Bowel Disease or Autism in a 14-Year Prospective Study," *Lancet* 351, no. 9112 (May 1998).
23. "Your Comments on MMR: Every Parent's Choice," *Panorama,* BBC News, February 4, 2002, 16:06 GMT (www.news.bbc.co.uk).
24. "Blair 'Should Admit MMR Jab,'" BBC News, December 23, 2001, 12:00 GMT.
25. From Albert Enayat's recollection—Merck officials did not return calls seeking comment.
26. National Vaccine Information Center, "Parent Groups and Vaccine Policymakers Clash over Research into Vaccines, Autism and Intestinal Disorders," press release, March 3, 1998.
27. Ibid.
28. Ibid.
29. New Jersey Center for Outreach and Services for the Autism Community (COSAC), "New Law Concerning Second Dose of MMR Vaccine," www.njcosac.org/govwatch, July 1, 2004.
30. Joan Lowy, Scripps-Howard News Service (SHNS), FEAT Daily Online Newsletter, May 31, 1999.
31. California Department of Developmental Services, "Changes in the Population of Persons with Autism and Pervasive Developmental Disorders in California's Developmental Services System: 1987 through 1998, a Report to the Legislature," March 1, 1999.

32. U.S. Department of Education, "Comparison of the 16th and 20th Annual Report to Congress on the Implementation of the Individuals with Disabilities Education Act," *Epidemic Statistics on Autism 1992–1997,* May 11, 1999.

33. E. R. Ritvo, M.D., "No Epidemic of Autism," University of California Los Angeles, Department of Physiological Science, Faculty Page, April 30, 1999.

34. Mark Blaxill, "Dr. Wakefield Moves Orlando 'to Tears,'" FEAT Daily Online, May 10, 1999, http://health.groups.yahoo.com/group/-AuTeach/messages.

35. William Egan, FDA, letter to drug companies, April 29, 1999.

36. Jon Christian Ryter, "Warning on Thimerosal Will Be Played Down by National Vaccine Program Office of the CDC on Friday," FreeRepublic.com, July 1, 1999.

3: MERCURY RISING

37. "Thimerosal in Vaccines: A Joint Statement of the American Academy of Pediatrics and the Public Health Service," *Morbidity and Mortality Weekly Report* 48, no. 26 (July 9, 1999): 563–65.

38. Board on Health Promotion and Disease Prevention, Institute of Medicine, *Immunization Safety Review: Vaccines and Autism* (Washington, DC: National Academics Press, 2004), 134–35.

39. Committee on the Toxicological Effects of Methylmercury, Board of Environmental Studies and Toxicology, Commission on Life Sciences, National Research Council, *Toxicological Effects of Methylmercury* (Washington, DC: National Academies Press, 2000).

40. Portia Iverson, contacted through her husband, John Shestack, did not respond to queries seeking comment on this account by Albert Enayati.

41. J. A. Lowell et al., "Mercury Poisoning Associated with High-Dose Hepatitis-B Immune Globulin Administration after Liver Transplantation for Chronic Hepatitis B," *Liver Transplantation and Surgery* 2, no. 6 (November 1996): 475–78.

42. European Agency for the Evaluation of Medicinal Products, Human Medicines Evaluation Unit, "Safety Working Party Assessment of the Toxicity of Thimerosal in Relation to Its Use in Medicinal Products," September 8, 1998.

43. Phyllis Schlafly, "Emerging Scandal in Vaccine Mandates," Eagle Forum, http://www.eagleforum.org, July 28, 1999.

44. FreeRepublic.com, July 1, 1999.

45. "Uproar over a Little-Known Preservative, Thimerosal, Jostles U.S. Hepatitis B Vaccination Policy," *Hepatitis Control Report* 4, no. 2 (Summer 1999): 1–40.

46. T. Tsubaki and K. Irukayama, eds., *Minamata Disease* (London: Elsevier, 1977); and A. Igata, "Epidemiological and Clinical Features of Minamata Disease," *Environmental Research* 63, no. 1 (1993): 157–69.

47. L. Amin-Zaki, "Intra-uterine Methylmercury Poisoning in Iraq," *Pediatrics* 54, no. 5 (1974): 587–95.

48. Ibid.

49. Ibid.

50. Irina D. Cinca et al., "Accidental Ethyl Mercury Poisoning with Nervous System, Skeletal, Muscle, and Myocardium Injury," *Journal of Neurology, Neurosurgery, and Psychiatry* 43 (1979): 143–49.

51. Information on acrodynia was taken from: Charles Rocaz, *L'Acrodynie infantile* (Paris: G. Doin, 1930); J. Warkany and D. H. Hubbard, "Acrodynia and Mercury," *Journal of Pediatrics* 42 (1953): 365–86; and a Pink Disease Support Group Web site, http://www.users.bigpond.com/difarnsworth/pcheek42.htm.

52. H. Thiele, "Pink Disease—Heather's Story," Pink Disease Support Group Web site, http://www.users.bigpond.com/difarnsworth.

53. S. Bernard et al., "Autism: A Novel Form of Mercury Poisoning," *Medical Hypothesis* 56, no. 4 (2001): 462–71.

54. U.S. Food and Drug Administration, Center For Evaluation and Research, "Mercury in Plasma-Derived Products," updated September 9, 2004, posted on CBER Web site at http://www.fda.gov/cber/blood/ mercplasma.htm.

55. U.S. Environmental Protection Agency, National Center for Environmental Assessment, "Reference Dose for Methylmercury," external review draft, *Federal Register* 65, no. 210 (October 30, 2000): 64,702–3.

56. Robert J. Peterson, "What Is Chelation Therapy?" http://www.americanchelation.com.

57. "Uproar over a Little-Known Preservative, Thimerosal, Jostles U.S. Hepatitis Vaccination Policy," *Hepatitis Control Report* 4, no. 2 (Summer 1999).

58. Ibid.

59. Neal A. Halsey, M.D., "Limiting Infant Exposure to Thimerosal in Vaccines and Other Sources of Mercury," *Journal of the American Medical Association* 282, no. 18 (November 10, 1999).

60. U.S. Food and Drug Administration, Center for Food Safety and Applied Nutrition, Office of Seafood; "Mercury in Fish: FDA Monitoring Program (1990–2003)," http://vm.cfsan.fda.gov, March 2004.

61. S. Bernard et al., "Autism: A Novel Form of Mercury Poisoning," *Medical Hypothesis,* 56(4) (2001): 462–71.

62. Albert Enayati, interview with the author, June 15, 2003. The FDA would not permit Dr. Egan to be interviewed for this book.

4: RED FLAGS ON THE HILL

63. Paul Offit, in an interview with the author in August 2004, conceded that Merck bought and distributed copies of his book, though he said he did not know how many copies the company bought, nor was he involved in the sale.

64. Offit, in an August 2004 interview with the author, said the funds went to the laboratory of his research and development partner (who also shares the patent) and not to Offit directly.

65. U.S. House of Representatives, Committee on Government Reform, "Conflicts of Interest in Vaccine Policy Making," Majority Staff Report, June 15, 2000.

66. Centers for Disease Control and Prevention, National Immunization Program, "Rotavirus Fact Sheet," http://www.cdc.gov/nip/publications/fs/rotavirus.htm.

67. U.S. House of Representatives, Committee on Government Reform, "Conflicts of Interest in Vaccine Policy Making," Majority Staff Report, June 15, 2000.

68. Dr. Paul Offit, interview with the author, Atlanta, Georgia, June 19, 2003.

69. U.S. House of Representatives, Committee on Government Reform, "Conflicts of Interest in Vaccine Policy Making," Majority Staff Report, June 15, 2000.

70. Neal A. Halsey, M.D., "IVS Perspective on the Use of Thimerosal-Containing Vaccines," slide show presentation from "Workshop on Thimerosal and Vaccines," Institute for Vaccine Safety, Johns Hopkins Bloomberg School of Public Health, August 11–12, 1999.

71. U.S. Food and Drug Administration, "Mercury-Containing Drug Products for Topical Antimicrobial Over-the-Counter Human Use; Establishment of a Monograph," proposed rules, *Federal Register* 47/436-01, January 5, 1982.

72. U.S. Food and Drug Administration, "Status of Certain Additional Over-the Counter Drug Category II and III Active Ingredients," final rule, *Federal Register* 63, no. 77 (April 22, 1998): 19,799–802.

73. *Physicians' Desk Reference* 2003 (Montvale, NJ: Thomson Healthcare, 2003).

74. J. Warkany and D. M. Hubbard, "Acrodynia and Mercury," *Pediatrics* 42 (1953): 365–86.

75. California Department of Developmental Services, "Changes in the Population of Persons with Autism and Pervasive Developmental Disorders in California's Developmental Services System: 1987 through 1998, a Report to the Legislature," March 1, 1999.

76. Barbara Feder Ostrov, "Alarming Rise in Autism in State Is Genuine, Researchers Conclude," *Mercury News,* October 18, 2002.

77. Centers for Disease Control and Prevention, National Vaccine Program Office, "CDC Examines Autism Among Children: Fact Sheet," www.cdc.gov.

78. Committee on Government Reform, 106th Congress, 1st Session, *Congressional Record,* serial no. 106–84 (August 1999): 75–80.

79. National Vaccine Information Center, "Parents and Researchers Call for Action to End Gaps in Knowledge about Autism and the Vaccine Connection," press release, April 6, 2000.

80. Philip J. Hilts, "After Disputes, House Panel Asks for Study of a Vaccine," *New York Times,* April 7, 2000.

81. "Autism: Present Challenges, Future Needs—Why the Increasing Rates?" 106th Congress, 2nd Session, *Congressional Record,* serial no. 106–80 (April 2000): 1–7. U.S. House Government Reform Committee video.

82. All testimony from "Autism," *Congressional Record,* April 2000.

83. Dialogue from the April 7, 2000, meeting between parents and directors at the National Institutes of Health was taken from a written account of the proceedings by Karyn Seroussi, a parent, and posted on the FEAT Daily Newsletter on April 11, 2000. Her account has been confirmed by other parents in attendance.

84. Karyn Seroussi e-mail to the author, November 3, 2004, 5:20 A.M.

5: HIDDEN AGENDAS

85. http://intl.elsevierhealth.com//journals/MeHy/Default.cfm.

86. Rep. Henry A. Waxman, "Bad Information Can Be Deadly; Vaccines: An Unsubstantiated Link to Autism Is Hampering Efforts to End Childhood Diseases," OpEd, *Los Angeles Times,* April 17, 2000.

87. Rep. Dan Burton, "Is It Harmful to Publicly Discuss the Possible Autism-Vaccine Link?", *Los Angeles Times,* April 24, 2000.

88. Information about the May 16 meeting at the NIH comes from e-mail accounts of the event sent out by participants shortly afterward, and from interviews with parents. The NIH did not respond to requests to confirm or deny these accounts.

89. Information about the May 16 meeting at the FDA comes from e-mail accounts of the event sent out by participants shortly afterward, and from interviews with parents. The FDA did not respond to requests to confirm or deny these accounts.

90. This figure came from an interview on June 17, 2003, with Stuart Burns from Rep. Dave Weldon's office. The CDC would not return calls to confirm.

91. National Network for Immunization Information, www.immunizationinfo.org.

92. Robert L. Davis et al., "Infant Exposure to Thimerosal-Containing Vaccines and Risk for Subsequent Neurologic and Renal [Kidney] Disease," abstract and poster, joint meeting of the American Academy of Pediatrics and the Pediatric Academic Societies, Boston, May 12–16, 2000.

93. All references in this section are from Board on Environmental Studies and Toxicology, Commission on Life Sciences, National Research Council, *Toxicological Effects of Methylmercury, Committee on the Toxicological Effects of Methylmercury* (Washington, DC: National Academy Press, 2000).

94. Information about the June 15 teleconference meeting with the CDC comes from e-mail accounts of the event sent out by participants shortly afterward and from interviews with parents. The CDC did not respond to requests to confirm or deny these accounts.

95. Rep. Dan Burton, "Opening Statement 'FACA: Conflicts of Interest and Vaccine Development: Preserving the Integrity of the Process,'" Committee on Government Reform, 106th Congress, 2nd Session, *Congressional Record,* serial no. 106–239, (June 15, 2000): 4–8. Other remarks at hearing: Ibid.

96. Steven G. Gilbert and Kimberly S. Grant-Webster, University of Washington, School of Public Health, "Neurobehavioral Effects of Developmental Methylmercury Exposure," *Environmental Health Perspectives* 103 (supplement 6) (September 1995): 135–42.

97. Davis quote is from Lyn Redwood interview with the author, June 15, 2003. Davis declined to be interviewed for this book. But he did send an e-mail confirming the content of the phone conversation.

98. All remarks made at the meeting come from Centers for Disease Control and Prevention, "Verbatim Transcript of the ACIP Conference," June 21, 2000.

6: SAFE MINDS

99. All quotes from the Committee on Government Reform hearing are from "Mercury in Medicine—Are We Taking Unnecessary Risks?" 106th Congress, 2nd Session, serial no. 106–232, (July 18, 2000).

100. Lyn Redwood, interview with the author, April 14, 2003.

101. Ibid.

102. http://www.safeminds.org. Baskin is no longer on the Safe Minds board.

103. Committee on the Toxicological Effects of Methylmercury, Board on Environmental Studies and Toxicology, Commission on Life Sciences, National Research Council, *Toxicological Effects of Methylmercury* (Washington, DC: National Academy Press, 2000).

104. References to amalgams, mercury toxicity and Alzheimer's disease taken from Boyd Haley, e-mail to Barbara Snelgrove, subject: "Alzheimer's Society Position on Dental Amalgam," June 28, 2000, 3:00 P.M.

105. Dr. Jane M. El-Dahr, "Thimerosal Containing Vaccines and Neurodevelopmental Outcomes," National Academy of Sciences, Institute of Medicine, Immunization Safety Review Committee, July 16, 2001.

106. David J. Thomas, "Effects of Age and Sex on Retention of Mercury by Methylmercury Treated Rats," *Toxicology and Applied Pharmacology* 62(3) (March 15, 1982): 445–54.

107. William J. Walsh, "New Research Suggests Cause of Autism," press release, PRNewswire, May 10, 2001; also from author's interview with Walsh, June 22, 2003.

108. Coalition for Safe Minds, letter to Dr. Jane Henney, FDA Commissioner, July 31, 2000.

109. Kathryn C. Zoon, Director, Center for Biologics Evaluation and Research. FDA, letter to Lyn Redwood, Safe Minds, August 16, 2000.

110. Safe Minds, letter to Dr. Jane Henney, FDA Commissioner, August 22, 2000.

111. Based on e-mails between Lyn Redwood, Mark Blaxill, and Sallie Bernard, August 2000.

112. Based on author's interview with Lyn Redwood, June 16, 2003. Also taken from Verstraeten e-mail to Lyn, August 2, 2000, 9:03 A.M. EDT.

113. Lyn Redwood, interview with the author, June 16, 2003. Also from Verstraeten e-mails, June–July 2000. Verstraeten declined to be interviewed for this book.

114. Jim Vandehei and Laurie McGinley, "Bush Nominates Drug-Industry Insider to Head Office of Management and Budget," *Wall Street Journal,* December 26, 2000.

7: MOUNTING EVIDENCE

115. Institute of Medicine, Immunization Safety Web site, http://www.iom.edu/focuson .asp?id=4189nfo.

116. Eric Fombonne, M.D., "Is There an Epidemic of Autism?" *Pediatrics* 107(2) (February 2001): 411–12.

117. Mark F. Blaxill, unpublished letter to the editor of *Pediatrics,* posted on FEAT newsletter, February 8, 2001.

118. Bernard Rimland, Autism Research Institute, "The Autism Explosion, the Vaccine Connection, and the Autism Research Institute's Mercury Detoxification Consensus Conference, February 9–11, 2001, Dallas, TX," press release, February 12, 2001.

119. Department of Health and Human Services, Health Resources and Services Administration, National Vaccine Injury Compensation Program Fact Sheet, http://www.hrsa.gov/ osp/vicp/fact_sheet.htm.

120. Department of Health and Human Services, Vaccine Injury Trust Fund, "Income Statement for Period 10/01/00 through 09/30/10," final unaudited.

121. *Joseph Counter et al. v. Abbott Laboratories, et al* (Case No. GN100866), 200th District Court of Travis County, Texas, March 28, 2001.

122. Waters & Kraus, "First Mercury Poisoning/Vaccine Case Filed," press release, March 23, 2001.

123. Cliff Shoemaker, a lead petitioner's attorney in the vaccine court cases, interview with the author, July 17, 2003.

124. Department of Health and Human Services, Vaccine Injury Trust Fund, "Income Statement for Period 10/01/00 through 09/30/10," Final unaudited.

125. Rep. Ron Lewis and Rep. Karen Thurman, "Dear Colleague" letter, April 20, 2001.

126. *A Bill to Amend the Public Health Service Act with Respect to the Vaccine Injury Compensation Program,* introduced in the U.S. House of Representatives by Rep. Dave Weldon and Rep. Jerrold R. Nadler, February 14, 2001, *Congressional Record,* February 14, 2001.

127. Rep. Dave Weldon and Rep. Jerrold R. Nadler, "Dear Colleague" letter, March 1, 2001.

128. Safe Minds, letter to Ms. Lyn Armstrong, Freedom of Information Act Office, CDC, May 21, 2001.

129. A. T. Kravchenko et al., "Evaluation of the Toxic Action of Prophylactic and Therapeutic Preparations on Cell Cultures of Different Types and Origin," *Zh Mikrobiol Epidemiol Immunobiol 5* (May 1982): 53–57. (Translation from the Russian by Safe Minds.)

130. W. Slikker, Jr., "Developmental Neurotoxicty of Therapeutics: Survey of Novel Recent Findings," *Neurotoxicology* 1, no. 2 (February-April 2000): 250.

131. Fritz Lorscheider, et al., "How Mercury Causes Brain Neuron Degeneration," *NeuroReport* 12, no. 2 (April 2001): 285–88. Also from "How Mercury Causes Brain Neuron Degeneration," CD-ROM, University of Calgary Medical School.

132. Frank Schmuck, e-mail to Lyn Redwood, January 18, 2001, 10:17 A.M.

133. Updated safety guide for laboratory researchers on thimerosal, National Institute of Environmental Health Sciences, 2001, http://ntp-server.niehs.gov/cgi/iH_Indexes/ALL_SRCH/iH_ALL_SRCH_Frames.html.

134. Mark F. Blaxill, "The Global Crisis in Autism Science" (draft working paper), June 2001.

135. Boyd E. Haley, Professor and Chair, Department of Chemistry, letter to Committee on Immunization Safety Review, Institute of Medicine, May 14, 2001.

136. Lyn Redwood, President, Safe Minds, letter to Committee on Immunization Safety Review, Institute of Medicine, June 8, 2001.

137. Dr. Jane El-Dahr, e-mail to Lyn Redwood and Sallie Bernard, subject: "CDC Thimerosal Study," March 25, 2001, 7:42 P.M.

138. Massachusetts Division of Insurance, "Governors Cellucci, Almond Announce Agreement—Harvard Pilgrim Receiverships in Both States Will Coordinate Efforts," press release, March 20, 2000.

139. Lynn Armstrong, letter to Elizabeth Birt, June 15, 2001.

140. Paul A. Stehr-Green, [*Rapporteur*] "Summary and Conclusions—Review of Vaccine Safety Datalink Information on Thimerosal-Containing Vaccines," June 7–8, 2000.

141. http://www.simpsonwood.org.

142. "Scientific Review of Vaccine Safety Datalink Information," June 7–8, 2000, Simpsonwood Retreat Center, Norcross, Georgia (Minutes).

143. Mark Blaxill, "The Governance Problem—Summary of Highlights of Scientific Review of Safety Datalink Information," Schafer Autism Report, May 2001.

144. Sallie Bernard, e-mail to Dr. Kathleen Stratton, subject: "Thimerosal Review," June 15, 2001.

145. *Lyndelle H. and William Thomas Redwood v. American Home Products Corp., et al.,* Superior Court of Fayette County, State of Georgia, July 13, 2001.

146. All testimony given at the meeting is from "Thimerosal-Containing Vaccines and Neurodevelopmental Outcomes—Public Meeting, July 16, 2001," National Academy of Sciences, Institute of Medicine, Immunization Safety Review Committee, transcript of the meeting.

147. Laszlo Magos, M.D., "Answers to Questions on the Toxicity of Ethylmercury," statement prepared for the Institute of Medicine Immunization Safety Review Committee, July 2, 2001.
148. P. Grandjean, M.D., "Presentation to Immunization Safety Review Committee. Faroe Islands Study," Cambridge, Massachusetts, July 16, 2001.

8: DAMN LIES AND STATISTICS

149. Rep. Dan Burton, letter to Walter Orenstein, Assistant Surgeon General, Director of National Immunization Program, July 28, 2001.
150. Liz Birt, letter to Lyn Armstrong, Office of Communication, CDC, August 6, 2001.
151. William A. Pierce, Deputy Assistant Secretary for Public Affairs/Media, Department of Health and Human Services, Office of the Secretary, letter to Elizabeth Birt, June 3, 2002.
152. Immunization Safety Review Committee, Institute of Medicine, e-mail to Sallie Bernard and Lyn Redwood, subject: "Briefing Regarding the Immunization Safety Review Committee's Report on Thimerosal," October 1, 2001, 9:26 A.M.
153. Dr. Kathleen Stratton et al., Immunization Safety Review Committee, Board of Health Promotion and Disease Prevention, Institute of Medicine, "Immunization Safety Review: Thimerosal Containing Vaccines and Neurodevelopmental Disorders" (Washington, DC: National Academy Press, October 1, 2001).
154. National Academies, "Link between Neurodevelopmental Disorders and Thimerosal Remains Unclear," press release, October 1, 2001.
155. Sallie Bernard, e-mail to Lyn Redwood, subject: "Press Conference Transcript," October 1, 2001, sent on October 2, 2002, 1:39 P.M.
156. Kathleen Fackelmann, "Vaccines May Pose Mercury Hazard for Kids," USA Today, October 1, 2001.
157. Safe Minds, "Safe Minds Applauds IOM Recommendations—Asks for Recall of ALL Childhood Vaccines Containing Mercury and Supports IOM's Call for Immediate Research Funding," press release, October 1, 2001.
158. Lyn Redwood, letter to Dr. Kenneth I. Shine, President, Institute of Medicine, October 5, 2001.
159. American Academy of Pediatrics, "IOM Report on Vaccines Should Reassure Parents— Children Should Be Vaccinated," press release, October 1, 2001.
160. Lyn Redwood, letter to Louis Z. Cooper, M.D., President-Elect, American Academy of Pediatrics, October 5, 2001.
161. Thomas Verstraeten et al., "Thimerosal VSD study, Phase I—Update 2/29/00," internal report of the National Immunization Program, CDC, February 29, 2000. Obtained via Freedom of Information Act request.
162. Thomas Verstraeten, e-mail to Robert Davis and Frank Destefano, subject: "It Just Won't Go Away . . . ," December 17, 1999, 4:40 P.M.
163. Thomas Verstraeten, e-mail to Miles M. Braun, Frank Destefano, and Robert Davis, subject: "Thimerosal Additional Analyses," March 9, 2000, 9:36 A.M.
164. Thomas Verstraeten, e-mail to Frank DeStefano, subject: "Preemies," March 19, 2000, 10:27 A.M.
165. Colleen Boyle, e-mail to Frank DeStefano, Tom Sinks, and Thomas Verstraeten, subject: "Comments on Analysis" April 25, 2000, 3:55 P.M.
166. Thomas Verstraeten, e-mail to Tracy Lieu, Harvard Pilgrim Health Care, subject: "Vaccine Types Used at HPHC," May 21, 2000, 3:21 P.M.
167. Dr. Tom Saari, e-mail to Committee on Infectious Diseases, American Academy of Pediatrics, liaisons, and ex-officios, subject: "Thimerosal in Vaccines Conference Call," June 13, 2000, 12:37 P.M.
168. Thomas Verstraeten, e-mail to Philippe Grandjean, subject: "Thimerosal and Neurologic Outcomes," July 14, 2000, 10:42 A.M.

169. Frank DeStefano, e-mail to Walter Orenstein inquiring about inviting Safe Minds to Simpsonwood, May 22, 2000, 4:11 P.M.

170. Mark Blaxill, e-mail to Sallie Bernard, Lyn Redwood, and Liz Birt, subject: "CDC Analysis," October 17, 2001, 11:41 A.M.

171. Waters & Kraus, press release, October 16, 2001.

172. Minutes from meeting of the Advisory Committee on Immunization Practices, CDC, Atlanta, Georgia, October 17, 2001.

9: WAR ON FOUR FRONTS

173. Boyd Haley, interview with the author, May 14, 2003, and testimony before House Government Reform Committee, November 14, 2002.

174. Sveltana Lutchmaya, Simon Baron-Cohen et al., "Foetal Testosterone and Eye Contact in 12-Month-Old Human Infants," *Infant Behavior & Development* 25 (2002): 319–25.

175. Boyd Haley, e-mail to Lyn Redwood, subject: "Univ. of Washington chemistry Exam," July 22, 2002, 1:06 P.M.

176. Dr. Amy Holmes, e-mail to Lyn Redwood, Sallie Bernard, and others, subject: "Predicted Mercury Concentrations in Hair from Infant Immunizations: Cause for Concern," January 7, 2002, 10:56 A.M.

177. Amy S. Holmes, Mark F. Blaxill, and Boyd E. Haley, "Reduced Levels of Mercury in First Baby Haircuts of Autistic Children," *International Journal of Toxicology* 22, no. 4 (July–August 2003): 277–85.

178. Amy S. Holmes, M.D., "Autism Treatments: Chelation of Mercury," http://www.healing-arts.org/children/holmes.htm.

179. Interviews with author and Capitol Hill staff, in the office of Sen. Debbie Stabenow on January 8, 2003, and Sen. Ted Kennedy on July 10, 2003. Also discussed in memo to plaintiff families from Andy Waters, subject: "Legislative Concerns—Thimerosal," February 1, 2002.

180. *National Vaccine Injury Compensation Program Improvement Act of 2002,* HR 3741, 107th Cong., 2d sess., *Congressional Record* (February 14, 2002): 148 (E-154).

181. Centers for Disease Control and Prevention, "Data Sharing Principles and System—National Immunization Program (NIP)—Draft Proposal," February 21, 2002.

182. James A. Moody, letter to Public Health Service Freedom of Information Office, February 27, 2002.

183. A. K. Winship, "Organic Mercury Compounds and Their Toxicity," *Adverse Drug Reactions and Acute Poisoning Review* 5, no. 3 (Autumn 1986): 141–80.

184. Liz Birt, letter to Rep. Dan Burton, March 7, 2002.

185. Waters & Kraus, "Eli Lilly Documents Reveal Dangers of Thimerosal," press release, March 17, 2002.

186. Committee on Government Reform, Subcommittee on Human Rights and Wellness, "Mercury in Medicine—Taking Unnecessary Risks," May 2003, 34.

187. "Plaintiff's Response to Eli Lilly and Company's Supplemental Motion for Summary Judgement," *Counter v. Abbot Laboratories, et al.,* District Court, Brazoria County, Texas, 23rd Judicial District, November 18, 2002.

188. Ibid.

189. Sen. Bill Frist, "Frist Introduces Bill to Improve Vaccine Availability," press release, March 22, 2002.

190. Jonathan D. Salant, "Medical Industry Gives to Sen. Frist—Donations to His Campaigns Near 20% of His Total," Associated Press, January 12, 2003.

191. Sen. Bill Frist, "Frist Introduces Bill to Improve Vaccine Availability," press release, March 22, 2002.

192. Scott and Laura Bono, interview with the author, June 19, 2003.

193. Laura Bono, letter to Sen. Jesse Helms (R-NC), April 10, 2002.

194. Beth Clay, interview with the author, August 2, 2004.

195. Rep. Henry Waxman (D-CA), letter to Rep. Dan Burton (R-IN), May 2, 2002.

196. Liz Birt, interview with the author, July 3, 2003.

197. Peter Patriarca, Director, Division of Viral Products, FDA, e-mail to Martin Meyers, Acting Director, National Vaccine Program Office, CDC, June 29, 1999, 11:48 A.M.

198. Peter Patriarca, e-mail to colleagues at FDA, subject: "Q and As—Sensitivity: Confidential," July 2, 1999, 10:24 A.M.

199. Susan Ellenberg, Ph.D., e-mail to colleagues at FDA, subject: "Status Report on Thimerosal in Vaccines," June 28, 1999, 9:48 P.M.

200. "The Autism Epidemic—Is the NIH and CDC Response Adequate?" Hearing before the Committee on Government Reform, House of Representatives, 107th Cong., 2d sess., April 18, 2002. U.S. Government Printing Office via GPO Access: http://www.gpo.gov/congress/house.

201. Valeri Williams, "Congressman Calls for Criminal Penalties at Vaccine Mercury Hearings," WFAA-TV, Dallas, Texas, June 20, 2002. Source: http://www.mercola.com. NOTE: A spokeswoman for WFAA-TV said that Williams was not fired, her contract expired, and she chose not to renew it. WFAA-TV has removed all transcripts and videos clips of Williams's work at the station from its Web site.

202. Valeri Williams, "Mercury in Childhood Vaccines: What Did the Government Know?" WFAA-TV, Dallas, Texas, June 19, 2002. Source: http://www.mercola.com.

203. White House, Office of the Press Secretary, "Appointments: President Bush to Appoint the Following Individuals to Serve as Members of the President's Homeland Security Advisory Council," press release, June 11, 2002.

204. Christopher Logan, "Inside the White House Advisory Group: Influential Business Leaders, Former Officials, Sit at the Homeland Security Table," Congressional Quarterly, October 18, 2002.

205. Eli Lilly, "Taurel to Serve on President's Homeland Security Advisory Council; Cassell to Advise HHS and Help Direct the Pharmaceutical Industry," press release, June 11, 2002; Source: Business Wire, "Lilly Commits Two Senior Officials to War on Terrorism," June 11, 2002. 5:40 A.M.

206. Christopher Logan, interview with the author, July 23, 2003; Capitol Hill staff in the office of Sen. Debbie Stabenow (D-MI), interview with the author, January 8, 2003; staff in the office of Sen. Ted Kennedy (D-MA) interview with the author, July 10, 2003.

207. Sheryl Gay Stolberg, "A Capitol Hill Mystery: Who Aided Drug Maker?" New York Times, November 29, 2002.

208. Maureen Groppe, "New Senate Leader Backs Drug Makers; Colleagues Expect First to Alter Measure Protecting Vaccine Producers from Lawsuits," Detroit News, December 24, 2002.

209. Jim VandeHei and Juliet Eilperin, "Drug Firms among Big Donors at GOP Event," Washington Post, June 19, 2002.

210. Jeff Swiatek, "Lilly in Lawyer's Cross Hairs Again—Lawsuits Suggest Vaccine May Be Linked to Autism," Indianapolis Star, July 14, 2002.

211. Autism General Order #1. "IN RE: Claims for Vaccine Injuries Resulting in Autism Spectrum Disorder or a Similar Neurodevelopmental Disorder, Various Petitioners v. Secretary of Health Human Services," Office of Special Masters, U.S. Court of Federal Claims, July 3, 2002.

212. Simon Baron-Cohen, "Argument for autism as a genetic 'epidemic'—Have the Airplane and the Computer Changed the Architecture of the Mind? And Is That Why Autism Is on the Increase?" http://www.edge.org, 2002.

213. Mark Blaxill, e-mail to the editor, www.edge.org, subject: "A response to Baron-Cohen's Essay on Autism: 'Geeks Get Lucky?'" January 21, 2002, 10:30 A.M.

214. Mark Blaxill, e-mail to Simon Baron-Cohen, subject: "Reply re Edge," January 21, 2002, 6:06 P.M.

215. Sen. Bill Frist, "Frist Urges Action to Alleviate Nation's Vaccine Shortage—Cites HHS Secretary's Advisory Commission's Recent Support for Senate Legislation," press release, June 24, 2002.

216. Tom Powers, e-mail to autism community, July 23, 2002, posted on Web site of National Vaccine Information Center, http://www.909shot.com.

217. Sallie Bernard, "Re: SAFE MIND's response to Frist Bill," Statement from Safe Minds, July 2002.

218. Laura Bono, e-mail to members of U.S. Senate, subject: "Oppose Frist Bill 2053," July 30, 2002, 10:43 A.M.

219. Eric Sapp, aide to Sen. Ted Kennedy, interview with the author, July 10, 2003.

220. Mark Geier, interview with the author, July 9, 2003.

221. Mark R. Geier, M.D., and David A. Geier, "Thimerosal in Childhood Vaccines, Neurodevelopmental Disorders, and Heart Disease in the United States," *Journal of American Physicians and Surgeons* 8 no. 1 (Spring 2003): 6–11.

10: HOMELAND INSECURITY

222. K. M. Madsen, M.D., et al., "A Population-Based Study of Measles, Mumps, and Rubella Vaccination and Autism," *New England Journal of Medicine* 347, no. 19 (November 7, 2002): 1477–82.

223. Safe Minds, "Denmark Study on Autism and MMR Vaccine Shows Need for Biological Research," letter to *New England Journal of Medicine* and press release, November 6, 2002.

224. Arthur Allen, "The Not-So-Crackpot Autism Theory," *New York Times Magazine*, November 10, 2002.

225. Lyn Redwood, e-mail to Dr. Neal Halsey, subject: "NYT Article," November 12, 2002, 4:59 P.M.

226. Dr. Neal Halsey, e-mail to Lyn Redwood, subject: "NYT Article," November 12, 2002, 6:52 P.M.

227. Neal Halsey, M.D., letter to the editor, *New York Times Magazine*, "Proposed title: Misleading the Public about Autism and Vaccines," November 11, 2002. Source: Vaccine Safety Institute, http://www.vaccinesafety.edu.

228. Anonymous (listed as a "Congressional Staff Source"), "The Homeland Security Bill Fiasco," November 15, 2002. Source: Mercury Policy Project, http://www.mercurypolicy.org.

229. Jonathan Weisman, "A Homeland Security Whodunit," *Washington Post,* November 28, 2002.

230. "A Reformer's Unending Quest," *Christian Broadcast Network,* January 8, 2002, transcript of interview with Rev. Pat Robertson. Source: http://www.cbn.com.

231. Dan Morgan, "Homeland Bill Rider Aids Drugmakers, Measure Would Block Suits Over Vaccines," *Washington Post,* November 15, 2002.

232. Christopher Logan, "Inside the White House Advisory Group: Influential Business Leaders, Former Officials, Sit at the Homeland Security Table," *Congressional Quarterly,* October 18, 2002.

233. This account, for example, was confirmed with staff in the office of Senator Debbie Stabenow (Democrat, Missouri) and Ted Kennedy (Democrat, Massachusetts).

234. Mark Blaxill, e-mail to Safe Minds parents, subject: "Serious concerns with this Press Release," November 17, 2002, 2:11 P.M.

235. Safe Minds and Mercury Policy Project, "Thimerosal Liability Shield Rider in Homeland Security Bill Opposed by Lawmakers and Activists as Unfair and Irresponsible," press release, November 18, 2002.

236. Rep. Henry Waxman, letter to Mitchell E. Daniels, Jr., November 15, 2002.

237. Sen. Debbie Stabenow, "Sen. Debbie Stabenow Calls for Removal of Provision in Homeland Security Bill Designed to Protect Eli Lilly and Co. from Lawsuits," press release, November 15, 2002.

238. Sen. Debbie Stabenow, interview with the author at press conference, Capitol Hill, January 8, 2003.

239. Sen. Bill Frist, "Homeland Security Debate: Vaccines II," Senate Floor Statement, November 18, 2002, http://frist.senate.gov.

240. Rep. Dan Burton, "Dear Colleague" letter, November 18, 2002.

241. "Showdown Could Impact Homeland Security Bill," Associated Press, November 18, 2002.

242. Lyn Redwood, interview with the author, June 18, 2003.

243. Dana Bash, "Last-Minute Deal Helped GOP Win Key Vote—Moderate Republicans Objected to Three Provisions," CNN, November 25, 2002.

244. "Senate Approves Homeland Bill," CNN, November 20, 2002.

245. Sen. Tom Daschle, "Statement to Reporters concerning the Thimerosal Liability Shield Provision in the 2002 Homeland Security Act," November 20, 2002.

246. Robert Pear and Richard A. Oppel, Jr., "Drug Industry Seeks Ways to Capitalize on Election Success," New York Times, November 21, 2002.

247. Bob Herbert, "Whose Hands Are Dirty?" New York Times, November 25, 2002.

248. Todd Zwillich, "U.S. Government Asks Court to Seal Vaccine Records," Reuters Health, November 19, 2002.

249. Motion for Protective Order, "In RE: Claims for Vaccine Injuries Resulting in Autism Spectrum Disorder or a Similar Neurodevelopmental Disorder," Various, petitioners v. Secretary of Health and Human Services, Office of Special Masters, U.S. Court of Federal Claims, November 19, 2002.

250. "Revisit GOP Efforts to Frustrate Autism Legal Claims," editorial, Newsday, December 3, 2002.

251. As quoted in Rep. John Conyers, "Conyers Criticizes Bush Administration Decision to Seal Thimerosal Records," press release, November 27, 2002.

252. Sen. Patrick Leahy, letter to U.S. Attorney General John D. Ashcroft and Secretary of Health and Human Services Tommy G. Thompson, December 9, 2002.

253. Eli Lilly, "Lilly Launches New Era in Attention-Deficit/Hyperactivity Disorder Treatment with First FDA-Approved Nonstimulant Medication," press release, published on Business Wire, January 14, 2003, 9:08 A.M. ET.

254. Michael E. Pichichero et al., "Mercury Concentrations and Metabolism in Infant Receiving Vaccines Containing Thimerosal: A Descriptive Study," Lancet, 360 no. 9347 (November 30, 2002): 1737–40.

255. Donald G. McNeil, Jr., "Study Suggests Mercury in Vaccines Was Not Harmful," New York Times, December 4, 2002.

256. Laurie Barclay, M.D., "Mercury in Vaccines: A Newsmaker Interview with Michael E. Pichichero, M.D.," Medscape Medical News, December 4, 2002.

257. Safe Minds, "Safe Minds Assessment of the Pichichero Thimerosal Study," press release, December 3, 2002.

258. Dr. Neal A Halsey and Dr. Lynn R. Goldman, letter Lancet, January 17, 2003.

259. Arianna Huffington, "Washington's Hottest Whodunit—Who Turned the Homeland Security Bill into the Eli Lilly Protection Act?" http://www.tompaine.com, December 6, 2002.

260. Transcribed videotape from ABC Good Morning America, December 3, 2002.

261. "The Truth about Thimerosal: Democrats and Trial Lawyers Play Politics with Vaccine Liability," Review and Outlook, Wall Street Journal, December 5, 2002.

262. Order, "In RE: Claims for Vaccine Injuries Resulting in Autism Spectrum Disorder or a Similar Neurodevelopmental Disorder," Various Petitioners v. Secretary of Health and Human Services, Office of Special Masters, U.S. Court of Federal Claims, December 19, 2002.

263. Mercury Policy Project and Safe Minds, "Bush Admin. Withdraws Motion to Seal Thimerosal Documents in Current Cases: Advocacy Groups Question Whether Future Cases Will be Subject to the Secrecy Order," press release, December 19, 2002.

264. Sen. Joseph I. Lieberman, "Lieberman Seeks to Strike Republican Special-Interest Provisions Added to Homeland Security Act Last Year," press release, January 7, 2003.

265. Notes taken at autism parents rally on Capitol Hill, Washington, D.C., January 8, 2003.

266. From video footage shot outside Senate Majority Leader Bill Frist's Health Committee office, January 8, 2003, in addition to interviews with Dawn and Rodney Roark, Laura Bono, and Albert Enayati.

267. "Senate Drops Vaccine Measure in Homeland Act," Reuters, published on *New York Times* Web site http://www.nytimes.com, January 10, 2003.

268. Rob Wells, "Lilly Hopes Congress Will Act on Vaccine Protections," *Dow Jones Business News*, January 10, 2003, 6:48 P.M. ET.

269. Thomas P. Wyman, "Lilly Vaccine Issue Will Get Front-Door Hearing It Deserves," Op-Ed, *Indianapolis Star,* January 14, 2002.

270. Karin B. Nelson, M.D. and Margaret L. Bauman, M.D., "Thimerosal and Autism?" Commentary, *Pediatrics* 111, no. 3 (March 2003): 674–79.

271. Safe Minds, "Link between Mercury-based Vaccine and Autism Sparks Concern, Spawns Pediatrics Science Article," press release, March 4, 2003.

272. Mark F. Blaxill, Lyn Redwood, and Sallie Bernard, "There Is No 'Typical and Characteristic' Pattern of Mercury Poisoning," Safe Minds' response to Nelson and Bauman, May 30, 2003.

273. L. Magos et al., "The Comparative Toxicology of Ethyl- and Methylmercury," *Archives of Toxicology* 57 (1985): 260–67.

274. *Pediatrics* reviewer's comments on Safe Minds' response to Nelson and Bauman, May 14, 2003.

275. "Study Fails to Show a Connection between Thimerosal and Autism," unsigned editorial, American Academy of Pediatrics Web site, http://www.aap.org, May 16, 2003.

276. Mark and David Geier, letter to Sen. Hillary Clinton, March 22, 2003.

277. S.754, Improved Vaccine Affordability and Availability Act of 2003, introduced by Sen. Bill Frist, April 1, 2003, http://frist.senate.gov.

278. Full page ad, *Roll Call,* March 19, 2003, sponsored by the Autism Autoimmunity Project and others.

279. National Vaccine Information Center, "Parents of Vaccine Injured Children Win Removal of Compensation Bill from Bioterrorism Legislation," press release, March 19, 2003.

280. Barbara Loe Fisher and Kathi Williams, of NVIC, pulled out of the "Dodd Compromise" at the last minute.

281. Ray Gallup, e-mail to autism parents, subject: "Cure Autism Now supports the Bill by Senator Frist," March 20, 2003, 9:35 P.M.

282. Albert Enayati, e-mail to Jon Shestack, subject: "Conference Call," March 20, 2003, 11:04 P.M.

283. Jon Shestack, e-mail to Albert Enayati et al., subject: "Conference Call," March 20, 2003, 11:23 P.M.

284. FAQ: S.754, Improved Vaccine Affordability and Availability Act, Introduced April 1, 2003, Office of Senator Bill Frist.

285. Mark Benjamin, "Deal on Frist Vaccine Bill May Be Set," United Press International, April 8, 2003.

286. Ibid.

287. Sheryl Gay Stolberg, "Vaccine Liability Compromise Collapses," *New York Times,* April 9, 2003.

288. "Senate Delays Action on Nullifying Suits," Associated Press, reported on *ABC News,* April 9, 2003.

289. Jonathan E. Kaplan, "Lobbyists Target Burton," *The Hill,* January 29, 2003.
290. Statement by Dan Burton at Autism One Conference, Chicago, May 3, 2003, Office of Rep. Dan Burton (R-IN).
291. "Mercury in Medicine: Taking Unnecessary Risks," A Report Prepared by the Staff of the Subcommittee on Human Rights and Wellness, Committee on Government Reform, U.S. House of Representatives, Chairman Dan Burton, May 2003.
292. Bobbie Manning, interview with the author, July 25, 2003.
293. Scott Rothschild, "Parents Seek State Aid in Autism Suit—Scientist Says Mercury Damage 'a Bigger Epidemic than 9–11 and AIDS,'" *Lawrence (Kansas) Journal-World,* July 18, 2003.

11: "PROOF" ON BOTH SIDES

294. Paul Stehr-Green et al., "Autism and Thimerosal-Containing Vaccines: Lack of Consistent Evidence for an Association," *American Journal of Preventive Medicine* 25, no. 2 (August 2003): 101–6. Reprinted with permission of the *American Journal of Preventive Medicine.*
295. K. M. Madsen et al., "Thimerosal and the Occurrence of Autism: Negative Ecological Evidence from Danish Population-Based Data," *Pediatrics* 112, no. 3 (September 2003): 604–6.
296. Safe Minds, "Vaccine Health Officials Manipulate Autism Records to Quell Rising Fears over Mercury in Vaccines," press release, PRNewswire, September 2, 2003, 8:06 A.M. ET.
297. Statement by Mark Blaxill, Director, Safe Minds, "Danish Thimerosal-Autism Study in Pediatrics Misleading and Uninformative on Autism Mercury Link."
298. K. M. Madsen et al., "A Population-Based Study of Measles, Mumps, and Rubella Vaccinations and Autism," *New England Journal of Medicine* 347, no. 9 (November 7, 2002): 1481.
299. Donald G. McNeil, Jr., "Study Casts Doubt on Theory of Vaccines' Link to Autism," *New York Times,* September 4, 2003.
300. Anders Hviid et al., "Association between Thimerosal-Containing Vaccine and Autism," *Journal of the American Medical Association* 290, no. 13 (October 1, 2003): 1763–66.
301. Sallie Bernard, letter to the editor, *Journal of the American Medical Association* 291 (2004): (13): 180.
302. Anders Hviid and Mads Melbye, MD, Ph.D., Department of Epidemiology Research, Statens Serum Institut, Copenhagen, letter to the editor, *Journal of the American Medical Association* 291 (2004): 180–81.
303. Mark and David Geier, Rep. Dave Weldon (R-FL), and Stuart Burns, interviews with the author, June–August 2003.
304. Ibid.
305. Thomas Verstraeten, MD, et al., "Safety of Thimerosal-Containing Vaccines: A Two-phase Study of Computerized Health Maintenance Organization Databases," *Pediatrics* 112, no. 5 (November 2003): 1039–46.
306. The information used in the section of Safe Minds' dissection of Verstraeten et al. was derived from various sources, including (1) Mark Blaxill, Lyn Redwood, and Sallie Bernard, interviews with the author in July 2003 and September 2003; (2) Mark Blaxill, e-mail to Lyn Redwood and others, subject: "Tom and IOM," October 29, 2003, 7:07 A.M.; (3) Lyn Redwood, e-mail to Sallie Bernard, Mark Blaxill, and others, subject: "VSD Comments," October 29, 2003, 9:03 A.M.; and (4) Safe Minds, "Analysis and Critique of the CDC's Handling of the Thimerosal Exposure Assessment Based on Vaccine Safety Datalink (VSD) Information," October 2003.
307. Lyn Redwood, letter to Dr. Kathleen Stratton, February 16, 2004.
308. Safe Minds, "CDC Manipulated Data in Study on Link between Children's Vaccines and Autism; CDC's Earlier Results Showing Significant Link Covered Up—Exposed by Freedom of Information Act Documents," press release, November 3, 2003.
309. Rep. Dave Weldon, letter to Dr. Julie L. Gerberding, October 31, 2003.

310. Paul Simao, "Study Finds No Link between Vaccines, Autism," Reuters, November 3, 2003.

311. "Study Disputes Vaccine, Autism Link; Little Evidence Found That Vaccinations Cause Problems," Associated Press, November 3, 2003.

312. Kelly Patricia O'Meara, "Vaccines May Fuel Autism Epidemic," *Insight on the News,* June 9, 2003.

313. Steve Wilson, Christine Lasek (Web producer), "Autism and Informed Inoculation: Part 2," WXYZ-TV News, Detroit, November 5, 2003, http://www.wxyz.com.

314. Dr. Neal Halsey et al., "Comments on Verstraeten et al., Safety of Thimerosal-Containing Vaccines from Nov 5, 2003 *Pediatrics,*" letter to *Pediatrics Post Publication Peer Review,* December 17, 2003.

315. M. Waly, R. C. Deth, et al., "Activation of Methionine Synthase by Insulin-like Growth Factor-1 and Dopamine: A Target for Neurodevelopmental Toxins and Thimerosal," *Molecular Psychiatry,* advance online publication, January 27, 2004, http://www.nature.com/mp.

316. Allan Goldblatt, interview with the author, April 20, 2004.

317. Jill James, interview with the author, August 4, 2004.

318. Dr. Jim Neubrander, interview with the author, August 9, 2004.

319. Jeff Bradstreet, M.D., "Biological Evidence of Significant Vaccine Related Side-effects Resulting in Neurodevelopmental Disorders," presentation to the Vaccine Safety Committee of the Institute of Medicine, February 9, 2004.

320. "The Politics of Autism—Lawsuits and Emotion vs. Science and Childhood Vaccines," editorial, *Wall Street Journal,* December 29, 2003.

321. Safe Minds, "Statement by Safe Minds on 'The Politics of Autism,'" press release, December 29, 2003.

322. Charles Laurence, "Wall Street Journal Besieged in MMR 'Autism Link' Row," *Telegraph* (UK), February 15, 2004.

323. http://www.talkaboutparenting.com.

12: SHOWDOWN

324. Neil Munro, "Missing the Mercury Menace?" *National Journal,* January 3, 2004.

325. Mark and David Geier, interviews with the author, May and July 2003. NOTE: The editorial manager of *Expert Review of Vaccines* told the author that the piece was ultimately unanimously rejected by the Editorial Advisory Board for being "scientifically inaccurate."

326. Mark R. Geier and David A. Geier, letter to *Pediatrics Post Publication Peer Review,* February 23, 2004.

327. Dr. Frank DeStefano, Phillip Rhodes, and Dr. Robert Davis, letter to *Pediatrics Post Publication Peer Review,* February 23, 2004.

328. Liz Birt, e-mail to Safe Minds members and supporters, subject: "Matthew," January 17, 2004, 12:22 A.M. CT.

329. Lyn Redwood, President, Safe Minds, letter to Dr. Kathleen Stratton, Institute of Medicine, January 15, 2004.

330. Rep. Dave Weldon, letter to Dr. Julie L. Gerberding, January 22, 2004.

331. Mark and David Geier, Rep. Dave Weldon, and Stuart Burns, interviews with the author, May and August 2004.

332. Guy Gugliotta, "Mercury Threat to Fetus Raised," *Washington Post,* February 6, 2004.

333. Elizabeth Weise, "Mercury Damage 'Irreversible'," *USA Today,* February 9, 2004.

334. Sharon Kirkey, "Vaccine Additive Linked to Brain Damage in Children; Mercury-Based Preservative Tied to Autism, ADHD, U.S. Researchers Say," CanWest News Service, reported in the *Vancouver Sun,* February 5, 2004.

335. Ibid.

336. All quotes from the February 9, 2004, IOM meeting: Immunization Safety Review Committee, Institute of Medicine, "Vaccines and Autism," February 9, 2004.

337. Boyd Haley, e-mail to Safe Minds parents and others, subject "IOM Thought for the Day," February 12, 2004, 12:32 P.M.
338. Alicia Ault, "Federal Panel Hears Testimony on Vaccinations and Autism," *New York Times,* February 10, 2004.
339. "Autism and Vaccines—Activists Wage a Nasty Campaign to Silence Scientists," Review & Outlook, *Wall Street Journal,* February 16, 2004.
340. "MMR Study Called 'Poor Science,' " Reuters, posted on CNN.com, February 23, 2004.
341. Cecelia Boyer, Office of the Vice President, letter to Rev. Lisa Karen Sykes, August 8, 2001.
342. "Introduction to the OSC," Office of Special Counsel Web site: http://www.osc.gov.
343. Rev. Lisa Skyes et al. letter to Special Counsel Scott Bloch, April 9, 2004.
344. Lisa Sykes, interview with the author, August 8, 2004.
345. Myron Levin, "U.S. Decision to Allow Mercury in Kids' Flu Shots Raises Alarms," *Los Angeles Times,* April 1, 2004.
346. Rep. Dave Weldon, "Weldon/Maloney Bill Eliminates Mercury Exposure for Children and Developing Fetuses," press release, April 5, 2004.
347. Melissa Ross, "Calls for Congressional Investigation into Thimerosal," First Coast News, WJXX ABC-25 and WTLV NBC-12, Jacksonville, Florida, Web site transcript, http://www.firstcoastnews.com.
348. Rick Rollens, "New Autism Data: Slight Decrease May Reflect Mercury Removal from Vaccines," Schafer Autism Report, April 18, 2004.
349. Jill James et al., "Metabolic Biomarkers of Increased Oxidative Stress and Impaired Methylation Capacity in Children with Autism," presentation at Defeat Autism Now! conference, McLean, Virginia, April 15–19, 2004.
350. Brenda Kerr, interview with the author, May 14, 2004.
351. Dr. P. Offit and Dr. J. Golden, "Thimerosal and Autism," letter to *Molecular Psychiatry* advance online publication, April 27, 2004, http://www.nature.com/mp.
352. Dr. Thomas Verstraeten, letter to *Pediatrics,* April 2004.
353. Lisa Sykes, interview with the author, August 8, 2004.
354. Details about the meeting with Dr. Julie Gerberding come from Laura Bono and Lyn Redwood, interviews with the author, June 2004.
355. Laura Bono, e-mail to parents and researchers, subject: "Meeting Notes and Debriefing Impressions—CDC Meeting with Dr. Gerberding in Congressman Weldon's Office—May 12, 2004," 10:39 P.M.
356. Institute of Medicine, Committee on Immunization Safety, "Executive Summary," in *Immunization Safety Review: Vaccines and Autism* (Washington, DC: National Academies Press, 2004): 1–20.
357. Lyn Redwood, e-mail to Lenny Schafer, subject: "Heads Up—IOM," May 18, 2004, 7:15 A.M.
358. No Vaccine Link to Autism Found—Time to Find Real Culprit, Concludes Institute of Medicine Report," Associated Press, from http://www.msnbc.com, May 19, 2004, 12:14 P.M.
359. McCormick quote confirmed by Lyn Redwood and Sallie Bernard; transcript of the May 18, 2004, conference call not posted on the IOM Web site.
360. Safe Minds, "Safe Minds Outraged That IOM Report Fails American Public," press release, May 18, 2004.
361. Safe Minds, "Collusion Seen After Release of Flawed Vaccine-Autism Report," press release, May 19, 2002.
362. Rep. Dave Weldon, "Weldon Calls IOM Conclusions Premature and Hastily Drawn," press release, May 18, 2004.
363. Richard Deth, e-mail to Lyn Redwood and others, subject: "IOM," May 20, 2004, 10:10 A.M.
364. Jill James, e-mail to Lyn Redwood, subject: "IOM," May 19, 2004, 9:35 A.M.
365. Boyd Haley, e-mail to Lyn Redwood, subject: "IOM," May 21, 2004, 8:29 P.M.

13: PAYING THE PIPER

366. Special Counsel Scott J. Bloch, "OSC Forwards Public Health Concerns on Vaccines to Congress," press release and letter, May 20, 2004.
367. Autism Research Institute, Autism Society of America, Cure Autism Now, National Autism Association, National Alliance for Autism Research, Safe Minds, Unlocking Autism, and NoMercury. org, "Joint Statement on the Institute of Medicine Report 'Vaccines and Autism,'" May 18, 2004.
368. Rep. Dave Weldon, "Something Is Rotten, but Not Just in Denmark," remarks at Autism One conference, Chicago, May 29, 2004.
369. *Molecular Psychiatry,* "Thimerosal, Found in Childhood Vaccines, Can Increase the Risk of Autism-Like Damage in Mice," press release, June 9, 2004.
370. Safe Minds, "New Columbia University Study Confirms IOM Vaccine-Autism Report Is Wrong," press release, June 9, 2004.
371. Thomas H. Maugh II, "New Finding on Vaccines and Autism," *Los Angeles Times,* June 10, 2004.
372. Laurie Barclay, "Mercury Linked to Autism-Like Damage in Mice," http://www.WebMD.com, June 9, 2004.
373. Mark and David Geier and Nancy Hokkanen, interviews with the author, July 2004.
374. Sen. John Edwards, letter to North Carolina Attorney General Roy A. Cooper, III, November 10, 2003.
375. David Geier, interview with the author, May 14, 2004.
376. Myron Levin, "Opposition to Mercury Ban Waning," *Los Angeles Times,* June 23, 2004.
377. Ibid.
378. Safe Minds, "Autism and Vaccine Initiatives—Research Priorities," "wish list" prepared for Rep. Dave Weldon, June 2004.
379. Rick Rollens, e-mail to Lyn Redwood, subject: "New Autism Cases Declining," July 14, 2004, 7:42 P.M.
380. "Minutes to Safe Minds Call with Rick Rollens to Discuss the Recently Released California Data," July 17, 2004.
381. State of California, Department of Finance, Demographic Research Unit, May 2004.
382. Safe Minds, "Latest Report Shows Steady Decline in Autism," press release, PRNewswire, July 19, 2004, 1:37 P.M. ET.
383. "PCIE/ECIE Mission and Organization," PCIE Web site, http://www.ignet.gov.
384. Teri Small and other parents, letter to Dara Corrigan, HHS Office of Inspector General, and Special Counsel Scott Bloch, April 15, 2004.
385. Teri Small and Mark Geier, interviews with the author; letters to and from the parents; and Teri Small, e-mails to the author.
386. Michael E. Little, HHS Deputy Inspector General for Investigations, letter to Rev. Lisa Sykes, July 19, 2004.
387. "Summary Statistics Thimerosal study—Site: All Total SS 363203," National Immunization Program, CDC, undated.
388. David Geier, e-mail to Safe Minds, subject: "Context of New CDC VSD Thimerosal Data Sent," July 21, 2004, 2:10 A.M.
389. For the autism relative risk of 11.35, it should be noted that there were only two outcomes in this category; also, the 95% CI is 2.70–47.76, which is quite wide, indicating a lack of sufficient statistical power for this subset.
390. Coalition for Mercury-Free Drugs, "Citing Recent Proof of Harm, Parents and Scientists Petition FDA for a Ban on Adding Mercury to Drugs, and Giving Mercury-Containing Drugs to Pregnant Women, Newborns and Children," press release, August 4, 2004.
391. Lisa Sykes and Kelli Ann Davis, interviews with the author, August 2004.
392. Paul G. King, e-mail to Lyn Redwood and other parents, subject: "Press Release," August 7, 2004, 5:55 A.M.

393. "Statement of Task—Review of the National Immunization Program's Research Procedures and Data Sharing Program," IOM Web site, August 8, 2004, http://www.iom.edu.

394. Teresa Binstock, e-mail to autism parents and others, subject: "IOM Registration," August 11, 2004, 9:35 A.M.

395. Myron Levin, "Taking It to Vaccine Court," *Los Angeles Times*, August 7, 2004.

396. "Vaccine Scrapped over Autism Fear," BBC News, August 7, 2004.

397. Roger Highfield, "Scientists Applaud Move Away from Use of Mercury," *Telegraph* (UK), October 8, 2004.

EPILOGUE

398. Andy Waters, interview with the author, September 9, 2004.

399. "5th Circuit: Thimerosal Claims against Lilly not Barred," *Mealey's Litigation Report: Thimerosal & Vaccines*, e-mail Bulletin, August 17, 2004.

400. "Ruling Concerning Motion for Discovery from Merck, RE: MMR vaccine," In Re: Claims for Vaccine Injuries Resulting in Autism Spectrum Disorder or a Similar Neurodevelopmental Disorder, *Various Petitioners v. Secretary of Health and Human Services*, Office of Special Masters, U.S. Court of Federal Claims, July 16, 2004.

401. Rep. Dave Weldon, interview with the author, June 10, 2004.

402. Leigh Pruneau, IRB Administrator, Kaiser Permanente Northern California, letter to Dr. Mark Geier, subject: "A Series of Studies to Analyze the Vaccine Safety Database (VSD)," July 19, 2004.

403. Safe Minds, National Autism Association, et al., "Joint Statement regarding the Vaccine Safety Datalink Project," press release, August 18, 2004.

404. Rep. Dave Weldon, memo to the CDC, subject: "VSD Data Access by Dr. Geier," November 6, 2003.

405. Rep. Dave Weldon, interview with the author, August 4, 2004.

406. Lynn Armstrong, FOIA Officer, CDC, letter to Brian Hooker, July 30, 2004.

407. Myron Levin, "Ban on Mercury in Shots Is Passed," *Los Angeles Times*, August 27, 2004.

408. Rep. Dave Weldon, interview with the author, August 4, 2004.

409. Rep. Dan Burton, interview with the author, July 23, 2003.

410. Robert Pear, "In Shift, Bush Moves to Block Medical Suits," *New York Times,* July 25, 2004.

411. Center for Responsive Politics, http://www.opensecrets.org, October 4, 2004.

412. Jim Moody, interview with the author, July 9, 2003.

413. John O'Brien, Communications Director, American Academy of Pediatrics, letter to David Kirby, October 3, 2003.

414. CDC Office of the Director, "Vaccine Safety: Public Comment Sought on CDC's Vaccine Safety," http://www.cdc.gov/od/vaccsafe.

415. "Safety of Thimerosal-Containing Vaccines: A Two-Phased Study of Computerized Health Maintenance Organization (HMO) Databases," Q&A on the VSD, http://www.cdc.gov.

416. Jeanie Lerche Davis, "Preservative in Childhood Vaccines Not a Cause of Autism, Researchers Find," WebMD, September 7, 2004.

417. Dr. Walter Orenstein, interview with the author, August 2, 2004.

418. Dr. Marie McCormick, interview with the author, July 26, 2004.

419. Dr. Paul Offit, interviews with the author, June 19, 2003, and July 27, 2004.

420. Boyd Haley, interview with the author, July 13, 2003.

421. Richard Deth, interview with the author, June 9, 2004.

422. Mark Blaxill, "Generation Zero: Thomas Verstraeten's First Analyses of the Link between Vaccine Mercury Exposure and the Risk of Diagnosis of Selected Neuro-Developmental Disorders Based on Data from the Vaccine Safety Datalink: November–December 1999," September 2004.

423. Rick Rollens, e-mail to the author, October 15, 2004, 12:22 A.M.

424. Bernard Rimland, interview with the author, August 10, 2004.

425. Rashid A. Buttar, DO, "Autism, the Misdiagnosis of Our Future," testimony before the U.S. House Subcommittee on Health and Wellness, Committee on Government Reform, May 6, 2004.

426. "Heyltex Corporation, letter to Heyl Pharmacy Clients," August 31, 2004.

427. J. B. Handley, e-mail to the author, October 29, 2004, 3:53 P.M.

428. Richard Deth, interview with the author, June 9, 2004.

429. Dr. Jim Neubrander, interview with the author, August 8, 2004.

430. www.accessdata.fda.gov.

431. Influenza Virus Vaccine (Fluvirin®) 2003–2004 Formula—Chiron Corp. Product Insert.

432. PubMed, http://www.ncbi.nim.nih.gov/entrez/query.fegi?cmd=Retrieve&db=pubmed&dopt=abstract&listvids=7773382&itool=iconabstr.

433. H. M. Aucken and T. L. Pitt, "Antibiotic Resistance and Putative Virulence Factors of Serratia Marcescens with Respect to O and K Serotypes," *Journal of Medical Microbiology.*

434. Vaccine Fund, "Children's Vaccine Advocates to Meet in The Netherlands to Share First-Year Successes," press release, November 17, 2000.

435. "Growth Rate for Vaccine Market in China—15%," *Isis Monthly Market Watch* 1, no. 3 (March 20, 2004): 10.

436. "More Children Suffer from Autism," Xinhua News Agency, posted on Xinhuanet, http://news.xinhuanet.com/english, August 11, 2004.

Acknowledgments

There are two people who deserve to be thanked first and foremost, and they are my good friends the award-winning author David France and the multi-talented journalist Jay Blotcher. With their knowledge, experience, and good humor, David and Jay were my guides and inspiration as I worked on this project. David's early reading of the manuscript and Jay's later reading, and the long hours that each spent making suggestions, changes, and other edits, were the mark of true friends and committed comrades.

Of course, this book could never have been completed without the support and cooperation of dozens of parents of autistic kids, and their families. These parents opened their homes, and their lives, to me, and they always made me feel like a welcome and honored guest.

Lyn and Tommy Redwood and their children Drew, Hanna, and Will were wonderful subjects and gracious hosts. Lyn, especially, dedicated herself to this project with untiring enthusiasm and incalculable assistance.

Other families who graciously allowed me to enter and record their private worlds were Liz Birt and her kids Sarah, Matthew, and Andrew; Scott and Laura Bono and their children Dillan, Ashley, and Jackson; Mark and Elise Blaxill and their daughters Sydney and Michaela; Jeff and Shelley Segal and their twins Josh and Jordan; and Rick and Janna Rollens and their boys Steven and Russell.

And though I did not have a chance to visit Sallie Bernard and her family at home, I thank Sallie Bernard, her husband, Thomas, and her family for countless hours of help and guidance on the book. Other parents I want to thank include Albert Enayati, Heidi Roger, Lori McIlwain, Jo Pike, Robert Krakow, Lisa Sykes, Teri Small, Laura Weinberg Aronow, Bobbie Manning, Kelly Kerns, Daniele Sarkine Burton, Lujene and Alan Clark, Linda Weinmaster, Nancy Hokkanen, Kelli Ann Davis, Brian Hooker, Brenda Kerr, Phil Ehart, and J. B. Handley. Wendy Fournier deserves credit for designing the Web site that will be a companion to this book.

There were friends and family, too, who saw me through this project, the most difficult endeavor of my life. Special thanks go to Tim Horn, who helped, encouraged, and supported me in ways that he will never know. Special mention is also deserved for Patty Glynn Lenartz and her husband, Bob Lenartz, who furnished food, wine, and love, and David Fromm, who kept me from going completely insane. My good friend Matthew Singer read primordial drafts and provided invaluable commentary. My sister Nancy Bue supported me with love, kind words, and the occasional loan. And her kids, Michael and Jennifer, are the best. Lou Pansulla lent me his ears, money, and a whole lot more. Support and advice was also given freely by Gabriel Rotello, Doug Fredman, Ted Loos, Lizzy Bowman, Jonathan Starch, Laura Perry, James Rexroad, Shimon Attie, Georges Piette, George Calderaro, Rob Arnold, and Na'an Nadar. I thank Yuri Sivo for bringing the autism epidemic to my attention. And I deeply thank Peter Downes for helping me to celebrate the book's completion.

I also want to thank my New York literary agent, Todd Shuster, for believing in me and in this book from the very beginning. The project would have been unthinkable without his kindness, professionalism, good humor, and support. I also want to thank Scott Gold, in Todd's office. Out in Los Angeles, I offer my heartfelt appreciation to Nancy Nigrosh, Max Roman, and Justin Winters at Innovative Artists. And Tom Acitelli, my transcriber, never missed a beat and did an impeccable job, always on time. PR gurus Jane Rohman and John Bianco, meanwhile, provided pro-bono direction that has been priceless and tremendously successful, and Peggy Klaus graciously supplied expert and gratis media training.

St. Martin's Press has been stellar, a wonderful company to work with. My editor, George Witte, demonstrated patience and compassion and helped guide a first-time author through the choppy waters of publication. His former deputy, Marie Estrada, deserves a special mention for her quiet, solid support, and outside attorney Heather Florence showed patience, respectfulness, and eagle-eyed attention to detail. Publicity experts Elizabeth Coxe and Vicki Lame worked wonders to get the book noticed.

A small army of researchers have not only worked tirelessly on the thimerosal issue, but provided me with invaluable assistance throughout the course of my research and writing. Special thanks goes to Jill James, of Arkansas Children's Hospital Research Institute, for helping a writer with a degree in liberal arts decipher some terrifically complicated data on biochemistry. The list of other researchers seemed to grow by the month. They include: Boyd Haley of the University of Kentucky; Mark and David Geier of Silver Spring, Maryland; Dr. Neal Halsey of Johns Hopkins University; Richard Deth of Northeastern University; Bill Walsh of the Pfeiffer Treatment Center; Allan Goldblatt of Long Island, New York; Bernard Rimland of the Autism Research Institute; Dr. Stephanie Cave of Baton Rouge; Dr. Jane El-Dahr of Tulane University; Dr. Jeffrey Bradstreet of the International Child Development Resource Center; Mady Hornig of Columbia University; Dr. Jim Neubrander; Dr. Sidney Baker; Rashid A. Buttar, D.O.; Dr. Marie McCormick of the Institute of Medicine's Immunization Safety Committee; Dr. Paul Offit of Philadelphia Children's Hospital; Dr. Richard Clover of the American Academy of Family Physicians; and Dr. Walter Ornstein of Emory Vaccine Center.

A number of people in politics and political activism were also essential to this effort. Chief among them are Rep. Dan Burton (R-IN) and his press secretary Nick Mutton. The support of Beth Clay, who worked for Burton when I started this book and now has her own consulting company, was priceless. Rep. Dave Weldon (R-FL) was instrumental to this book, and his aide Stuart Burns went beyond the call to help whenever he could. Other elected officials who went out of their way to help include Sen. Debbie Stabenow (D-MI) and her assistant Dave Lemmon, Eric Sapp, formerly of Sen. Ted Kennedy's staff, and the offices of Sen. Patrick Leahy (D-VT) and John Conyers (D-MI).

Among the activists who helped me, I want to single out Barbara Loe Fisher of the National Vaccine Information Center, Michael Bender of the Mercury Policy Project, and Cheri Jacobus, a Republican activist and media consultant from Washington.

Many attorneys also deserve thanks. Chief among them is Jim Moody of Washington, who never failed to provide crystal-clear insight into a very murky story. Andrew Waters of Dallas was also tremendously cooperative, as well as Tom Yost of Baltimore, Cliff Shoemaker of Virginia, and Mike Williams of Portland, Oregon.

Finally, I want to thank whoever it was that placed the furtive Lilly rider into the Homeland Security Act of 2002. Without them, I might never have heard of thimerosal, and this book would not have been written.

Index

size of fund, and payouts, 158
statute of limitations for filing with, 2,
 157, 158–59, 203
Vaccine Injured Children's Compensation Act
 of 2001 (VICCA), 159
Vaccine Injury Compensation Program
 (VICP), 72, 156–57, 198, 202–3, 207,
 210–11, 222, 227–28, 229, 251,
 260–64, 268, 298, 328, 394, 396, 400
vaccines
 components of, 36, 84, 97, 109
 live viruses in, 28, 33–35
 multidose, xv, 84–85, 417–18
 need for, in confronting bioterrorism, 6,
  202–4
 preservatives in, 2, xv, 84–85, 417–18
 shortage of, due to litigation, according to
  Frist, 226–28
 U.S. exports to Third World countries,
  417–18
vaccines, thimerosal-containing
 adverse outcomes not seen, 246–49
 adverse outcomes seen, 229–30
 FDA petitioned to recall, 145–46, 368–69,
  383–85
 legislation to ban (Weldon-Maloney),
  334–36, 398
 mercury levels in, in excess of federal
  safety limits, 3
 mercury poisoning from, 4
 phasing out of, and decrease in autism
  cases, 374–76
 recall, urged, 45, 84, 109, 114–15
 recalled in UK, 391
 suits over, 1–7, 162–63
Vaccine Safety Datalink (VSD), 115, 126,
 129, 135, 140, 142, 159–60, 164,
 176–77, 184, 190–91, 195–96, 198,
 204–5, 213–14, 230–31, 257, 268,
 270, 279–89, 291–92, 300–303,
 305–6, 313–16, 317–18, 331–32,
 341–43, 347, 348, 349, 352, 362, 372,
 378, 380, 385–87, 395, 396–97, 401,
 407
 CDC analysis of, final version, 283–86
 CDC offer to open to outside research,
  with conditions, 167–68, 204–5
 CDC offer to reanalyse, 185
 CDC refusal to release, 184
 CDC restriction of access to, 140, 213–14,
  280–83, 287–88, 305–6, 403
 confidential version (February 2000),
  190–97, 202

destruction of data in, 396
earliest memos (1999) showing a thimerosal-
 autism link, 380–82
early indications of a thimerosal-autism
 connection, 191–92, 257, 380–83
errors in analysis of, 147–50, 164–67,
 179–80, 193–94, 284–88, 302, 408–9
errors in data chosen for analysis, 195–96,
 271, 302, 364
Geiers' attempt to access, 230–31, 279–83,
 305–6, 310, 328
generations of analysis of, 283, 291,
 313–16, 382–83, 407–9
"Generation Zero," 407–9
manipulation of analytical results, alleged,
 164–67, 284–86, 287–88
narrowed scope of, to show no thimerosal-
 autism link, alleged, 364
standards for data sharing, to be proposed
 by IOM, 385–87, 396–97
Vaccines and Related Biological Products
 Advisory Comittee (VRBPAC), 123
Vaccines: What Every Parent Should Know
 (Offit), 79
Vancouver Sun, 307
Vanderbilt University, 276
Verstraeten, Dr. Thomas, 116, 126–27, 142,
 157, 160, 165, 171, 174, 176, 192–93,
 196, 283–89, 301–2, 331, 341–43, 347,
 351, 355, 363, 364, 370, 382, 386,
 394, 396, 401, 407–9
 alleged conflict of interest of, 286–87, 402
 e-mails on VSD study, 192–93, 382
 "it just won't go away" e-mail, 192, 382
 meeting with Lyn Redwood, 148–50
 self-admitted errors in VSD analysis, 171–72
 self-defense of VSD study, 341–43
 "signal will simply not just go away"
  statement at Simpsonwood meeting, 171
 testimony at IOM 2001 meeting, 176–77
 VSD study, 126–30, 147–48, 279, 401–2
Virginia, 269
viruses, live, in vaccines, 28, 33–35
vision problems, 20–21
vitamin B-1, 339
vitamin B-12, 183, 297, 337, 338, 339, 344

Wakefield, Dr. Andrew, xvi, 28–29, 32–33,
 37, 43, 57, 60, 74, 85, 91, 92, 94, 99,
 100, 101–2, 109, 328–29
 ridicule of and alarm at findings, 32–34
Waldie, Jerome, 89
Walker-Smith, Dr. John, 73

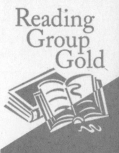

Reading
Group
Gold

EVIDENCE OF HARM

by David Kirby

*A
Reading
Group Gold
Selection*

For more reading group suggestions
visit www.readinggroupgold.com

 ST. MARTIN'S GRIFFIN

A Note from the Author

It has been one year since I turned in the epilogue to this book, and much has happened during that time. Equally important, much has *not* happened. We are not much closer to solving the all-important question at hand—did thimerosal in vaccines contribute to the dramatic increase in autism and other disorders, or did it not?—than we were a year ago. I am hopeful that the coming year will yield more clues to the riddle that is autism.

In the meantime, the smoldering dispute between those who reject the hypothesis and those who embrace it seems to have intensified, if anything. Most of the scientists, pediatricians, and public health officials that I have spoken to loathe this subject, and truly want it to go away. But given the tenacity, resourcefulness, and unbounded energy of thousands of parents and their allies who are convinced of a link, this story, rather like Thomas Verstraeten's thimerosal signal, will not "just go away."

Many in the autism community had hoped that this fall would have been the autumn of autism, a season of reckoning. Over the spring and summer of 2005, after all, high-level meetings were held with leading senators and their staffs. And the mainstream American media seemed to begin to notice the controversy, however reluctantly and not always in the most positive light, at least from the parental point of view. By the end of the summer, it looked like the controversy was about to gain the attention it deserved—within the mass media and inside the nation's capital. Thimerosal, it seemed, was finally going to become a major news story in America.

But then hurricane Katrina hit and, suddenly, all bets were off. The category 5 storm, which chewed up the Gulf Coast and nearly finished off New Orleans, devoured airtime and newsprint and bumped every other story off the media radar screen. And throughout the fall, Washington was dominated by political turmoil and scandal. Autism never really had a chance.

What follows is an abbreviated version of the major autism-related events in science, the media, and politics that took place over the past twelve months.

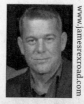

New Studies Cited by Supporters of the Theory

Inorganic Mercury in Primate Brains—(University of Washington—National Institutes of Environmental Health Sciences—Published in *Environmental Health Perspectives*)

Lead researcher Thomas Burbacher et al. confirmed that, in primates, injected ethylmercury from vaccines clears from the blood more quickly than ingested methylmercury, which in turn was concentrated in the brain more than the ethyl form. However, once ethylmercury does enter the brain, it converts to inorganic mercury at two to three times the rate of methylmercury. Organic mercury had a half-life in the brain of just thirty-seven days. Inorganic mercury, however, has been shown to have a brain half-life of up to twenty years. A previous study by the same team found that inorganic mercury trapped in the brain caused changes in brain tissue, including neuro-inflammation, which is significant, given the finding of "big brains" in autistic children.

Autism and Environmentally Induced Brain Swelling—(Harvard University—Published in *The Neuroscientist*)

Dr. Martha Herbert's study may help refute the notion that the brains of autistic children are simply wired differently and she notes, "neuroinflammation appears to be present in autistic brain tissue from childhood through adulthood." The study suggests that chronic disease or an external environmental source (like heavy metals) may be causing the inflammation.

Immune-Related Inflammation in Autistic Brains—(Johns Hopkins University School of Medicine—Published in *Annals of Neurology*)

This study produced new data showing that the autistic brains studied demonstrate clear signs of inflammation, which was apparently associated with activation of the brain's immune system. Compared with controls, the brains of deceased autistic people showed ongoing inflammation in various sections of brain, produced by cells known as microglia and astroglia. The findings support the contention of some researchers that immune-triggered brain inflammation, possibly as a result of heavy metal exposure, is involved in autism. The study did not determine, however, whether the inflammation is a result of disease, a cause of it, or both.

Autism and Immune Dysfunction—(University of California—M.I.N.D.® Institute—Presented at the 2005 International Meeting for Autism Research) Children with autism have markedly different immune profiles from normal kids, this study reported. Autistic children were found to have increased autoimmunity, extremely high levels of certain immune cells and cytokines, and an imbalance of the TH1 vs. TH2 immune response. Though not part of this study, the researchers failed to note that many of these abnormal conditions also appear in the literature on mercury toxicity.

U.S. Education Figures Show True Increase, No Diagnostic Substitution—(Johns Hopkins Bloomberg School of Public Health—Published in *Pediatrics*)
The rate of increase in reported cases of autism among children born every year in the United States was relatively stable until the 1987 birth cohort, when rates suddenly began to spike, and then continued to rise among children born in each subsequent year. A second spike in the rate of increase was noted in 1992, a few years after which, the rate began to level off. It is interesting to recall that, between 1987 and 1992, with the introduction of new thimerosal-containing vaccines, total mercury exposure from infant immunization went from 75 to nearly 240 micrograms. Meanwhile, the article said, reported incidents of mental retardation and other childhood disorders remained constant, meaning that "diagnostic substitution" was not an explanation for the rise in autism cases. (See *Harvard Mental Health Letter*'s rebuttal in the following section).

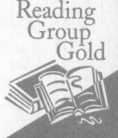

Coal Emissions a Risk Factor for Autism?—(University of Texas—
Published in *Health and Place*)
Mercury released primarily from coal-fired power plants may be contributing to an increase in the risk of autism. The study found that autism increased in Texas counties as mercury emissions rose. For every thousand pounds of environmentally released mercury, there was a 61 percent increase in autism rates. The study looked at Texas county-by-county levels of mercury emissions and compared them to the rates of autism and special education services in 1,200 Texas school districts. One county with low mercury emissions but significant autism rates was found to harbor one of the nation's largest mercury mines. One author said the study showed a potentially "important connection between environmental exposure to mercury and the development of autism."

Home Videos Demonstrate Autistic Regression—(University of
Washington—Published in *Archives of General Psychiatry*)
In this blind study, researchers analyzed videotapes from children with early onset autism, children with parentally reported regressive autism, and typical children, taken at one year and at two years of age. Children who went on to regress into autism spectrum disorder (ASD) actually babbled and spoke more at one year than other ASD children, and even more than typical children. But by two years of age, language and attention levels in the two ASD groups lagged well behind the typical children. The study "validates the phenomenon of regression in a subgroup of children with ASD," it said. But regressive children did not always experience normal development on all fronts. "The data from parental interviews suggests the existence of nonspecific behavioral anomalies in these children before developmental regression, such as sleep problems and sensory hypersensitivity," the authors noted.

Earlier Studies Are Finally Published

Meanwhile, since the Institute of Medicine's final report on thimerosal came out in May 2004 (in which the IOM ruled against a link and determined that biological evidence was "theoretical only") many of the biological studies that were largely overlooked by the IOM were published in respected, peer-reviewed journals. These included: Dr. Mady Hornig's mouse study, conducted at Columbia University and published in *Molecular Psychology;* Dr. Richard Deth's study of methylation problems possibly caused by interference from thimerosal, conducted at Northeastern University (among others) and published in *Molecular Psychiatry;* and Dr. Jill James's study of glutathione deficiencies in autistic children and subsequent treatment with a methyl B-12 "cocktail," conducted at the University of Arkansas— Arkansas Children's Hospital and published in the journal *Biology.*

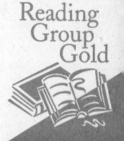

The Science

New Studies Cited by Opponents of the Theory

Rise in Minnesota Autism Cases Due to Better Diagnostics—(Mayo Clinic College of Medicine—Published in *Archives of Pediatrics & Adolescent Medicine*)

The authors investigated the incidents of "research identified" autism in Olmsted County, Minnesota, between 1976–1997. They determined that the age-adjusted incidence was 5.5 per 100,000 children from 1980–1983 and 44.9 per 100,000 from 1995–1997, an 8.2-fold increase. However, the authors stated, "Broader, more precise diagnostic criteria for autism were introduced in 1987," and the 1991 federal special education laws "improved the availability of educational services for children with autism." Although it was "possible that unidentified environmental factors have contributed to an increase in autism," the study said, "the timing of the increase suggests that it may be due to improved awareness, changes in diagnostic criteria, and availability of services, leading to identification of previously unrecognized young children with autism." The authors did not provide evidence to support such an assertion. Nor did they explain why, after reviewing the medical records of local teenagers and reassigning some of them with newly "research identified" autism diagnoses, they had still failed to account for what Mark Blaxill labeled the "hidden horde."

No Association Between Rho-D Immune Globulin and Autism—(University of Missouri—Presented at the American College of Medical Genetics)

Pediatrics professor Judith Miles determined the blood type and Rho-D immune globulin exposure of mothers of autistic children evaluated at the university from 1995 to 2004. She analyzed data from 200 autism families and 50 control families and found no significant difference in exposure to Rho-D immune globulin during pregnancy between autism mothers (12.9 percent; 26/201) and Down's syndrome mothers (15 percent; 4/27), and exposure of nonautistic and autistic siblings was similar (12.9 percent vs. 12.6 percent.) "We conclude that there is no indication that pregnancies of children with autism were any more likely to be complicated by Rh immune globulin/thimerosal exposure than those of

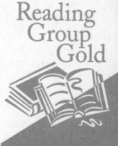

controls," Miller wrote, "which suggests no etiologic role for thimerosal in the development of autism." The study was funded by Johnson & Johnson, maker of Rho-Gam brand immune globulin, which used to contain thimerosal. The company has been named as a defendant in a number of thimerosal-autism lawsuits.

No Autism Epidemic—(Published in *Harvard Mental Health Letter*)

The respected newsletter published a review of two studies that argue against an actual increase in the number of diagnosed ASD cases in the United States and United Kingdom. The U.S. data, collected by the Department of Education, showed a rate of 4 cases of autism per 10,000 children in 1993 and 25 cases per 10,000 in 2003—a six-fold increase. "But these findings contain internal inconsistencies," the newsletter said. "Apparently, as many children are being newly diagnosed at age 15 as at age 8, yet the symptoms of autism appear before age 3, and most studies show that the diagnosis is usually made before age 8." Diagnostic standards in U.S. schools "have varied by time and place," it added. With greater awareness and more special education services, diagnoses were "increasingly extended to children with milder symptoms and less serious disabilities."

In the UK, researchers found that the rate of diagnosis of pervasive development disorder (PDD) in the county of Staffordshire among children born in 1992–1995 was nearly identical as children born in 1997–1998, about 6 per 1,000. The rate of full-blown autism was also the same in both groups, about 1 in 500. Of course, children born in 1992 were exposed to roughly the same amount of thimerosal in vaccines as those born in 1998.

Another interesting note: The rate of ASD in the U.S. and UK is the same, about 6 per 1,000 children. The rate of full-blown (DSM IV) autism, however, is twice as high in America (4 per 1,000) than in Britain (2 per 1,000). In addition, it is interesting to note that British children received roughly half the mercury in their vaccines in the first six months of life (75 mcg) than their American counterparts.

The California Numbers

The quarterly net gain of autism cases entering California's Department of Developmental Services' regional intake centers has continued to decline, but neither side has seized upon the data as evidence of much of anything. The bottom line is, it is probably still a little too early to determine if a real trend is at work here or not. The figures remain murky and confusing.

Even though there was a spike in cases in late 2004, it was not a record year. In fact, according to state data, 2002 was the year with the greatest net gain in autism diagnoses, as an additional 3,259 cases entered the system. In 2003, this number dropped to 3,125, while 2004 finished the year with a net gain of 3,074 cases.

So far, 2005 has also seen a decline in the numbers. For the first half of 2005, there was a net gain of 1,470 cases, compared to 1,518 in the same period in 2004, the *Los Angeles Times* reported in July. By the third quarter of 2005, the numbers had fallen even more dramatically, with a net gain of just 678 autism cases, compared with 734 cases in the second quarter of 2005, a 7.5 percent decline. So far this year (during the first three quarters of 2005), California had a net gain of 2,148 cases, down from 2,267 cases in the first three quarters of 2004, and 2,449 cases in the same period of 2003.

But looking at net increases among 3–5 year olds only, the numbers have gone up and down. (90 percent of all autistic children are younger than 6 years of age before they enter the system, which does not count children under 3.) For example, the third quarter of 2003 registered a net gain of 92 autism cases, which rose to a gain of 103 cases in the same quarter of 2004, and then fell back to 93 cases in the same quarter of 2005:

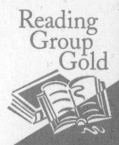

QUARTER	Total # children 3–5 years old in DDS system	Net gain from previous quarter	Change in net gain
1Q 2003	4,228	189	+81
2Q 2003	4,466	238	+49
3Q 2003	4,558	92	−146
4Q 2003	4,611	53	−39
1Q 2004	4,793	182	+129
2Q 2004	4,894	101	−81
3Q 2004	4,997	103	+2
4Q 2004	5,156	159	+56
1Q 2005	5,307	151	−8
2Q 2005	5,446	139	−12
3Q 2005	5,539	93	−46

The Science

In July, Dr. Robert Hendren, executive director of the M.I.N.D.® Institute, told the *Los Angeles Times* that, "perhaps, whatever caused [the number of cases] to go up—environmental insult, or whatever— —is no longer present." But he added, "It's all specula- tion. I wish we had good studies." Dr. Hendren's cau- tion is easily understood.

Autism in the News

One year ago, in November of 2004, when the hardcover edition of this book was completed, the subject of thimerosal and autism was rarely reported upon within the national media. But over the past twelve months, we have seen this story ebb and flow within the vagaries of the 24-hour news cycle, with peaks that included Don Imus and *Meet the Press,* and long, silent valleys, including the past few months in which the hard to pronounce word "thimerosal" was virtually lost amid glaring headlines about hurricanes, court appointments, leaks, and indictments.

The controversy over thimerosal and autism as a national media story really took off in earnest in February 2005, when the president of NBC Universal, Bob Wright, sent a memo to the entire staff of the media conglomerate saying that his young grandson had just been diagnosed with autism, and that the network would begin reporting more on the autism epidemic, including its possible causes and potential treatments. At the same time, Wright and his wife Suzanne announced the formation of a multimillion dollar research charity called "Autism Speaks."

During sweeps week in late February, NBC gave more airtime to autism in five days than all the other networks combined had likely aired in their history on air. *The Today Show* dedicated two segments each morning to the subject, including a piece about the thimerosal hypothesis and chelation as a possible autism treatment, in which I was briefly interviewed. Other NBC stories, which ran in conjunction with a *Newsweek* cover story on autism that week, included pieces on *Dateline NBC,* on sister networks MSNBC and CNBC, and a major report on the *NBC Nightly News with Brian Williams,* in which health reporter Robert Bazell stated that vaccines had been "cleared" as a cause of autism.

People paid attention, and one of them was Don Imus, the cantankerous but irresistible sage of the morning airwaves, whose highly rated radio show, *Imus in the Morning,* is also broadcast live on MSNBC. Throughout much of 2005, Imus took up the question of thimerosal and autism, typically bringing up the subject whenever a powerful lawmaker appeared on his show. Senator Rick Santorum (R-PA) was regularly peppered with thimerosal questions from the man in the cowboy hat, who also interviewed me three times during the spring. Imus also got Brian

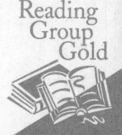

Williams, the NBC news anchor, and Tim Russert, of NBC's *Meet the Press* (though not Chris Matthews of MSNBC's *Hardball*) to agree that more coverage of thimerosal should be done. Both men would later keep their commitment to broadcasting thimerosal segments.

In June, 2005, syndicated talk show host Montel Williams aired an hour-long segment about *Evidence of Harm* that included Lyn and Tommy Redwood, Representative Dave Weldon and me, as well as Dr. Andy Shih, an opponent of the thimerosal theory and director of research of the National Association for Autism Research (NAAR.) That same week, Ron Reagan and Monica Crowley invited me onto MSNBC's *Connected,* along with Dr. Louis Cooper, former head of the AAP. Meanwhile, Dr. Paul Offit, who refused to appear live with me, was interviewed separately, at his request. Many other local television news outlets covered the story, as well as political talk show hosts on the radio. Widely supportive coverage of the theory ranged from Janeane Garofalo on the left to G. Gordon Liddy on the right, and most everyone in between.

In June 2005, lawyer and environmental activist Robert F. Kennedy, Jr., published a scathing indictment of thimerosal and the federal response to parental concerns about its use in vaccines, simultaneously on the political Web site *Salon.com* and in the magazine *Rolling Stone.* Kennedy ignited a mass-media bonfire that smoldered for months and was fanned by his appearances on *Imus in the Morning, The Daily Show with Jon Stewart,* and MSNBC's *Scarborough Country,* in an extraordinary segment in which the conservative host told the liberal guest that his own son had Asperger's Syndrome.

Scarborough said that one day, he was sure, thimerosal would be revealed as the cause.

Also in June, *The New York Times* published a harsh assessment of the thimerosal theory and the Mercury Moms who were propelling it, making them out to look like religious zealots with zero scientific knowledge, up against the best and brightest of the scientific and public health communities in America. Oddly, perhaps because it ran on a Saturday, the front-page article seemed to have limited impact on the debate. In fact, a more balanced piece, by the Associated Press, was published the same weekend. The wire-service story was picked up by dozens of papers, including many of the big city dailies.

ABC News, meanwhile, produced its own dismissive piece on thimerosal and vaccines, which aimed its criticism mostly at Kennedy (whose piece, it should be noted, included some errors that required corrections). The ABC story was capped by a quasi lecture from health reporter Dr. Timothy Johnson, who belittled Kennedy for being a lawyer, not a member of the scientific world, and therefore someone who should keep quiet on a subject that he was unqualified to address. Kennedy and the mercury-autism theory got a thorough thrashing in an article published on *Slate.com* titled "Sticking up for Thimerosal." It was authored by Arthur Allen, the same journalist who had written the lengthy thimerosal-autism article in *The New York Times Magazine* in November 2002.

But not everyone was harsh on Kennedy. *NBC Nightly News* produced a very balanced piece on Kennedy's activism, and *CBS Evening News* delivered a respectful and in-depth interview with Kennedy, conducted by Sharyl Attkisson. Kennedy was also invited to publish op-ed pieces supporting the theory—and accusations of a government cover-up—in the *Boston Globe* and *USA Today.* Also at *USA Today,* health reporter Anita Manning wrote a highly balanced article on the controversy in early July, as did Maggie Fox, at Reuters. Meanwhile, Fox Television local affiliates covered the story with exceptional dedication and fairness, and at least three famous Americans, in addition to Joe Scarborough, publicly announced in the media their personal belief that thimerosal had caused autism in their children. They were football star Doug Flutie, actor Aidan Quinn, and singer-guitarist Stephen Stills.

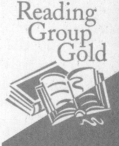

Also during the spring and summer of 2005, a new
pro-chelation parents group founded by J. B. Handley,
Generation Rescue, purchased full-page ads in *USA
Today* and *The New York Times* promoting the mercury-autism link and chelation (and *Evidence of
Harm*). For its part, Unlocking Autism placed a series
of hardball ads reminding George W. Bush of his
2004 campaign statement that thimerosal should be
removed from all childhood vaccines. The ads, all
bearing the tag line "Giving Mercury to Children on
Purpose Is Stupid," appeared on billboards and in
local newspapers in a number of states.

Some of journalism's most in-depth and original
reporting on autism was conducted in 2005 by a
United Press International reporter named Dan
Olmsted, who continues to doggedly pursue the story
in his regular column, "The Age of Autism." Among
Olmsted's most important work is research into the
reclusive Amish community in America, and why
these families—who tend to spurn vaccines in large
numbers, for religious reasons—seem to have much
lower rates of autism than the general population.
Olmsted has been attacked for not being "scientific."
But he is a reporter, not an epidemiologist. He
deserves credit for opening up an intriguing avenue
of autism research previously overlooked. It is possible that private research funds will be made available for study of the Amish and other unvaccinated
populations. Many critics of Olmsted's reporting
suggested that the Amish might have particularly
insular genes that protect them from autism. If that
is the case, then couldn't this knowledge conceivably
go a long way toward identifying the cause of this
disorder?

The *Los Angeles Times'* Myron Levin continued his

own hard-nosed reporting on the thimerosal controversy in 2005. In February, Levin dropped a bombshell, of sorts, when he reported on a leaked memo from Merck & Co., dated March 1991. The memo warned company executives that six-month-old children who were vaccinated on schedule would be exposed to mercury at levels up to eight-seven times the limit in guidelines on mercury from fish. "When viewed in this way, the mercury load appears rather large," Dr. Maurice R. Hilleman, an internationally renowned vaccinologist, had written to Merck's vaccine division. "The memo was prepared at a time when U.S. health authorities were aggressively expanding their immunization schedule by adding five new shots for children in their first six months. Many of these shots, as well as some previously included on the vaccine schedule, contained thimerosal," wrote Levin, who received the leaked memo from Washington, D.C., attorney Jim Moody, the legal adviser to Safe Minds. Levin made the point that federal officials did not do the math, and publicly announced that vaccine mercury levels had indeed exceeded safety guidelines, until July 1999.

In March, Levin reported that Merck & Co. had continued to market thimerosal-containing hepatitis-B vaccine "for two years after declaring that it had eliminated the chemical." Back in September of 1999, Merck issued a press release saying, "Now, Merck's infant vaccine line is free of all preservatives," Levin reported. But, he wrote, Merck continued to distribute mercury containing hepatitis-B vaccine, along with the new product, until October 2001. The thimerosal containing doses had expiration dates of 2002. But most doctors assumed that hepatitis-B shots were suddenly all mercury-free. So, apparently, did the CDC. On the day after Merck issued its press release, the CDC announced a revised policy on the birth dose of the vaccine. In July 1999, the "Joint Statement" on thimerosal had said that parents could postpone the hepatitis-B series, which began with the birth dose, until six months of age, when babies are larger. But now that Merck had "removed" the preservative, CDC again recommended that birth dose for hepatitis-B.

In early August, NBC's *Meet the Press* made history in the annals of autism *and* journalism by bringing together two parties, face-to-face, for the first time, to rationally discuss the evidence for and against a link between mercury in vaccines and autism. Tim Russert invited Dr. Harvey Fineberg, president of the Institute of Medicine, and me to appear on the highly rated and influential program. Russert indicated that he would revisit the controversy again at some later date.

Another remarkable event, which received zero coverage in the mainstream media, was a public statement put out in July 2005 by the nation's three largest private autism research funders: Cure Autism Now, the National Association for Autism Research, and Autism Speaks, newly formed by NBC president Bob Wright and his wife Suzanne. Until recently, none of these groups had expressed any extraordinary interest in pursuing the thimerosal-autism theory. But this new statement asserted that autism "may be triggered by environmental factors." Mercury, it said, "including the preservative thimerosal, is among the environmental factors currently under scientific investigation." The groups vowed to "support and fund research that investigates all theories surrounding potential causes of autism, including whether there is a link between mercury and autism, and we invite researchers to submit proposals in this area."

There was terribly sad news, as well. In August, it was reported that Abubakar Tariq Nadama, an autistic five-year-old had died while undergoing chelation therapy at a private doctor's office in western Pennsylvania. Some opponents of the thimerosal-autism theory have pointed to his death as proof that the very idea of chelation is not only bogus, but dangerous. Supporters of chelation noted that Abubakar was given EDTA, and he was receiving it intravenously. EDTA is used mostly for the treatment of lead

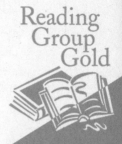

poisoning, and not typically for mercury cases. Also, most autistic children receive chelation in the oral or transdermal form, and not through IV administration. Of course, only through clinical trials of chelation will we settle the debate about the safety and efficacy of chelation therapy and autism. Now, the first ever trial of chelation as therapy for autism is about to get underway at Arizona State University, in a privately funded study being conducted by Dr. Jim Adams.

Finally, in the November/December issue of the *Columbia Journalism Review,* assistant editor Daniel Schulman wrote an exhaustive assessment of how the media have covered the thimerosal issue in the past few years. It was the most comprehensive article of its kind ever published. When the IOM issued its report in May 2004, dismissing the theory, Schulman wrote, "For a time it appeared the controversy over thimerosal would end there. It didn't. Over the past seven months, it has gained traction again, leaving journalists in an awkward position. The thimerosal question—scientifically, politically, and emotionally complex—is proving to be a test for journalism, and the successes and failures are evident in the coverage."

Schulman noted that the "bulk of the scientific establishment" denied a link, and that many scientists "view believers as crackpots, conspiracy theorists, or zealots." Perhaps that's why some journalists who tried to cover the story, "have been discouraged by colleagues and their superiors," he wrote. One reporter said that pursuit of the story was a "nearly career-ending" move. After arguing with superiors who believed that coverage would "legitimize a crackpot theory," the reporter decided against pursuing any more thimerosal stories. Whether thimerosal is ultimately linked to autism or not, Schulman wrote, "there will be consequences—for the public health apparatus and vaccine manufacturers, for parents and their children, even for journalists. But with science left to be done and scientists eager to do it," he added, "it seems too soon for the press to shut the door on the debate.

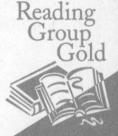

Parents Keep Up the Heat

Nearly all of the parents mentioned in this book continue to organize themselves politically and most
have made repeated trips to Washington or their
state capitals to lobby on several counts—everything
from opening the Vaccine Safety Datalink database
to funding more scientific research into mercury and
autism to investigating allegations of malfeasance
and conflicts of interest to removing mercury from
vaccines. Groups like the National Autism
Association, Unlocking Autism, NoMercury,
Generation Rescue, Defeat Autism Now!, and Autism
One have, if anything, stepped up their efforts on the
above-mentioned fronts. Some parents, like Bobbie
Manning, Lujene Clark, and Robert Krakow have
started a new autism political-action committee,
A-CHAMP, which raises money for sympathetic political candidates and helps organize action in
Washington.

Safe Minds continues its efforts to investigate a
connection between mercury and neurodevelopmental disorders, including autism. During 2005, the
group met extensively with top officials at the
National Institute of Environmental Health Sciences
(NIEHS), which culminated in an "Environmental
Factors Symposium," held near Washington in
August. Safe Minds and the National Autism
Association brought in over a dozen top researchers
"to present the latest findings linking autism to environmental factors, with a focus on mercury," according to Lyn Redwood. Safe Minds is presently writing
an update to the current NIH autism research program, supplementing its environmental initiatives,
Lyn said. Safe Minds also renewed its research funding from the Department of Health and Human

*The Politics
of Mercury*

Services (HHS) this year, and was awarded an additional $198,000 in September, which the group has earmarked for the continuation of the work of Mady Hornig and Thomas Burbacher (who still has brain and other tissue from his primate study, which could be used to look for signs of neuroinflammation and other possible effects of mercury).

A broad-based coalition of autism groups also held two rallies in Washington this year: a large and rather raucous gathering in July, which received ample media coverage, and a smaller, wet, and rainy event in October, held on the same weekend as the 75th Annual Convention of the American Academy of Pediatrics, in downtown Washington. Generation Rescue had bought space for a booth at the convention, and two dozen activists were scheduled to staff the booth throughout the weekend. Most of them, however, were blackballed by the AAP and blocked from entering the convention hall.

Lyn and Tommy Redwood, and their son Will, now eleven, were among those ejected from the premises. "Will was so excited about being able to hand out information at the booth, and he was very upset and started crying when security escorted us from the building," Lyn recalled. "He was so upset. He viewed the AAP reps and security folks as bullies. Will knows a lot about bullies from school. As John Gilmore, a father from New York, said at the rally: 'Why is the AAP afraid of Will Redwood? He was diagnosed autistic and, with treatment for mercury toxicity, has basically recovered. This is a huge threat. He is, in essence, proof that our contentions are correct.'"

Finally, Lyn and other activists have also had to address the issue of Will's baby haircut, which showed very elevated levels of mercury, and helped convince Lyn that mercury was implicated in her son's autism. The problem is, the baby haircut study conducted by Holmes et al. showed the exact opposite: children with autism had excreted very little mercury in their baby haircuts as compared to controls. How to explain this contradiction? It's not easy, and it certainly points to an inconsistency in the hypothesis. Asked about it, Lyn and Mark Blaxill offered the following possible explanations for the admitted anomaly:

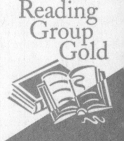
1. Will received inordinately high levels of mercury. Lyn received two injections of thimerosal containing Rho-D immune globulin while pregnant (with 65 mcg mercury each), and a third shot before breast feeding. Lyn also ate ample seafood while pregnant and nursing and had several dental amalgams. Moreover, the Redwoods live in an area powered by two coal-fired electric plants. All this in addition to the 235 mcg of ethylmercury baby Will received in his shots.

2. Will was diagnosed with a relatively moderate case of PDD-NOS, and not full-blown autism. The Holmes baby-hair study showed that milder autism cases had higher mercury levels than severe ones, though nowhere near as high as Will's levels.

3. A similar study, still unpublished, showed that a small number of ASD children, inexplicably, had elevated mercury levels in their hair as well.

4. The lab that analyzed Will's haircut may have committed human error.

Of course, the other explanation is that mercury levels in baby haircuts have no relation to autism whatsoever, though the data—except for Will's haircuts—indicate otherwise.

State and Federal Bills
In the past year, four states—Delaware, Illinois,

The Politics
of Mercury

Missouri, and New York—passed their own version of a mercury-in-vaccines ban, joining the ranks of Iowa and California, which passed their own bills in 2004. Interestingly, when the New York bill was passed and sent to the desk of Republican governor George Pataki, the state chapter of the AAP lobbied openly and insistently (and unsuccessfully) for the governor to veto the bill—even though the AAP had also joined a lawsuit against the Federal Environmental Protection Agency, whose proposed new rules would allow coal-fired power plants to buy and sell "pollution" credits. The AAP said that areas around some plants could become mercury "hot spots," placing pregnant women and small children at increased risk of damage. Meanwhile, on the national level, in addition to the House bill sponsored by Representative Dave Weldon to outlaw the use of mercury in vaccines, a similar bill was introduced in the Senate by Chuck Hagel, the Republican from Nebraska who has been mentioned as a possible candidate for the 2008 presidential election.

Not all Senate action has been welcomed by the mercury moms (and increasingly, dads). In October, Senator Richard Burr (R-NC) introduced Senate bill 1873, the "Biodefense and Pandemic Vaccine and Drug Development Act of 2005," which passed out of the U.S. Senate HELP Committee one day after it was introduced. Senator Burr told the Committee that the legislation "creates a true partnership" between the federal government, the pharmaceutical industry, and academia to walk the drug companies "through the Valley of Death" in bringing new vaccines to market. Burr said it will give the Department of Health and Human Services "additional authority and resources to partner with the private sector to rapidly develop drugs and vaccines." The bill would give the HHS secretary exclusive authority to decide whether a manufacturer violated laws mandating drug safety and would bar the right to challenge his decision in court. The bill would also establish the Biomedical Advanced Research and Development Agency (BARDA), as the sole government agency in charge of advanced research and development of drugs and vaccines in response to bioterrorism and natural disease such as the flu—or even childhood illnesses like whooping cough or measles. BARDA would operate in secret, exempt from the Freedom of Information Act and the Federal Advisory Committee Act.

Access to the Vaccine Safety Datalink

In late June 2005, Don Imus extracted an announcement from Senator Chris Dodd that the Connecticut Democrat and his Republican counterpart, Lamar Alexander of Tennessee, were considering thimerosal hearings in the subcommittee they head. And Imus was told by Senator Rick Santorum (R-PA) that an official investigation of the matter was already underway by Senator Mike Enzi (R-WY), chairman of the powerful Health, Education, Labor and Pensions Committee.

Senator Joe Lieberman (D-CT) stunned the autism community by pledging, on Imus's show, to take up the debate over mercury and autism, and demand more transparency from government researchers. He also expressed compassion for affected families. "I'm going to be a battler for them," he said of the parents. "I think they have a just cause and, you know, I don't care how many respected institutions are on the other side." Lieberman's chief goal was to open up the relatively secretive Vaccine Safety Datalink (VSD) database to qualified researchers outside the CDC, in order to reanalyze the original data, or run new studies comparing children who received mercury-free vaccines with those who received the highest levels of thimerosal.

Lieberman's call for transparency in the handling of the VSD data was backed up by none other than the IOM, in a report issued on February 17, 2005. "The VSD is a tax-supported public resource (and) the public deserves access to the data," concluded the report, from the hearings held on data sharing in 2004. "The public is entitled to transparency and independence in the processes that permit or restrict access. It is possible to facilitate public access and

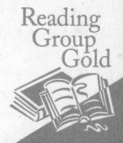

Reading
Group
Gold

The Politics
of Mercury

483

transparency while also protecting patient privacy." The report continued: "The lack of transparency of some of the processes also affects the trust relationship between the National Immunization Program (NIP) and the general public. The dataset from which the final results were obtained should be available to other researchers who may verify and extend the results through an audit or broader reanalysis."

As of this writing, Senator Lieberman was preparing to introduce language into a Senate appropriations bill that would increase access by outside researchers to the Vaccine Safety Datalink. "I believe that we must at least consider an association between thimerosal exposure and autism," Lieberman said in October. "Some experts suggest this VSD database could provide answers regarding the thimerosal-autism link. My staff and I have talked with two former NIEHS directors. They support additional effort to study the association between thimerosal and autism. They assure me that NIEHS would be able to administer a grant for carefully selected expert independent researchers to join in the study of the VSD with the CDC." He added that NIEHS could put together "a panel of toxicologists, doctors, expert representatives from the autism community, and public health advocates to advise the study."

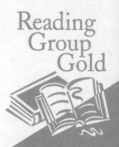

📖 *Questions for the Future*

To date, not a single potential whistle-blower has completed the process needed to attain federal protection status, and it seems as if little has happened with preliminary, internal investigations that were underway within the vast HHS bureaucracy in 2004 (see Epilogue). For now, at least, it looks like most of the action will be in the U.S. Senate.

Over the summer, a number of parents, often accompanied by Jim Moody and sometimes, myself, spent time in Washington briefing political leaders on the many unanswered questions of the debate. The group met with Chairman Enzi and his staff, with the staff of Majority Leader Bill Frist and Senator Joe Lieberman. We met Illinois Democrat senators Barak Obama and Richard Durbin and briefed their staffs, and with a very high ranking HHS official, who recognized that this story is important. Everywhere, we met intelligent, compassionate people—Republicans and Democrats—committed to getting the difficult answers the public deserves. Meanwhile, several groups have started to push for a new IOM hearing, with a new committee that would review new evidence and issue a new report. I personally support this effort, and I know there is support for the idea in certain sectors of Congress.

Speaking of Congress, if hearings are one day held on Capitol Hill, there are several questions that really should be asked. Among them:

Why hasn't the loss of original datasets been investigated?

Federal law requires that all publicly funded data and datasets (patient groupings) be properly maintained, and it's a felony to deliberately lose or destroy such records. In its investigation, the IOM committee that

485

looked into VSD data sharing heard a top CDC official testify that some of the original datasets "hadn't been archived in a standard manner." Those sets, she added, "may not allow all the reanalyses that one might want to do, or in fact may not be available at all." In other words, publicly funded records were lost or destroyed, perhaps criminally. The IOM committee, citing the Federal Information Quality Act, recommended that vaccine officials "seek legal advice" on the matter. Have they?

Why was crucial information about a key study omitted from press releases—*twice*?

Last April, Thomas Burbacher and other researchers at the University of Washington published a study in the NIEHS journal *Environmental Health Perspectives* that compared injected thimerosal and ingested methylmercury in infant primates. The investigators found that ethylmercury in the brain degrades into inorganic mercury much faster than methylmercury. But nothing about inorganic mercury was reported in the press release, or in media accounts. Dr. Burbacher requested a revision, but even when a corrected release was issued, it still omitted crucial details furnished by Burbacher. The revised release did note that inorganic mercury affects white brain matter in primates, and that similar trends were seen in autistic children. But it still omitted Burbacher's observation that thimerosal deposited significantly higher amounts of inorganic mercury in the brain. This omission essentially made the revision senseless. The press releases weren't issued by NIEHS, but rather by a PR firm in Research Triangle Park, North Carolina, whose clients have included Eli Lilly and Pfizer.

Did the CDC exert undue pressure on the IOM?

The IOM's Fineberg steadfastly denied this allegation on *Meet the Press*, but transcripts from private meetings suggest otherwise. So far, two transcripts and some handwritten notes have been leaked. In one transcript, committee chairwoman Marie McCormick comments that "[the CDC] wants us to declare" that vaccines are safe "on a population basis." Fineberg complained that McCormick's words were taken out of context. He added that she had argued in favor of addressing vaccine safety on an *individual* basis, as well on the population level, to better address parental concerns. But Fineberg's protestations raise a host of new questions. Why is McCormick, a scientist, so fixated on the reaction of parents? Who overruled her efforts to address individual risks, and why? And in what context, exactly, would the words "[the CDC] wants us to declare" be acceptable, given that the CDC was paying for the study? Furthermore, what does committee staff director Kathleen Stratton mean when she says, "the line we will not cross in public policy is to pull the vaccine, change the schedule," before any evidence was presented?

At times, tensions rose between committee members and Stratton and McCormick, who seemed to be framing the agenda according to what "they" (presumably the CDC) desire. This clearly ruffled some feathers. Committee member Gerald Medoff, rather derisively said, "You just want us to say the evidence favors rejection of the hypothesis?" to which McCormick answered, "Yes, that's what they want to say." And Stratton at one point informed the members that, "There are pros and cons of letting them determine the topic—to be expedient, it is better that they determine it." Panelist Alfred Berg grumbled, "They are paying for it," to which Stratton replied reassuringly, "We can shape it a little. We have—you know, what are the boundaries. Does that make you feel any better?"

Apparently it did not. "Now I am curious what other parts of the methods [the] CDC has figured out for us," Berg said. Later, he called the CDC "one of the malefactors on this issue, because they are always pushing to go beyond the data." Wouldn't these exchanges indicate at least some undue influ-

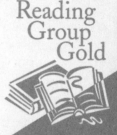

Questions for the Future

ence from the CDC? And while we're on the subject, what is written on the one-page document contained within "Task Order 74" (the directive from the CDC to the IOM) that the government refuses to make public? Shouldn't taxpayers know what the CDC is doing with their dollars?

Why did the IOM base its decision almost entirely on epidemiology?
Epidemiology alone is "not acceptable" to disprove causation, according to the Federal Court System. But the IOM and other thimerosal naysayers routinely point to epidemiology *exclusively* as proof against an association, despite a growing body of biological evidence to the contrary. Why base such a critical decision on population studies alone, especially when the integrity of those studies is questioned by the lead investigators themselves? For example, Danish authors conceded that they "may have spuriously increased the apparent number of autism cases," and the lead author of the U.S. study claimed there was no "evidence against an association," and insisted that his conclusions were "neutral."

Were there IOM conflicts of interest that should have been revealed?
Last summer, Harvey Fineberg issued a statement defending the vaccine safety committee and asserted that the CDC and NIH "had no relationship with the committee." This is simply untrue. Of course the agencies had a "relationship" with the committee. Panel member Rebecca Parkin, for example, was a former CDC epidemiologist with an active research grant from a CDC agency at the time of her committee appointment. Chris Wilson had done a stint at the Public Health Service, which oversees the CDC and NIH, and McCormick's department at the Harvard School of Public Health reportedly received a CDC grant just months before the last IOM report. One member of the peer-review committee that assessed the final IOM report was Scott Ratzin, vice president of Johnson & Johnson—a lawsuit defendant that had made a thimerosal-laden immune-globulin product for injection into pregnant women.

Reading Group Questions

1. First and foremost: do *you* believe there is a link between mercury in vaccines and autism? If you don't believe that mercury is a cause of autism, what other environmental factors might have triggered an increase of cases in the 1990s?

2. As best you can, place yourself in the position of the various mothers and fathers who are profiled in this book. How do you think you would have reacted to finding out your child had autism? Which parents' situation did you most identify with, and why?

3. What do you think of the Safe Minds parents? Could you see yourself ever becoming an activist, like they did? Or would you deal with the issues more privately? Do you believe one or the other of these is the "right" way to handle the situation?

4. Several issues are clouded by the fact that significant information in this debate is not made public (e.g., the internal IOM transcripts; research done by Eli Lilly). Should this information be made public? Where do you suggest the balance between full disclosure and the right to privacy be weighted?

5. Do you believe privately funded studies are useful? If so, what do you say to charges of "bad science" and the suggestion that these studies just seek to support their theory? If not, how and where do you see studies finding funding?

6. Are concerns over patient confidentiality a legitimate reason for denying access to the raw Vaccine Safety Datalink (VSD) data? Why or why not?

7. What do you think the government's role and responsibility should be in addressing the issue? Are they doing a good job, a bad job, or somewhere in between? What do you think are the major positives and negatives of government involvement?

8. Related to the question above, should states and/or the federal government pass bans on thimerosal in vaccines? Why or why not?

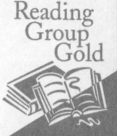

9. It has been argued that some experts who sit on vaccine advisory panels to the FDA and the CDC have a conflict of interest since they have financial relationships with pharmaceutical companies. How should this be handled?

10. What are your opinions about the highly controversial chelation therapy (the two-step process that "scrapes" metals from cells)? If a member of your family was thinking about having this treatment for autism, would you be encouraging or discouraging? Why?

11. Has this book caused you to think twice about the thimerosal content of the vaccines you and your family have received? Has it caused you to rethink any other part of your life, like lowering the levels of mercury to which you and your family are exposed?

12. What would you like to see pursued at this point—in terms of the relation between autism and thimerosal and the way federal officials have handled the controversy?